Essentials of Nursing Care

Essentials of Nursing Care

Edited by

CHRIS BASSETT RN, BA(HONS), RNT
Lecturer in Nursing, University of Sheffield

W
WHURR PUBLISHERS
LONDON AND PHILADELPHIA

© 2003 Whurr Publishers Ltd
First published 2003
by Whurr Publishers Ltd
19b Compton Terrace
London N1 2UN England and
325 Chestnut Street, Philadelphia PA 19106 USA

British Library Cataloguing in Publication Data

A catalogue record for this book
is available from the British Library.

ISBN 1 86156 332 9

Printed and bound in the UK by Athenaeum Press Ltd, Gateshead,
Tyne & Wear.

Contents

Contributors

Chris Bassett BA(Hons), RN, RNT, lecturer in nursing at the University of Sheffield.

Jane Bassett RN, RM, DipAcupuncture, nurse practitioner (pain) at Bassetlaw Hospital.

Lee Cutler MA(Ed), BSc(Hons), RN, consultant nurse in ITU at Doncaster and Bassetlaw Hospitals.

Robert Donald BA(Hons), MA, RN, clinical educator at the Sheffield Kidney Institute, Northern General Hospital, Sheffield.

Helen Hand MA(Ed), BSc, CertEd, DPSN, RN, lecturer in nursing at the University of Sheffield.

Jill Jesper DipCounselling, MMedSci, BSc(Hons), RNLD, lecturer in nursing at the University of Sheffield.

Margaret R Kay MSc, BSc(Hons), RN, lecturer in nursing at the University of Sheffield.

Phil Murch BA(Hons), RN, lecturer practitioner in GITU/HDU at Northern General Hospital and the University of Sheffield.

Sarah Starr RGN, MA(Ed), BA(Hons), RGN(T), nurse consultant in critical care, Princess Alexandra Hospital. Harlow.

Mandy Street BMedSci(Hons), DPSN, RN, sister on the General Intensive Care Unit, Rotherham General Hospital.

Catherine Waskett BSc(Hons), RN, lecturer in nursing at the University of Sheffield.

Dedicated to two dear old ladies for their loyal support,
Alice (died April 2002) and Jess.

Preface

The challenge of becoming a nurse has always been a considerable one. The work is often difficult emotionally and, at times, extremely hard physically. Over the years, nurse education has evolved through many forms, and in recent years has become technically based and scientifically challenging.

The philosophy of education has also changed in many ways, with the focus of the training/education process changing between a predominantly practical nursing focus and one based on what some might argue is an overly theoretical programme. Having worked in the nursing profession for well over 20 years and seen at first hand the effects of the differing approaches to education, I believe I am well placed to argue for a much more practically based and care-centred way of providing nursing care to patients.

There has also been a movement from what was until ten years ago a course delivered at certificate level to one that is now at diploma/degree level. This has in itself made a marked difference to the way that nursing is thought of and, of course, carried out at the 'sharp end'. Prior to the advent of the 'Project 2000' course, the 'hands-on' style of apprenticeship dominated. This style of education was very much based on rote learning. I remember memorizing endless patient scenarios and writing essays describing the ways the nurse must provide what was predominantly a medically based series of inputs, with little or no attention paid to, or real credit given for, the individualization of care for the patient. At the time, it was thought that this was sufficient for nurses. They were neither expected nor wanted to act in an autonomous or even semi-autonomous way, the patients seemed to get what they needed and things moved along in comfortable kind of way. This was, of course, until the 'modernizers' gained the ascendancy. The 'modernizers' were not really a distinct group of people. Rather, the modernization movement seemed to encapsulate an unholy alliance of academics, quasi-academics, governmental and quasi-governmental people (the regulatory bodies), and frustrated senior nurses, all of whom had a vague feeling that nursing and nursing education needed lifting to a higher academic level. This time also saw an acceptance that many members of the public saw nursing as a poorly paid and low-status job, both of which were true, and still are. With the demographic time bomb ticking, upgrading the training to a full diploma was seen by the government as a way of attracting the dwindling supply of 18–21-year-olds into nursing courses.

So dawned Project 2000. The ENB and UKCC set guidelines outlining the need for knowledgeable 'doers', and nursing academics designed educational (the word training was banned, as it harked back to the earlier days) curricula to teach the new nursing students 'new nursing'. It was, of course, at this time that the pendulum began its inevitable swing towards the other end of the theory/practice continuum. The academics felt that this was a good time to use all the wonderful new things they had learnt in their own rush for greater status in getting degrees. Most nurse teachers had studied and gained often odd hybrid degrees in the social sciences, psychology, anatomy and physiology, and pure education. Very few had nursing degrees that were based on real principles of nursing care, due mainly to the paucity of such courses in Britain at that time. So, as a consequence of this, Project 2000 dawned with pre-registration courses consisting of strange amalgams of socio/psychological, anato/physiological material, strongly underpinned by pure, often totally theoretical and dogmatic, educational ideology. Little wonder, therefore, that the new courses were generally fraught with difficulty and were accompanied by a general uneasy feeling that they produced qualified nurses who were not really fit for purpose, i.e. able to provide focused, humanistic and effective healthcare for patients. In the very recent years, there has been a gradual acceptance that the Project 2000 courses as they were first created did not work, and research carried out by governmental bodies and patient groups seems to support this notion. Finally, new curricula were designed and at last the pendulum is beginning to move back again to the practice end of the continuum. It is my belief that nursing has become overly 'academized' and what is needed is a real refocusing on how we can make patients feel better and double quick, which is what they want. Of course for this, we need smart, well-taught and thinking nurses to provide the care, so let's get to it and soon. That is where the idea for this book arose; I saw a real need for a book that meets student nurses' need for accessible nursing information.

This text draws together acknowledged experts in their respective fields and, using a very patient-focused approach, provides the reader with the concise, practical and readily usable information they need to give the patient tangible and effective care. The book uses a system-based approach to work through the entire body, and includes the vital area of psychological care.

Chris Bassett
October 2002

CHAPTER ONE

The cardiovascular system

MANDY STREET

Introduction

This chapter explores the function of the heart and considers the most commonly encountered diseases related to the cardiovascular system. It is designed to equip the nurse with the knowledge she or he needs to inform the care that a patient with a cardiovascular disease requires. The chapter begins with an overview of the heart, and then focuses primarily on the most commonly encountered conditions: myocardial infarction, hypertension and the often poorly understood condition of 'shock'.

Action point 1

Write down all you know about the structure and function of the heart.

Cardiovascular anatomy and physiology

The heart is a muscular organ located in the mediastinal space of the chest. The average healthy adult heart is approximately the size of a clenched fist, about 12 cm long and 9 cm wide, and weighs 250–400 g. The anterior of the heart consists of the right ventricle (RV) and the right atrium (RA). The left atrium (LA) lies posterior, with the left ventricle (LV) lying around the lateral surface (Figure 1.1).

The heart has four layers. The pericardium is a thin sac that covers the heart. The space between the pericardium and the epicardium contains 10–30 ml of thin, clear serous fluid. Its main function is to lubricate the

1

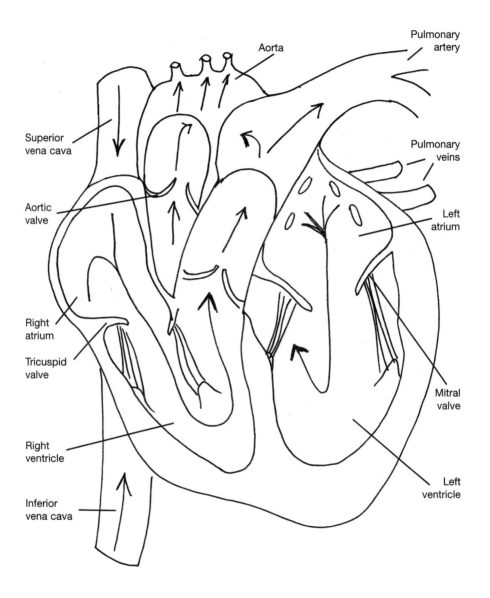

Figure 1.1 The structure of the heart.

moving surfaces of the heart. It prevents ventricular dilatation and helps to hold the heart in position.

The epicardium is a layer of mesothelial cells forming the visceral or heart layer of the serous pericardium. Branches of the coronary circulation, lymph vessels and nerves are contained within this layer. The epicardium completely encloses the external surface of the heart. The serous parietal pericardium lines the thicker, tougher, fibrous pericardial membrane.

The myocardium is composed of cardiac muscle cells, connective tissue and small blood vessels. Myocardial tissue consists of working myocardial cells for contractile force, nodal cells for pacemaker function and Purkinje cells for rapid conduction of electrical impulses.

The endocardium is a layer of endothelial cells with some collagen and elastic fibres. It is continuous with the tunica intima of the blood vessels.

Conduction tissue

The electrical activity (stimulation) of the heart is coupled with the mechanical activity (contraction). The electrical activity occurs before contraction, as the specialized nodal tissue depolarizes (discharges) spontaneously, generating impulses that are conducted to the larger mass of myocardium. This inherent property of nodal tissue is called automaticity. The conduction system of the heart comprises of the sinoatrial (SA) node, the atrioventricular (AV) node, the AV bundle (bundle of His), the right and left bundle branches, and the Purkinje fibres.

Cardiac structures

The heart is made up of a fibrous skeleton. Dense, fibrous, connective tissue rings (annuli fibrosi) surround the cardiac valves and provide internal support for the heart.

Primarily, the heart is divided into two anatomically distinct sides, the right side and the left side. Each side is further subdivided into upper and lower chambers (atria and ventricles). The atria receive blood from various parts of the body, while the ventricles pump blood to various parts of the body.

The wall thickness of each of the four chambers reflects the amount of pressure generated by that chamber. The two thin-walled atria act as reservoirs for blood that is primarily being funnelled into the ventricles. They add a small force to the moving blood. The wall of the LV, which creates the greatest amount of force to the blood flow, is two to three times as thick as that of the RV. The ventricles consist of figure-of-eight, muscle fibre path spirals attached to the fibrous skeleton. This arrangement allows circumferential movement and therefore ventricular contraction.

The RA receives deoxygenated blood from the inferior vena cava (from the lower body), the superior vena cava (from the upper body) and the coronary sinus (from the coronary veins). Blood flows from the RA into the RV and is ejected through the pulmonary system into the pulmonary circuit.

The RV is a thin-walled chamber that makes up the inferior portion of the heart's apex. Blood is pumped from the RV to the lungs, where it is reoxygenated.

The LA is slightly thicker than the RA. It receives oxygenated blood from the lungs through four pulmonary veins and then empties into the LV. The LV is three to five times thicker than the RV, because it has to be able to pump blood against the resistance of the entire circulation. The LV is the main pump of the heart. It propels blood through the aorta into the arterial system.

The valves

Atrioventricular valves

The tricuspid (RV) and bicuspid (LV) (mitral) are inflow valves. They comprise several components which function together as a unit: the atria, the valve rings of the fibrous skeleton, the valve cusps, the chordae tendinae, the papillary muscles and the ventricular walls. The tricuspid valve separates the RA and RV and has three cusps. The mitral valve separates the LA and LV and has two cusps. Fibrous cords called chordae tendinae connect the valves to the wall surfaces. The papillary muscle bundles extend from the walls to the chordae tendinae.

During diastole, the AV valves open passively as pressure in the atria exceeds that of the ventricles. The valve cusps part, forming a funnel, and blood flows through the funnel into the ventricle. Towards the end of diastole the increasing pressure in the ventricle and the decreasing flow of blood help the valves to close. The papillary muscles and chordae tendinae prevent the valves from opening in systole.

Semilunar valves

The pulmonary and aortic valves are outflow valves, and are composed of three cup-shaped cusps which attach their base to the fibrous skeleton. The aortic cusps are thicker than the pulmonary cusps. During systole, the cusps are thrust upwards as blood flows from the ventricles under great pressure. Decreasing flow of blood towards the end of systole helps to close the valves, and the strength of the valves helps to prevent backflow.

The coronary arteries

The two main coronary arteries (right and left) branch from the aorta at the sinus of Valsalva. They extend over the epicardial surface of the myocardium, branching several times. They plunge inwards through the myocardial wall. Branches to the epicardial surface exit first, so blood supply to the endocardium is easily compromised. The arteries branch and become arterioles and capillaries.

Right coronary artery (RCA)

This supplies the RA and RV and the inferior and posterior surfaces of the LV. It supplies the SA node, AV node and bundle of His in 90% of cases.

Left coronary artery (LCA)

Left main stem
This arises from the aorta behind the left cusp of the aortic valve. It divides into two branches – the left anterior descending coronary artery (LAD) and the left circumflex coronary artery.

Left anterior descending artery
This supplies portions of the left (anterior wall) and right ventricular myocardium and much of the interventricular septum. It appears to be a continuation of the left main stem.

Circumflex artery
This supplies blood to the LA and LV, and some to the SA node. It exits at right angles from the left main coronary artery.

The coronary veins

Most of the drainage is through the epicardial veins. They feed into the great cardiac vein, which becomes the coronary sinus and empties into the RA.

The cardiac nerves

Sensory nerve fibres from the ventricular walls, pericardium and coronary arteries transmit impulses to the central nervous system (CNS). The autonomic nervous system regulates the heart. Sympathetic stimulation accelerates the firing rate of the SA node, enhances AV conduction and increases force of contraction. Parasympathetic stimulation (vagus nerve) works in the opposite way.

The cardiac cycle

The cardiac cycle refers to one mechanical beat that commences with ventricular relaxation (diastole) and ends at the conclusion of systole (contraction).

Diastole comprises 60% of the cardiac cycle. The ventricles fill, and towards the end of diastole the atria contract, forcing blood into the ventricles. This additional blood contributes 30% to the cardiac output (CO). The AV valves then close.

Systole comprises 40% of the cardiac cycle. The ventricles contract under great pressure and rapidly propel blood into the aorta and pulmonary artery. The semilunar valves close and the cycle begins again.

The vascular system

The arterial system

The arterial system is responsible for ensuring that a blood supply rich in nutrients is able to reach the peripheral vascular beds.

The structure of the arteries

The walls of the arteries comprise three distinct layers: the intima, media and adventitia. The intima (inside layer) is a single layer of endothelial cells with a layer of elastic membrane to separate it from the medial layer. Endothelial cells are smooth and so reduce the risk of the blood clotting as it passes over the intima.

The media is composed of smooth muscle. Arteries are thicker than veins because their medial layer contains more smooth muscle, collagen and elastic fibres in order to propel blood to the organs. The adventitia (outer layer) contains connective tissue, collagen and elastic fibres.

Those arteries near to the heart are known as elastic arteries, because of the great pressures that they have to endure as the LV contracts. Muscular (distributive) arteries, which have less supportive tissue, are present in the lower extremities of the body. Blood leaves the heart and flows along distributive arteries, which branch off to major organs. The diameter of the arteries gradually reduces as they approach the extremities. Arterioles are smaller and offer most resistance to flow. As they become capillaries, the muscular layer of the vessel disappears and the resistance becomes less. Capillaries permeate into the tissues and allow for the exchange of gases and nutrients before they connect with the venules and veins that return the blood to the heart.

The microvascular system

Capillary walls comprise a single-thickness layer of endothelial cells, surrounded by a basement membrane. They form a network between the arterial and venous systems (the capillary bed). Capillaries divide profusely, so that all tissue cells are in contact with a capillary to allow diffusion of molecules from the circulation. Forces control the flow of fluid and solutes in and out of capillaries.

The venous system

The venous system arises in the capillary beds, as the capillaries become venules. These then unite to form larger single veins and eventually become the inferior and superior vena cava. The anatomy of the vein is slightly different to that of the artery in that they are flat vessels when empty. Larger veins contain a subendothelial layer of supportive tissue to give extra strength. The intimal layer contains bicuspid valves that open towards the heart so preventing backflow of blood.

Veins are very compliant, acting as reservoirs should blood volume increase quickly. As the walls of the vessels distend easily, there is little change in venous pressure. Venous flow in the body depends on the position of the vessels. Blood from the legs relies on the calf muscle pump to exert pressure and force blood up towards the heart. Blood flow from the neck and head relies on gravity to return blood to the superior vena cava.

Lymph vessels

The lymph vessels are not dissimilar to veins, but they contain more valves. They join together to form larger vessels called lymphatics. Movement of fluid in the lymphatics relies on external compression from surrounding muscles. Lymph passes through lymph nodes in the neck, axilla, abdomen and groin. Debris and bacteria are attacked by phagocytes.

Action point 2

Think of a patient with cardiovascular problems who you have looked after. How was he or she assessed, what was he or she like and what was your role in the process?

Assessment of the cardiovascular system

As with any system, the assessment of the patient is a vital nursing responsibility. Cardiovascular assessment is dictated by the need to prioritize patient care according to the clinical state of the patient. A primary assessment involving a rapid, accurate history of the signs and symptoms of the presenting complaint will enable potentially lifesaving interventions to be administered quickly. Once the patient is stabilized, a secondary assessment with a more detailed history can be carried out.

Primary assessment

This should be approached in a structured manner and cover the entire body, from top to toe. The assessment should be repeated regularly. Frequent reassessments will enable subtle changes in the patient's condition to be detected quickly and thus allow further interventional strategies to be started as soon as possible.

Objective assessment

This includes all the investigations and physiological measurements undertaken to elicit a diagnosis and assist with treatment plans. It may include blood pressure (BP), pulse, electrocardiogram (ECG), oxygen (O_2) saturation, echocardiogram, Doppler (an instrument that measures blood flow in arteries), cardiac monitor, haematological tests, ultrasound, x-rays, angiograms, perfusion scans, urine output and central venous pressure (CVP) measurements.

Subjective assessment

This includes how the patient looks, feels and sounds. It involves looking at the patient's general appearance, temperature, colour and consistency of the skin, mental state and breathing adequacy. Early signs of a deteriorating cardiovascular condition are unlikely to be identified by equipment and monitor readings alone. Much more information can be gleaned from touching, feeling, listening and looking at the patient.

Secondary assessment

Once the patient is stable, a much more detailed, systematic assessment of the history, formulation of the diagnosis and treatment/nursing management plan can be obtained. It should include an accurate history of the signs and symptoms of the presenting complaint, associated signs and symptoms, time of onset, manner of onset, frequency and duration of complaint, location, severity of complaint, aggravating or alleviating factors, and compensatory mechanisms. A nursing care plan can then be devised based on the condition and problems identified.

Physical assessment

The patient's physical condition should be assessed from top to toe, and should include the following.

General appearance

This can be assessed while taking the patient's history. General appearance and responses to questions will give clues to the patient's cardiovascular state. Of particular note should be build, skin colour and texture, and breathing status. Agitation, distress or anxiety may indicate pain or cerebral hypoxia. Appropriateness of weight may indicate signs of malnutrition or chronic heart failure encompassing peripheral oedema. The level of consciousness should be observed, as well as appropriateness of thought and conversation reflecting adequacy of cerebral perfusion.

Skin cyanosis

A bluish discoloration of the skin and mucous membranes occurs when the haemoglobin (O_2-carrying component) concentration is reduced.

Peripheral cyanosis

This implies a reduced blood flow to the facial periphery, e.g. nose, lips, earlobes or limbs. There are a number of causes:

- physiological – vasoconstriction, e.g. anxiety, cold temperatures
- pathological – conditions that reduce blood flow, e.g. shock (discussed later in this chapter).

Central cyanosis

This is seen in the buccal mucosa and indicates serious lung/heart disease. It usually occurs with peripheral cyanosis. Pulmonary oedema or disease prevents adequate oxygenation of blood as it passes through the lungs.

Pallor

This can be caused by: anaemia, in which reduced haemoglobin levels reduce the oxygen-carrying capacity of the blood; increased systemic vascular resistance (SVR); or reduced CO reducing blood flow to the periphery.

Carotid arteries

The carotid pulse is palpated in the lower third of the neck to avoid pressure on the carotid sinus baroreceptors, which reduce the heart rate if palpated. It is palpated only when there is a need to check for the presence of a major pulse to determine whether the patient is in cardiac arrest. It should be palpated only on one side of the neck to preserve circulation to the brain via the other carotid artery. The carotid pulse is felt in the groove between the thyroid cartilage and the sternocleidomastoid muscle of the neck. This is a skill requiring much practice.

Jugular veins

The neck veins are mostly visible when the patient is laid flat. They can be inspected for non-invasive estimates of intravascular volume and pressure. If they are distended and clearly visible it means the CVP is elevated, indicating potential heart failure or volume overload.

Temperature

Normal temperature is 37 degrees Celsius (°C). Hypothermia exists when the temperature is below 35°C. Pyrexia exists when the temperature rises above 37°C. Oral temperature averages 0.6°C below rectal temperature. The temperature is recorded peripherally; however, if hypothermia is suspected, a rectal (core) temperature should be taken.

Capillary refill

This is recorded to allow assessment of the arterial circulation. The nail bed is compressed for 5 seconds (s), which causes blanching. When the pressure is released the capillary should refill in less than 2 s.

Assessment of the heart

Auscultation of the heart will reveal the sounds of the closing of the mitral and tricuspid valves (systole) and the aortic and pulmonary valves (diastole). Extra heart sounds may be present in conditions such as left ventricular failure (LVF). It may also reveal the presence of pericardial friction rubs, denoting inflammation of the pericardium. A chest x-ray will demonstrate the size and shape of the heart, highlighting any structural abnormalities such as dissection of the aorta or ventricular hypertrophy.

Arterial pulse

Pulse rate

The most common peripheral site for assessment is the radial artery; others include the brachial or femoral arteries. A resting adult's pulse rate is 60–100 beats per minute (bpm). If the pulse rate is less than 60 bpm, this is called bradycardia and may be seen in quite healthy athletic individuals, post-myocardial infarction (MI) or as a result of drugs, e.g. beta blockers. If the pulse rate is greater than 100 bpm, this is called tachycardia and may be caused by fever, stress, metabolic conditions or exercise.

The pulse is created by cardiac contraction. Not all contractions are transmitted to the extremities, so the pulse rate should not be monitored using only a cardiac monitor.

Pulse rhythm

This may be classified as regular or irregular. There can be a normal variance with respiration. Irregular rhythms are not normal. (See below for cardiac rhythms and ECG monitoring.)

Pulse amplitude

The amplitude of the pulse reflects pulse pressure. Small, weak pulses have a low pulse pressure, indicating reduced stroke volume (SV – the amount of blood ejected from the ventricle with each contraction) and increased SVR (vascular tone of the arteries). Patients with small, weak pulses might be in cardiogenic or hypovolaemic shock.

Large, bounding pulses have an increased pulse pressure resulting from increased SV and low SVR. Patients with septicaemia, thyrotoxicosis or pyrexia may have large, bounding pulses.

Procedure for monitoring arterial pulse

Compress the radial artery using the pads of the index and middle fingers. Feel for a place where there is maximum volume. If it is regular, count the number of pulsations in 15 s and multiply by 4. If it is irregular, you need to palpate for a full minute.

Action point 3

Are you fully familiar with taking a patient's blood pressure? There are many key concepts that you must be aware of. What are they?

Blood pressure

The blood pressure (BP) is the result of the CO SVR. The systemic arterial BP can be measured directly or indirectly.

A direct measurement requires the insertion of a catheter directly into an artery and is performed in a critical care environment where it can be closely monitored.

Indirect BP measurement is easier and a lot more common. It is carried out using a sphygmomanometer. Peak systemic arterial BP incorporates the systolic and diastolic BP.

Systolic BP is the result of left ventricular pressure during systole, i.e. when ventricular contraction exerts sufficient pressure to open the valves and eject blood. Diastolic BP is the result of pressure produced by the vascular tone of the arteries and an intact aortic valve, which remains closed to allow ventricular filling.

Blood pressure manometers

Sphygmomanometers

A sphygmomanometer measures the BP indirectly. It comprises an inflatable rubber bladder inside a non-distensible covering (cuff). The size and placement of the bladder is crucial for accuracy. Bladder width should be 40% of the circumference of the limb. Bladder length should be 80% of the limb circumference. This will reduce inaccurate measurements.

Aneroid manometers (manual)

An aneroid manometer consists of a round gauge calibrated in millimetres of mercury (mmHg), an inflation system (bulb), exhaust valve and tubing. Mercury manometers are now seldom used in clinical practice because of the risk of mercury leakage.

Electronic devices

Electronic devices should be checked with a mercury manometer. They consist of a self-inflation/deflation system, and the rules of measurement are the same as for manual manometers. They should not be used for patients with irregular heart rhythms or post-cardiac arrest because of the variability of pulse pressure, which may give inaccurate results.

Procedure for taking the blood pressure

- The patient should be relaxed and comfortable.
- Place the deflated cuff around the arm, 2.5 cm above the antecubital fossa.
- The bladder should cover the inner arm, with the arterial point on the cuff aligned over the brachial artery.
- Ensure the patient's arm is at heart level for accuracy, supported on a pillow.
- The patient should be lying or sitting and the position should be documented.
- Palpate the brachial artery.
- Close the exhaust valve to enable inflation of the cuff.
- Inflate the cuff until the brachial pulse can no longer be palpated.
- The cuff pressure is now greater than the arterial pressure. Increase inflation 20–30 mmHg above this point.
- Place the stethoscope diaphragm over the brachial artery.
- Slowly reopen the exhaust valve and reduce the cuff pressure until there is an audible pulse. These sounds are known as Korotkoff's sounds (Table 1.1) , and the point at which they are audible is the systolic pressure.
- Reduce the pressure further until the sounds become muffled.
- The point at which the pulse sound disappears is the diastolic pressure.
- Normal systolic BP = <160 mmHg, normal diastolic BP = <90 mmHg

Table 1.1 Korotkoff's sounds

Phase	Sound	Recording
I	First appearance of faint clear tapping sound	Systolic BP
II	Sounds of swishing quality	
III	Sounds become crisper and increase in intensity	
IV	Distinct muffling abruptly occurs, soft, blowing sounds	Diastolic BP in children < 13 years
V	Disappearance of sounds	Diastolic BP in adults

Variations in blood pressure

The systolic BP varies by up to 10 mmHg between the right and left brachial arteries. Standing causes a slight reduction in systolic BP (10–20 mmHg) and a slight increase in diastolic BP (5–10 mmHg).

Postural (orthostatic) hypotension involves a larger reduction in both systolic and diastolic BP. It is usually associated with symptoms of dizziness or syncope. It may be associated with hypovolaemia, poor vasoconstrictor mechanisms (e.g. immobility) or autonomic insufficiency (beta blockers).

Cardiac monitoring

The cardiac impulse

When an impulse from the SA node stimulates the Purkinje myocardial cells it causes a discharge of the electrical forces stored in the cell membrane. This electrical 'discharging' process is called depolarization and results in myocardial contraction.

After depolarization has occurred, the muscle cells recover and restore the electrical charges. This 'recharging' process is called repolarization. The next impulse from the SA node occurs when repolarization has been completed, after which activation can occur again. The combined periods of depolarization and repolarization constitute the electrical events of the cardiac cycle. Both processes are associated with chemical events that involve the exchange of sodium and potassium ions across the myocardial cell membrane. Electrical functioning of the heart is measured using the ECG. A brief description of the ECG follows. As a student nurse, you will not be expected to be able to interpret ECGs but it is useful to have some knowledge of a normal tracing.

The normal waves of the ECG

The ECG is characterized by five separate waveforms, designated P, Q, R, S and T (Figure 1.2).

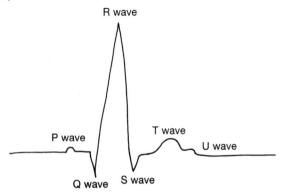

Figure 1.2 The normal ECG tracing.

The P wave

This is the first wave of the ECG and constitutes depolarization of the atria.

The PR interval

The impulse reaches the AV node, located low in the right atrium. Activation of the AV node does not produce an identifiable wave but contributes to the time interval between the P and QRS.

The PR interval signifies the time taken for the impulse to spread across the atria and through the AV node.

The QRS complex

Once the impulse has traversed the AV node, it enters the bundle of His. Current flowing through the septum and ventricles via the bundle branches represents the QRS complex.

The conduction pathway terminates by dividing into the Purkinje fibres that distribute the depolarization wave rapidly through the ventricles.

The ST segment

This is the transient period when no further electrical current can be passed through the myocardium. It is measured from the beginning of the S wave to the beginning of the T wave. It signifies a pause in the ventricular electrical activity before repolarization. It assists in the diagnosis of myocardial infarction and ischaemia.

The T wave

This represents repolarization of the ventricular myocardium to its resting electrical state. Myocardial ischaemia may interfere with the normal repolarization and cause the T wave to invert.

The QT interval

This signifies the total duration of depolarization and repolarization of the ventricular muscle. It is measured from the beginning of the QRS complex to the end of the T wave.

Procedure for cardiac monitoring

All patients who have cardiac problems will be attached to a cardiac monitor to enable the electrical condition of their heart to be assessed constantly by the nursing staff. The correct procedure is:

- *Explain the procedure* to the patient, including lead attachments, why the monitor is required and the effects, e.g. alarms sounding.
- *Prepare the equipment* required – cardiac monitor, monitor lead, gel electrodes, shaver and alcohol swabs if required.
- *Prepare the patient's skin* – shave hair from the site, cleanse the skin with an alcohol wipe to remove dead skin cells. Warn the patient of slight stinging.
- *Place the electrodes* on the prepared sites by peeling off the backing paper and placing them in the centre of the sites. Ensure that the entire adhesive is well secured to the skin. Electrodes should be placed on bony prominences to reduce muscle artefact (interference) and away from defibrillation sites.
- *Attach the lead* via the press stud or clip to the electrodes, according to the colour co-ordination:
    right arm – red
    left arm – yellow
    left leg – green/ black.

The 12-lead ECG

A more sophisticated method of monitoring the heart's electrical activity is to use a 12-lead ECG. This signifies that the heart is viewed from 12 different angles (or leads). The interpretation of the readings from an ECG is beyond the scope of this chapter.

Action point 4

Atheroma is major problem in Western society today and contributes greatly to cardiovascular disease. What is it, and what are the causes?

Development of atherosclerosis

Atherosclerosis is a major contributor to cardiac disease; it mostly affects the medium-sized arteries perfusing the heart, brain and kidneys, and the large arteries branching off the aorta.

Plaque formation

Plaques are fatty deposits that form in the blood vessels. Plaque formation occurs when plasma low-density lipoprotein (LDL) invades the intima, creating an inflammatory process. This evolves to form an advanced lesion, which recruits macrophages to form a lipid and cholesterol core inside the vessel. The accumulation continues until a raised fibrolipid plaque occurs, which may cause narrowing of the vessel lumen. The plaque is separated from the lumen by a very thin, easily ruptured sheet of fibromuscular tissue, which is at high risk of thrombotic (clot-developing) events. The plaque grows until the intimal lining tears or fissures. This attracts platelets, which stick to the damaged area.

Thrombosis development

The ruptured plaque encourages platelet adhesion, and clotting factors develop a thrombus, which becomes superimposed on the plaque. This grows and projects into the lumen, which further narrows, or it may block the vessel, causing a myocardial infarction (MI).

Atherosclerosis of the coronary circulation

Several factors can increase myocardial oxygen demand, including physical exercise, emotional stress, heavy meals and smoking, and when demand rises vasodilatation usually occurs to increase the supply of oxygen. When atherosclerosis is present, vasodilatation cannot occur, resulting in a greater demand than can be supplied. This creates myocardial ischaemia (reduced oxygen for cellular metabolism). Initially, this is reversible. However, if the supply is not increased or demand is not reduced, cell necrosis (cell death) may occur, as in MI.

Myocardial infarction

Infarction is identified pathologically as a centre of coagulation necrosis, i.e. all cells (interstitial, nervous, muscle) in this zone are electrically silent. It occurs when there is a thrombus in the coronary artery blocking the oxygen supply to part of the myocardium. Lack of oxygen (anoxia) then causes myocardial cell death. Anaerobic metabolism occurs, with a corresponding build-up of lactic acid, creating chest pain.

After 20 minutes, necrosis begins and spreads in a waveform from epi-cardium to endocardium. The infarcted area is primarily red, due to the 'stuffing in' of the red cells. The area later becomes pale as the necrotic mus-cle swells and squeezes out the extravasated blood, replacing it with fibrous scar tissue.

Signs and symptoms

Chest pain

Ischaemic pain is abrupt and present constantly. It is more severe than angina, and medication does not provide any relief. It is not always described as pain; sometimes pain equivalents are used, such as strangling, aching, squeezing, pressing, tightness, heaviness, crushing, constriction or indigestion.

The pain is located substernally, referred there by spinal nerve reflexes (see Chapter 7). Impulses from the myocardium travel via sympathetic nerve fibres to the thoracic sympathetic ganglia. These spinal nerves also supply the anterior chest wall and inner aspect of the arm and hand, hence a common sensation of tingling or aching in the arms and fingers.

Associated symptoms are almost always present as a result of sympathetic nervous activity from severe pain.

Associated symptoms

Dyspnoea

This is usually due to left ventricular failure causing pulmonary oedema. The lungs become congested with fluid, resulting in decreased O_2 levels, and the oedema narrows the larger airways, making respiration difficult.

Diaphoresis or sweating

Overstimulation of the CNS in response to the MI causes excessive sweating, and the patient becomes cold and clammy. The sweat glands are greatly stimulated and the peripheral blood vessels are constricted.

Nausea and vomiting

This is caused by overstimulation of the parasympathetic nervous system. The activity of the vagus nerve causes emptying of the stomach contents, and this symptom can last for up to 24 h.

Dizziness

This may be due to a low BP or pulse. Pain-relieving medications (glyceryl trinitrate or diamorphine) can also cause dizziness.

Diagnosis in acute MI

1. Patient history – assessment of signs and symptoms (i.e. pain – type, duration, severity, radiation, location, associated symptoms, precipitating factors) to enable accurate diagnosis.
2. Twelve-lead ECG – to identify site, size and time of MI.
3. Other investigations on admission – cardiac enzymes, lipids, full blood count.

The location of the MI influences the clinical course and outcome of the attack. A higher death rate is associated with anterior MI, because of the greater muscle loss involved.

Medical management

Medical management includes the following essential factors.

Pain relief

The patient will receive O_2 in high concentration via a non-rebreather mask. Intravenous (IV) diamorphine 5 mg is given and repeated every 5 min until the patient is pain-free. The dose will be dependent on the patient's pain score and sedation level. This reduces pain and anxiety, so reducing the workload of the heart and the infarct size. The goal is a total pain-free state. Nitrates may be given sublingually or intravenously for pain control once the patient is pain-free post-diamorphine.

Cardiac monitoring

This will monitor for arrhythmias or changes in the ECG. Monitoring must be continuous and an alarm facility must be used. Twelve-lead ECGs will be recorded on admission, and again if the patient experiences pain episodes post-treatment.

Reduction of infarction size

Thrombolytics may be used to reopen a blocked vessel by lysing (dissolving) the thrombus that is occluding it. The injured myocardium is then reperfused with blood, which salvages viable myocardium and limits the damage. The patient must be assessed for any conditions that may create a risk of bleeding and are thus a contraindication to thrombolytic treatment. Streptokinase is given for inferior MI, reteplase or tenecteplase is given for anterior MI of patients younger than 70 with fewer than 4 hours of chest pain. The main aim is recanalization of the occluded artery. For secondary management, select from a choice of beta blockers, angiotensin-converting enzyme (ACE) inhibitors, nitrates and calcium channel blockers (see the local coronary care unit (CCU) protocol).

Cardiac rehabilitation

This is usually an 8-week physical exercise and health education programme that focuses on behavioural and cognitive changes to adopt healthier approaches to lifestyle.

Acute coronary syndromes

Angina pectoris

Defined as 'strangling of the chest', angina pectoris is a symptom of coronary artery disease (CAD) rather than an actual disease process, i.e. it is a sensation experienced by the patient. It occurs as a result of myocardial ischaemia.

Classification of angina

Stable angina

This is characterized by transient episodes of substernal chest pain or discomfort. Usually there are no ECG changes present. Episodes are predictable and related to exercise or emotional distress, i.e. activities that increase myocardial oxygen demand. Fixed lesions of more than 75% are the culprits for this condition. Patients become accustomed to the pattern of pain and control it through rest or glyceryl trinitrate (GTN), a coronary vasodilator administered by sublingual spray or tablet. It can be managed with medication for long periods of time.

Unstable angina

This is characterized by a change in a previous pattern of angina, prolonged angina at rest or a new onset of severe angina. If the angina persists for more than 20 minutes despite the use of GTN, it is regarded as a medical emergency requiring immediate admission to hospital. It is a dangerous mid-zone between stable angina and MI. Associated symptoms may be present, including diaphoresis (profuse sweating), breathlessness, nausea and dizziness.

Priorities of assessment

This is characterized by two approaches.

Objective assessment

- Twelve-lead ECG – to assess myocardial ischaemia.
- Blood tests – test for troponin T, creatine kinase (CK), full blood count (FBC), urea and electrolytes (U&Es), and lipids.
- Oxygen saturation level ($SaO_2\%$) – helps to assess pulmonary oedema.
- BP and pulse – may be tachycardic or hypotensive with pain.

Subjective assessment

- Pain score 0 (no pain) up to 3 (severe pain).
- General appearance of patient.
- Assessment of pain description, i.e. type, location, duration, radiation, severity, associated symptoms, precipitating/relieving factors.
- Presence of anxiety.
- Temperature and texture of skin.
- Colour – cyanosis, pallor.
- Associated symptoms – mild to moderate, e.g. breathlessness (? LVF), nausea and vomiting, dizziness, diaphoresis (sympathetic nervous system [SNS] stimulation).

Medical management

In the pre-hospital stage the following treatments may be used:

- Oxygen therapy – high concentration, 60–100%, via a non-rebreather mask, to increase oxygenation and counteract ischaemia.
- Aspirin 300 mg – reduces platelet 'stickiness' to prevent thrombosis.
- Intravenous opiate and antiemetic – Cyclimorph (cyclizine), a strong analgesic, reduces catecholamine release, which reduces the workload of the heart; cyclizine 25–50 mg prevents nausea caused by CNS and intravenous opiate.

In-hospital treatment

This is usually the following treatment, sometimes known as 'MONA':

- **Morphine** – intravenous diamorphine 5 mg titrated until the patient is pain-free, dependent on pain score and sedation score.
- **Oxygen** – 60–100 % via a non-rebreather mask.
- **Nitrate** – tablet or spray. In continuing pain, intravenous GTN infusion 0.9–10 mg increased slowly, dependent on pain score and BP (causes hypotension).
- **Aspirin** 300 mg immediately, then 75–150 mg daily reduces risk of MI.

Additional treatments may include the following:

- Low-molecular-weight heparin (LMWH, e.g. Clexane). This is an anticoagulant to prevent thrombus development and is weight-adjusted.
- Glycoprotein inhibitors – a new treatment to reduce platelet adhesion.
- Anti-ischaemic medications, including:
    beta blockers: atenolol, bisoprolol, metoprolol

ACE inhibitors: lisinopril, perindopril, ramipril
nitrates: isosorbide mononitrate
calcium channel blockers: diltiazem, amlodipine.

Essential nursing care in myocardial infarction

There are many things the nurse can do to help a patient who is suffering from acute cardiac distress. The following activities are a guide to the care the patient will need.

Chest pain management

Take an in-depth history of the patient's condition and provide adequate analgesia to achieve a pain-free state. Place the patient on bed rest to reduce myocardial O_2 demand and workload. Reassess and monitor constantly for effective analgesic relief. Ensure the patient knows how important it is to express pain, so that other anti-ischaemic medications may be administered if necessary. Reduce anxiety from pain and the psychological effects of emergency admission. Stress reduction is paramount to reduce myocardial O_2 demand from catecholamine release, which increases heart rate and thus the workload of the heart. Reassurance in a calm, confident environment is the best approach.

Cardiac monitoring

- Continuously observe the patient for arrhythmias.
- Take BP, temperature, pulse and respiration every 5–15 min to 4-hourly, depending on his condition and the medications administered.
- Twelve-lead ECG on arrival, 90 min and 4 h post-thrombolysis.

Care of fluid balance

This is very important in MI because the compromised myocardium can easily be overloaded. Caution with fluid input and output monitoring should be maintained. You need to take care of the intravenous line; this is vital for emergency access in the event of a cardiac arrest and for administration of pain relief.

Care of reduced mobility

Bed rest should be maintained for 24 h to reduce myocardial O_2 demand.

The patient should mobilize slowly after being pain-free for 12 h, to help prevent complications of inactivity.

Care of hygiene needs

Help the patient to wash or bed bath while immobile, and provide oral hygiene for possible dry mouth from O_2 administration.

Health education needs

Identify risk factors and engage in interactive discussion with the patient and family to help them adopt a healthier lifestyle. Refer the patient to the cardiac rehabilitation service for long-term rehabilitation.

Care of family

Don't forget to offer support to the patient's distressed relatives.

Continuing care

It is important to see the patient's care as a continuum that is maintained throughout their stay in hospital and beyond. Daily living activities, e.g. hygiene, nutrition and mobility, will gradually be increased once a pain-free state has been achieved. Health education needs include risk factor identification and management, pain control and exercise tolerance.

Education on the different medications prescribed, their effects and side effects, and their importance to the patient's treatment is also important.

The patient may require further interventions, including an exercise tolerance test (ETT), coronary angiography or echocardiogram. The patient may require this as a hospital inpatient (if unstable) or after discharge as an outpatient once stabilized.

Complications post-MI

Action point 5

The condition of MI is a serious one and there is a risk of complications following the infarction. It is important to be aware of them. Can you think of the possible complications?

Arrhythmias

These can be of any origin. They occur from necrotic injury to the myocardium, which causes the myocardial cells to become electrically unstable. Ventricular fibrillation is the most common and is the reason for sudden death.

Cardiogenic shock

This is an extreme form of LVF. The myocardium is failing to generate adequate perfusion to the vital organs. This is covered in more detail later in the chapter.

Thromboembolism

A clot (thrombus) may occur in the LV, and this may break loose and form an embolus which may occlude elsewhere in the arterial system, causing ischaemia or necrosis of other organs.

Pericarditis

Inflammation of the pericardium occurs from a full-thickness infarct. The pericardium becomes tight, restricting and swollen. It causes extreme pain, which is sharp and stabbing in nature, becomes worse on lying flat and easier when sitting forward. The temperature spikes and a pericardial friction rub may be heard as the myocardium and pericardium rub over each other. Anti-inflammatory treatment is required.

Left ventricular rupture

Extensive damage to the myocardium creates an area of soft muscle. This may weaken, leading to rupture of the LV wall. Blood from the LV fills the pericardial sac and causes compression of the heart (cardiac tamponade). The heart is unable to contract adequately and death can occur within minutes.

Cardiac arrest

This is failure of the heart to pump sufficient blood to maintain cerebral perfusion and therefore life. There are three mechanisms that cause cardiac arrest:

1. ventricular fibrillation (VF) (shockable)
2. pulseless ventricular tachycardia (VT) (shockable)
3. asystole, pulseless electrical activity (non-shockable).

Defibrillation is the only treatment for VF or VT and should not be delayed. Brain death occurs from anoxia after 4–6 min. Cardiopulmonary resuscitation must be commenced immediately the patient is found to be pulseless. The main priorities of management are airway, breathing and circulation (ABC), with adjunctive adrenaline to assist with myocardial and cerebral perfusion.

Heart failure

Heart failure can be desribed as a pathophysiological state in which there is an abnormality of cardiac function that prevents the heart from pumping blood to the capacity required to meet the metabolic and physiological demands of the tissues. There may be a loss of functioning myocardium (from MI) or a mechanical/structural disruption (from the valves). It may be acute or chronic, depending on the speed at which the syndrome develops. It may affect the right or left side of the heart.

Acute heart failure

In acute heart failure the contractile state of the LV is markedly reduced owing to necrotic damage. The heart begins to fail as a pump. Blood remains in the LV after each contraction due to the inability of the weakened muscles to expel all the contents. This residual amount increases until the following volume delivery from the atria and lungs is unable to enter the LV, and the volume exceeds the capacity of the LV. This creates backward pressure to the atria, pulmonary venous system and lungs, creating venous and alveolar congestion.

Fluid is squeezed out from the blood through the capillary membrane into the alveolar space, creating pulmonary oedema. This prevents adequate gaseous exchange resulting in myocardial hypoxia, which exacerbates the ischaemia and causes further impairment of the LV. The fluid can be heard as crackles in the lung fields. Diuretics and vasodilators are required to reduce the preload, thereby reducing myocardial workload.

Chronic heart failure

This develops over time and results from advanced heart disease processes. It is represented by a chronic increasing inability of physiological compensatory mechanisms. It is caused by inadequate delivery of blood into the arterial system coupled with the failure of the ventricle to empty.

Right heart failure

This is created by ineffective contractile function of the RV, which may be caused by RV infarction, pulmonary embolus or as a secondary effect of LV failure. The right heart receives deoxygenated blood from the major organs. Signs and symptoms may include generalized weakness, peripheral or sacral oedema, jugular distension, hepatomegaly, liver tenderness, jaundice and cyanosis.

Investigations

A chest x-ray will be taken to examine for signs of pulmonary oedema, and an ECG will be taken to observe for tachycardia or ischaemia.

Following this, a series of blood tests will be carried out:

- U&Es to monitor for acute renal failure from impaired renal perfusion
- liver function test (LFT) to observe for liver failure from fluid congestion
- arterial blood gas analysis to observe oxygenation, including respiratory and metabolic function.

An echocardiogram may be taken to observe and assess cardiac function.

Medical management

The medical aims for this condition are to relieve symptoms and improve cardiac performance.

Acute

Manage fluid overload and improve CO by reducing SVR through vasodilatation, thus reducing circulating volume. Acute management of this serious condition is as follows:

- Oxygen therapy – high concentration > 60%.
- Diuretics – reduce preload through greater fluid excretion. Furosemide (frusemide) 40–80 mg i.v., Burinex (bumetanide) 2–4 mg i.v. and assess response.
- Opiates intravenously to reduce anxiety created by extreme dyspnoea. Breathing performance improved by reducing tachypnoea. This enables peripheral vasodilatation, reducing circulating volume and myocardial workload, and thereby improving myocardial oxygenation and function.

Diamorphine 2.5–5.0 mg, repeated as necessary according to response and dependent on respiration rate and sedation score.
- Nitrate intravenously – reduces circulating volume by peripheral vasodilatation. Nitrocine infusion 0.9–10 mg gradually titrated upwards in 0.3-mg increments according to response and BP. This requires constant close observation of the patient.

Chronic

Oral diuretics – furosemide or Burinex, doses same as for intravenously, dependent on response.

- ACE inhibitor – improves cardiac performance by reducing vasoconstriction. Lisinopril, ramipril, perindopril. Enables cardiac remodelling.
- Cardiospecific beta blocker, e.g. bisoprolol 2.5–5 mg.

Essential nursing care

Subjective aspects

LOOK – general appearance: distressed mentally, dyspnoeic, tachypnoeic, skin colour.
LISTEN – for breathlessness, noisy breathing (audible crackles from fluid in lungs).
FEEL – temperature and texture of skin (cold and clammy).

Objective aspects

- Vital signs – BP may be high from distress or low from reduced CO.
- Pulse rapid, weak and thready (compensatory).
- Respiratory rate – tachypnoeic > 30.
- O_2 saturations – 70–90% due to pulmonary oedema in alveoli.
- Blood tests – arterial blood gas analysis, U&Es, FBC, LFT, CK.
- ECG – demonstrates myocardial ischaemia.

Nursing care

The patient will feel breathless, so you must remember the care of the dyspnoeic patient. Sit the patient upright, well supported by pillows, in the orthopnoeic position. The pillow should be on the bed table, with the patient's arms over the top of the pillow to enable greater lung expansion.

High-concentration oxygen should be given via a non-rebreather mask with a reservoir, as prescribed. Another thing that might help is fan therapy to aid air circulation; this helps to satisfy 'air hunger' from dyspnoea.

You will need to administer medications and monitor their effect: diuretics, intravenous opiates, intravenous nitrates, ACE inhibitor in acute and chronic phase.

Monitoring cardiac performance is an important nursing function. Attach the patient to a cardiac monitor. The pulse may be tachycardic owing to compensatory mechanisms. The ECG may show ischaemic changes due to reduced myocardial oxygenation. The BP may be low due to poor cardiac performance or the effects of intravenous nitrates.

Other things to remember in caring for these patients are:

- Potential chest pain from ischaemic myocardium:
    assess chest pain type, duration, location and severity
    record ECG in pain
    administer analgesia – sublingual GTN and diamorphine depending on severity; intravenous nitrate to maintain pain-free state.
- Fluid balance/restriction:
    limit fluids to 1–1.5 l/day
    check balance twice daily – positive (more input than output), negative (more output than input)
    record excessive diaphoresis.
- Reduced mobility:
    pressure area care to improve tissue viability from poor skin texture and sedation from diamorphine
    hygiene – excessive diaphoresis and sedation; oral care – dry mouth from oxygen, reduced intake from nausea or sedation
    leg exercises – lack of movement from sedation.
- Maintenance of cardiac performance by adequate rest, drugs.
- Living with chronic heart failure (CHF) – education on minimizing oedema, coping with condition and breathlessness, measuring weight, nutrition (reducing salt intake), medications, exercise plan.

With good treatment and nursing care the patient can often make a good recovery following an MI, and return to a normal life.

Hypertension

Hypertension (HT) is the commonest cause of cardiovascular disease in developed countries, and is a potentially serious condition if untreated. Treatment is improving greatly with medication and, if used with lifestyle changes, patients can live long and healthy lives.

When does a patient have hypertension?

A systolic BP of >160 mmHg and a diastolic BP of >90 mmHg are considered to define HT.

Under normal conditions, BP measurements are made on three separate occasions before a diagnosis of HT is made.

Classification

Primary (essential) HT represents 95% of diagnosed cases. Primary HT exists where no cause can be identified and the origin is not known. It is usually genetic.

Secondary (malignant) HT exists in 5% of diagnosed cases, where a specific cause can be attributed.

Signs and symptoms

Hypertension has no real symptoms until target organ damage occurs. However, there may be increased incidence of nocturia, epistaxis (bleeding from the nose) and headaches in some hypertensive patients.

Effects of HT on the body

Large arteries

These can become dilated, particularly the aorta, which loses elasticity. Peripherally, arteries are elongated and tortuous. Atheroma development is apparent in vessels with increased pressure.

Small arteries

Thickening of the vessel wall (medial hypertrophy) occurs, creating increased resistance to flow.

The heart

Hypertension increases the load against which the LV has to contract, and this leads to LV hypertrophy (LVH). The muscle swelling causes a reduced filling capacity and so LVF may also be present. Coronary atheroma is frequently present with HT. MI is the most frequent cause of death and is three times more common than stroke.

Brain

The brain may suffer an increased prevalence of atheroma in the extra- and intracranial vessels, increasing the risk of cerebral infarction from thrombosis. There may also be aneurysm development, which can lead to intracerebral haemorrhage.

Kidneys

Renal failure is rare with primary hypertension. However, patients with HT and renal disease appear to have a worse prognosis. In HT, the elevated glomerular filtration pressure causes proteinuria. In accelerated HT, fibrinoid necrosis causes renal failure to progress rapidly (see Chapter 5).

The eyes

The retina is the only part of the body where arteries and arterioles can be seen non-invasively. Evidence of retinal damage indicates blood vessel damage elsewhere. Changes caused by HT can include focal spasms, haemorrhages, local infarctions and oedema of the optic fundus.

Investigations for hypertension

- ECG – to monitor for LVH, large QRS complexes.
- Bloods – measure U&Es, FBC, blood sugar, lipid, CK to look for cause.
- Mid-stream specimen of urine (MSU) to monitor for proteinuria, micro-albuminuria, casts, red cells and white cells, which may be present from increased renal pressure.
- Chest x-ray to monitor for LV enlargement or LVF.
- Ambulatory BP monitoring to observe for fluctuations in BP.
- Renal urography to detect possible renal artery stenosis.
- Renal ultrasound to check for renal cysts.
- Echocardiogram to monitor for LV wall thickness.

Priorities of treatment

1. Assess target organ involvement.
2. Assess other cardiovascular risk factors.
3. Assess presence of cardiovascular disease.
4. Find the cause of the HT.
5. Assess and treat co-morbid conditions.

Choice of drug treatment

Beta blockers, calcium channel blockers and diuretics are all used with good effect in this condition.

Nursing care of the hypertensive patient

As with any illness, assessment of the patient is an essential requirement. It helps the medical team to assess the effectiveness of drug therapy, and therefore accurate recording of BP and maintenance of goal BP is a vital nursing function.

Care of associated symptoms is also important. For example, a patient who suffers from dizziness should receive adequate rest and good BP control. Headaches can sometimes be a problem. Again, plenty of rest, BP control and analgesia will help. Epistaxis, if present, is a nursing priority, so rest, control of the bleeding and BP control are essential.

Education on condition and lifestyle is also important. Lifestyle changes may be required, as may dietary changes. Reducing intake of fat, salt and caffeine may all help. Exercise should be gradual; an exercise programme can be devised with the physiotherapist. Plenty of rest and stress relaxation therapy will help to reduce heart rate and contractility. Patients who are smokers will need to be helped to give up.

Finally, medication is very important. Explain the patient's drug regimen, how and why the drugs work, the side effects and the importance of compliance.

Shock

Shock is a potentially life-threatening condition that may occur in any patient suffering from cardiac disease. It can also be caused by other conditions. This chapter will now explore the issues surrounding shock.

Action point 6

What do you understand shock to be? Have you ever seen a patient suffering from this condition? What caused it and how were they treated?

Defining shock

Shock can be defined as a state of tissue perfusion that is inadequate to maintain the supply of nutrients and oxygen required for normal cellular function, resulting in generalized tissue hypoxia.

Pathophysiology

Cellular and systemic dysfunction occurs as a result of generalized hypoxia. Tissue hypoperfusion activates compensatory mechanisms that aim to restore adequate BP and volume to ensure sufficient perfusion of the vital organs. These mechanisms become counterproductive if the underlying problem is not resolved, and a vicious cycle of irreversible shock ensues.

Stages of shock

Initial stage

No signs or symptoms are present. Hypoperfusion causes anaerobic metabolism. The end products of this metabolism are lactic acid and pyruvic acid, which result in metabolic acidosis.

Compensatory stage

Physiological adaptations occur in an attempt to overcome the problem. Neural, hormonal and chemical mechanisms come into play to overcome the worsening effects of shock on the body.

Neural mechanisms
Hypotension stimulates the stress response (stimulation of the SNS). Catecholamines (adrenaline and noradrenaline) are released to vasoconstrict blood vessels to the skin, kidney and gastrointestinal (GI) tract to preserve the cardiac output to the heart and brain. Cardiac output is increased by an increased heart rate and BP, but this also increases the workload of the heart.

Hormonal mechanisms

- Adrenocorticotrophic hormone (ACTH) is released to stimulate the adrenal cortex to produce glucocorticoids and mineralocorticoids, which increase the blood sugar level.
- Aldosterone is released to increase reabsorption of sodium and chloride by the kidneys, to improve circulating volume and CO.

- Antidiuretic hormone increases renal water reabsorption to increase circulating volume.
- Noradrenaline's effects stimulate renin production, which, through angiotensin and aldosterone production, results in increased circulating volume and vasoconstriction.
- Thyroxine sensitizes beta-receptors to noradrenaline in the heart, which will increase the heart rate, BP, SV and CO.

Chemical mechanisms

Chemoreceptors in the aorta and carotid bodies sense decreased oxygen in the blood and so increase the respiratory rate to compensate. The increased carbon dioxide (CO_2) expiration results in respiratory alkalosis and cerebral hypoxia. Anaerobic metabolism leads to metabolic acidosis. The patient may be cold and clammy with decreased urine output and increased pulse rate, anxious, restless and confused.

Progressive stage

As the compensatory mechanisms start to fail and the shock cycle worsens, there is insufficient energy created within the cells by anaerobic metabolism to maintain normal function, and this results in irreversible cell damage.

The microcirculation collapses due to anaerobic metabolism, resulting in a sluggish circulation from vasodilatation. This leads to disseminated intravascular coagulation (DIC), where the clotting mechanisms do not function normally and clots form in the capillaries. Fibrinolytic (clot-dissolving) factors are activated when they are not required, resulting in uncontrolled haemorrhage.

Prolonged vasoconstriction eventually compromises the functioning of the vital organs, as outlined below.

Kidney

The kidney becomes unable to filter, excrete and reabsorb fluid, reducing urine output to less than 30 ml/h. Acute tubular necrosis results in raised creatinine and urea.

Pancreatic cells

These release amylase and lipase, which increase a myocardial depressant factor, decreasing myocardial contractility.

Lungs

Fluid and plasma proteins leak into the interstitium, creating pulmonary oedema from the altered osmotic pressure. This reduces gaseous exchange and increases acidosis.

Heart

Coronary perfusion and O_2 supply become inadequate to meet the demands of the myocardium, which is working harder to maintain the blood flow against increased vasoconstriction.

Intestines

Ischaemic damage to the internal mucosa releases bacteria and toxins from the gut into the central circulation.

Brain

Hypoxia creates varying responses, such as reduced mental state, behavioural changes and coma.

Refractory stage

Continued circulatory collapse, increased acidosis, sludging of the red cells and platelets, and decreased intravascular volume result in an extremely hypoperfused state. Inefficient ventilation leads to further inadequate oxygenation. Renal failure will create metabolic abnormalities and the brain becomes ischaemic and ceases to function, leading to unconsciousness and, ultimately, death.

Types of shock

Hypovolaemic shock

This is the most common type of shock and results from loss of fluid in the intravascular space, i.e. the circulation.

Aetiology

Absolute

External loss of fluid from the body, including whole blood, plasma, vomiting, diarrhoea, burns, diabetes, excessive diuretics.

Relative

Internal fluid shift occurs from the intravascular space to the extravascular space. It may be due to reduced intravascular integrity, increased capillary permeability or decreased colloidal osmotic pressure.

Pathophysiology

Decreased circulating volume results in reduced venous return, reducing preload (filling). Cardiac output is low, resulting in tissue hypoxia.

Compensatory mechanisms are activated when the BP starts to fall. If the loss is greater than 10%, and not replaced quickly, compensatory mechanisms will fail quickly. The nurse plays a key role in identifying the patient who is at risk of shock.

Action point 7

What do you need to watch for in your patient? Make a list and compare it with the following.

Signs and symptoms

- Anxiety, restlessness, confusion from reduced cerebral perfusion.
- Rapid, weak, thready pulse from reduced blood volume. Pulse increases to compensate.
- Cool, clammy skin from peripheral vasoconstriction and stimulation of sweat glands. There is delayed capillary refill.
- Decreased urine output from renal artery vasoconstriction and metabolic compensation.
- Rapid, deep respirations from SNS, hypoxia and acidosis.
- Reduced body temperature from altered metabolism, perfusion and heat loss from sweat.
- Thirst and dry mouth from fluid depletion and SNS stimulation.
- Fatigue resulting from inadequate perfusion of vital organs.
- Reduced pulse pressure (difference between systolic and diastolic BP) from reduced SV and increased peripheral vascular resistance (PVR).

Medical management

Because of its seriousness, the management of shock requires an aggressive approach. It is essential to correct the cause of hypovolaemia and restore tissue perfusion, which involves the following:

- identifying and stopping the fluid loss
- administering replacement fluid to restore circulating volume
- CVP measurement.

Investigations

These include arterial blood gas measurement, chest x-ray, U&Es, FBC, group and cross-match.

Nursing management

First it is essential to identify patients who are at risk. As shock is really a problem associated with fluid shifts in the body, it is important that fluid replacement and fluid balance are measured accurately. The patient will certainly need an intravenous infusion (IVI), and rate, flow and insertion site will all need to be observed.

The patient may be confused, so care of mental state is important, and orientation and reassurance are essential. Poor tissue perfusion means tissue viability is an issue. The patient will be cold and clammy, and the skin will be prone to pressure damage and shearing. The nurse will need to take care of the patient's hygiene needs, as the patient will suffer from excess sweating. Oral care will also be required. The patient will have a dry mouth due to high-flow O_2 increasing tissue oxygenation. The nurse will need to monitor O_2 saturations, and sit the patient as upright as possible.

Vital signs, BP, pulse, CVP and temperature must be recorded. If the patient is catheterized, the nurse will need to check the hygiene and patency of the urinary catheter.

Do not forget the care of the patient's family, who will be extremely worried.

Cardiogenic shock

Cardiogenic shock occurs when the heart fails to pump blood forward effectively, resulting in hypoperfusion and shock. It may occur after an MI, when the mortality rate is 65–90%. It may also be caused by metabolic imbalances (e.g. hypoxaemia, acidosis, hypoglycaemia, hypocalcaemia) or obstructions such as pulmonary embolism, tension pneumothorax or cardiac tamponade.

Pathophysiology

As a result of MI, myocardial contractility is impaired. A large reduction in functioning myocardium (40–50%) will result in a reduced CO that is insufficient to maintain adequate tissue perfusion. The LV does not empty adequately because of reduced contractility, so pressure in the LV, lungs and right heart will increase. This will create pulmonary oedema, as fluid is pushed back through into the alveolar spaces. This reduces oxygenation as fluid blocks O_2 uptake, reducing myocardial perfusion and further reducing CO. Heart failure, hypoxia and acidosis activate compensatory mechanisms to increase the CO of an already impaired myocardium.

Signs and symptoms

• Systolic BP <90 mmHg.

- Increased pulse rate, weak and thready pulse (reduced CO).
- Cold, clammy skin (SNS).
- Oliguria <20 ml/h (reduced renal perfusion).
- Confusion (cerebral hypoxia).
- Increased respiration rate to improve oxygenation.
- Chest pain (myocardial ischaemia).
- Arrhythmias (ischaemic myocardium).

Investigations

These include arterial blood gas measurement, chest x-ray, U&Es, FBC, group and cross-match.

Medical management

The aim is to treat the cause, enhance pump effectiveness and improve tissue perfusion.

- If MI is apparent – thrombolysis, and angioplasty to reduce the size of the infarct.
- Inotropic agents – sympathomimetics to increase the strength of myocardial contraction and BP. Dobutamine 2.5–20 μg/kg per min, incrementally titrated according to BP. Increases the workload of the heart by increasing heart rate and decreasing PVR.
- Diuretics – to reduce workload by reducing circulating volume and ventricular filling. Intravenous furosemide, dose dependent on the severity of pulmonary oedema – 40–250 mg (infusion). Intravenous bumetanide 2–4 mg.
- Vasodilators – to reduce preload and afterload via vasodilatation. GTN infusion improves coronary perfusion and reduces myocardial workload through vasodilatation.
- Intra-aortic balloon pump – a temporary measure to decrease myocardial workload by improving oxygen supply and reducing demand through counterpulsation.

Distributive shock

Distributive shock occurs when there is inadequate perfusion due to maldistribution of blood flow. Circulating volume and heart function are normal, but the blood does not reach the tissues because of acute vasodilatation. It is caused by different types of shock.

Septic shock

Pathophysiology

The mortality rate in this condition is between 40% and 70%. In health, the body has protective mechanisms to counteract infections. If these mechanisms fail, micro-organisms invade the body. When this happens, a general inflammatory response occurs (complement cascade) and immunogenic cells move to the site of infection.

Immunogenic cells adhere to foreign cells to destroy them. The foreign cells initiate toxin release, which damages endothelial cells. The immunogenic cells then release mediators (the second part of the inflammatory response), causing alterations in the vascular beds. This affects clotting, blood flow distribution, capillary permeability and, eventually, metabolic state. The immune system cannot cope and so fails to protect the body. The CNS and endocrine system cannot function correctly and a hypermetabolic state ensues. Vasodilatation occurs and there is maldistribution of blood flow, with increased capillary membrane permeability, microemboli formation and selective vasoconstriction.

Massive peripheral vasodilatation causes relative hypovolaemia and reduced tissue perfusion. Microemboli and increased blood viscosity reduce tissue perfusion further. Selective vasoconstriction causes hypoperfusion and organ dysfunction. Increased capillary permeability creates more fluid loss from the circulating volume. Eventually, maldistribution of blood flow and a hyperdynamic state reducing O_2 to the cells result in cell death.

Phases of septic shock

- Warm hyperdynamic state.
- Cold hypodynamic state.

Hyperdynamic state
- Fever and chills (infection).
- Low urine output (renal hypoperfusion).
- Tachycardia – full, bounding pulse (high CO/hypermetabolic state).
- Hypotension – vasodilatation, hypovolaemia, low SVR.
- Tachypnoea – compensatory for reduced O_2.
- Restlessness, agitation and confusion (cerebral hypoxia).
- Warm, flushed skin, sweating (infection).
- Haematology – raised white cell count (WCC) (infection), raised plasma viscosity (volume depletion), raised urea and creatinine (renal hypoperfusion and dehydration).

Hypodynamic state
- Occurs as shock progresses.
- Cold, clammy skin – vasoconstriction, catecholamine release.
- Hypotension – hypovolaemia.
- Low urine output (renal hypoperfusion).
- Tachycardia – compensatory for hypotension, rapid, weak and thready pulse.
- Depressed conscious level (cerebral hypoperfusion).
- Haematology – DIC from toxin release and activation of coagulation/fibrinolytic systems.
- Tachypnoea – hypoxia induced.
- Metabolic acidosis – build-up of lactic acid from anaerobic metabolism.

Medical management aims

1. Identify and treat infection.
2. Support cardiovascular system.
3. Enhance tissue perfusion to avoid organ dysfunction.
4. Initiate nutritional therapy.

Infection is present, so it is essential to find the source. Cultures of blood, urine, sputum, wounds and drains will be taken. When the pathogen is found, the aim is to eradicate the infection. Antibiotics will be given immediately, and surgery will be performed, if required, to remove the source.

Once this has been achieved, the priority will be support for the cardiovascular system, with the aim of enhancing tissue perfusion. Aggressive fluid delivery will be started to increase intravascular volume. Crystalloid (saline) or colloid (Haemaccel) will be used dependent on the patient's condition and fluid loss. In conjunction with this vasoconstrictor agents will be prescribed to reverse vasodilatation such as adrenaline. Positive inotropic agents (dobutamine) may also be given to increase myocardial contractility.

The patient may require intubation and mechanical ventilation to optimize oxygenation. Temperature control must be achieved to reduce metabolic demands. The patient will also require extra nutrition, and a high-protein feed will be started to enhance the immune system and promote wound healing.

Nursing management will follow the care of the shocked patient as described earlier in this chapter.

Anaphylactic shock

Anaphylactic shock is caused by an antigen–antibody response, and is life threatening if not dealt with immediately. The antigen (causative agent)

causes a hypersensitive reaction and may enter the body by injection, ingestion, through the skin or through the respiratory tract. It may include foods,
drugs, environmental agents, diagnostic agents, biological agents or venoms.
It is a severe allergy after a previously sensitized person has been exposed to
a substance.

The release of histamine and vasoactive substances from mast cells creates
massive vasodilatation and increased capillary permeability that redistributes
blood flow. Anaphylactic reactions are either immunoglobulin E (IgE) mediated or non-IgE mediated. As an antigen enters the body, a specific IgE
antibody is formed. It is stored by attaching to a mast cell. This is the primary
immune response. On subsequent exposure to the same antigen, the IgE
antibody reacts with it, causing a second immune response. This reaction
stimulates the release of biochemical mediators from the mast cells, trigger-
ing the shock cascade.

Non-IgE responses occur after direct activation of the mast cells to release
biochemical mediators. Reactions occur on initial exposure and are called
anaphylactoid reactions. Biochemical mediators create increased capillary
permeability, vasodilatation, bronchoconstriction, excessive mucus secretion, inflammation, coronary vasoconstriction, cutaneous reactions and
smooth muscle constriction (intestinal, bladder).

Peripheral vasodilatation causes reduced venous return and, along with
increased capillary permeability, results in loss of intravascular volume leading to hypovolaemia and hypoperfusion of tissues.

Signs and symptoms

This type of shock can affect a number of organ systems, and symptoms
occur within minutes of exposure to the antigen.

- Cutaneous symptoms occur first – erythema, urticaria of the skin, and
  angio-oedema of the face, oral cavity or lower pharynx. Fluid leaks into
  the interstitial space causing swelling. The patient feels warm.
- Cerebral – anxiety, restlessness, apprehension, deteriorating consciousness.
- Respiratory – laryngeal oedema, bronchoconstriction, stridor, wheeze,
  hoarseness, dysphagia, dyspnoea and chest tightness.
- Cardiovascular – hypotension from vasodilatation, tachycardia to compensate for hypovolaemia.
- Digestive – diarrhoea and vomiting, abdominal pain.
- Genitourinary – urinary incontinence, vaginal bleeding.

Medical management

The aim is to remove the offending antigen, but this may be impossible if it is already in the body. Stop the infusion if the patient is receiving any intravenous medications, blood or diagnostic therapies, as these may be the cause of the reaction. Reverse the effects of biochemical mediators and preserve the airway, breathing and circulation, with possible intubation and O_2. Administer:

- adrenaline 0.5–1.0 mg promotes bronchodilatation and vasoconstriction to inhibit further release of mediators – subcutaneous, intramuscular, nebulised or intravenous.
- hydrocortisone 200 mg to reduce inflammatory response.
- Piriton (chlorphenamine) 10 mg to reduce histamine response.

   Promote adequate tissue perfusion; again colloid or crystalloid infusions for volume replacement may be used. Inotropes may be given to increase myocardial contractility, and vasoconstrictor agents such as an adrenaline/noradrenaline infusion.

Nursing management

This is the same as for septic shock, plus the following:

- Care of urticaria – medications/creams to reduce itching.
- Monitor vital signs – BP, heart rate, CVP, temperature, respiratory rate and depth.
- Care of breathing – O_2 saturations, administer high-concentration O_2, protect the airway (oropharyngeal/nasopharyngeal), sit upright if BP can tolerate.

Summary

The cardiovascular system is a complex functioning system and you will need to read around the subject to gain more information. As with any nursing care, the key lies in assessing the patient effectively. Assessment is not a one-off activity carried out at admission; it is something that the nurse, at whatever level, should carry out at all stages of the patient's treatment. Early recognition of problems is essential when caring for a patient who has cardiovascular problems. If one can pre-empt a severe worsening of the patient's condition, then the chances of preventing a life-threatening situation will be increased.

Further reading

Albarran J, Kapeluch H (1994) Role of the nurse in thrombolytic therapy. British Journal of Nursing 3(3): 104–109.

Alexander MF, Fawcett JN, Runciman PJ (2000) Nursing Practice: hospital and home. The adult, 2nd edn. Edinburgh: Churchill Livingstone.

Anderson RH, Becker AE (1993) The Heart. Cardiac anatomy. London: Gower Medical Publishing.

Audit Commission (1999) Critical to Success: the place of efficient and effective critical care services within the acute hospital. London: Audit Commission.

Auter R (1998) Calculating patients' risk of DVT. British Journal of Nursing 7(1): 7–12.

Bassett C, Makin L (1999) Caring for the Seriously Ill Patient. London: Edward Arnold.

Beard JD (2000) ABC of arterial and venous disease. Chronic lower limb ischaemia. British Medical Journal 320: 854–857.

Bennett O (2001) Cardiovascular problems in the diabetic patient. Professional Nurse 16(9): 1339–1343.

Bloe C (2001) Nurse-initiated coronary thrombolysis. Nursing Times 97(15): 40–42.

Boehringer Ingelheim (1995) ECG Diagnosis. Myocardial Infarction – the need for early diagnosis. London: Boehringer Ingelheim.

Bojar RM (1994) Manual of Perioperative Care in Cardiac and Thoracic Surgery, 2nd edn. London: Blackwell Scientific.

Bright LD, Georgi S (1992) Peripheral vascular disease: is it arterial or venous? American Journal of Nursing 92(9): 34–47.

Brough EA (1998) Update. Deep vein thrombosis. Professional Nurse 13(10): 687–691.

Bucher L, Melander S (1999) Critical Care Nursing. London: Saunders.

Cowan T (1997) Compression hosiery. Professional Nurse 12(12): 881–886.

Dahlen R, Roberts S (1995a) Nursing management of chronic heart failure. Part 1. Intensive and Critical Care Nursing 11: 272–279.

Dahlen R, Roberts S (1995b) Nursing management of chronic heart failure. Part 2. Intensive and Critical Care Nursing 11: 322–328.

Davidson TI (1987) Fluid Balance. London: Blackwell Scientific.

Davies MJ, Woolf N (1990) Atheroma: atherosclerosis in ischaemic heart disease. 1. The mechanisms. London: Bayer Science Press.

Davies N (2001) When to use antihypertensives. Nursing Times 97(28): 41–42.

Davies N, Curtis M (2000) Providing palliative care in end stage heart failure. Professional Nurse 15(6): 389–392.

Department of Health (2000) National Service Framework for Coronary Heart Disease. Modern Standards and Service Models. London: HMSO.

Dougherty L (1992) Intravenous therapy. Surgical Nurse 5(2): 10–13.

Edhouse JA, Sakr M, Wardrope J, Morris FP (1999) Thrombolysis in acute myocardial infarction: the safety and efficiency of treatment in the accident and emergency department. Journal of Accident and Emergency Medicine 16: 325–330.

Edwards S (2001) Shock: types, classifications and explorations of their physiological effects. Emergency Nurse 9(2): 29–38.

Fahey TP, Peters TJ (1996) What constitutes hypertension? Patient based comparison of hypertension guidelines. British Medical Journal 313: 93–96.

Fife A (1998) Acute myocardial infarction. Nursing Standard 12(26): 49–54.

Flisher D (1995) Fast track: early thrombolysis. British Journal of Nursing 4(10): 562–565.

Gobbi M (2000) Fluid and electrolyte balance. In Alexander MF, Fawcett JN, Runciman PJ (eds) Nursing Practice: hospital and home. The adult, 2nd edn. Edinburgh: Churchill Livingstone.

Goldhill DR (1999a) The patient at risk team: identifying and managing seriously ill ward patients. Anaesthesia 54(9): 853–860.

Goodall S (2000) Peripheral vascular disease. Nursing Standard 14(25): 48–52.

Gordon K, Child A (2000a) Systems and diseases. Heart failure part 1. Nursing Times 96(12): 53–56.

Gordon K, Child A (2000b) Systems and diseases. Heart failure part 2. Nursing Times 96(16): 49–52.

Gordon K, Child A (2000c) Systems and diseases. Heart failure part 3. Nursing Times 96(20): 45–48.

Hagenoff BD, Feutz C, Conn VS, Sagehorn KK, Moranviulle-Hunziker M (1994) Patient education needs as reported by chronic heart failure patients and their nurses. Journal of Advanced Nursing 19: 685–690.

Hand H (2001a) Myocardial infarction part 1. Nursing Standard 15(36): 45–53.

Hand H (2001b) Myocardial infarction part 2. Nursing Standard 15(37): 45–53.

Haynes S (1989) Infusion, phlebitis and extravasation. Professional Nurse 5(3): 160–161.

Herbert LM (1997) Caring for the Vascular Patient. London: Churchill Livingstone.

Hinchliff SM, Montague SE, Watson R (eds) (1996) Physiology for Nursing Practice, 2nd edn. London: Ballière Tindall.

Hollingworth H (1998) Venous leg ulcers. Part 1. Aetiology. Professional Nurse 13(8): 553–558.

Houghton AR, Gray D (1997) Making Sense of the ECG – a hands on guide. London: Arnold Publishing.

Jackonen S (1997) Dehydration and hydration in the terminally ill: care considerations. Nursing Forum 32(3): 5–13.

Jackson RT, Sackett DL (1996) Guidelines for raised blood pressure: evidence based or evidence burdened? British Medical Journal 313: 64–65.

Jenkins DA, Rogers H (1995) Transfer anxiety in patients with MI. British Journal of Nursing 4: 1248–1252.

Johnson MI (1997) Treatment and prevention of varicose veins. Journal of Vascular Nursing 15(3): 97–103.

Joint European Society of Cardiology/American College of Cardiology Committee (2000) Myocardial Infarction Redefined – a concensus document of the Joint Society of Cardiology/American College of Cardiology Committee for the redefinement of myocardial infarction. Vienna: Elsevier Science, pp. 959–969.

Jolliffe J, Taylor R (1998) Physical activity and cardiac rehabilitation: a critical review of the literature. Coronary Health Care 2(4): 179–186.

Jones C (1992) Sexual activity after MI. Nursing Standard 6(48): 25–28.

Kaplan NM (1994) Metabolic Aspects of Hypertension. New York: Science Press.

Kern M (1998) The Cardiac Catheterisation Handbook, 3rd edn. New York: Mosby Wolfe.

Kumar P, Clarke M (1999) Clinical Medicine, 4th edn. London: WB Saunders.

Lee TH, Goldman L (2000) Evaluation of the patient with acute chest pain. New England Journal of Medicine 342(16): 1187–1195.

Lewin B, Robertson IM, Cay EL, Irving JB, Cambell M (1992) A self help post myocardial infarction rehabilitation package. The Heart Manual: effects on psychological adjustment, hospitalisation and GP consultation. The Lancet 339: 1036–1040.

London NJM, Donnelly R (2000) ABC of arterial and venous disease. Ulcerated lower limb. British Medical Journal 320: 1589–1591.

Lossnitzer K, Pfennigsdorf G, Brauer H (1984) Myocardium. Vessels. Calcium. An Illustrated Synopsis of the Principle of Calcium Antagonism. Ludwigshafen: Knoll AG.

Lydakis C, Lip GYH, Beevers M, Beevers DG (1997) Diet, lifestyle and blood pressure. Coronary Health Care 1: 130–137.

Maki DG, Goldman D, Rhame S (1993) Infection control in IV therapy. Annals of Internal Medicine 79(6): 867–887.

Mangan P, Kershaw B, Campbell J (1994) Professional cevelopment. Cardiac conditions. Knowledge for practice. Nursing Times 90(40): 1–3.

McBride A (1995) Health promotion in hospitals: the attitudes, beliefs and practices of hospital nurses. Journal of Advanced Nursing 20: 92–100.

McLeod AL, Fox AA (2001) Management of unstable angina. Trends in Cardiology and Vascular Disease Jan/Feb: 18–23.

McMurray JJV, Stewart S (1998) Nurse led multidisciplinary intervention in chronic heart failure. Editorial. Heart 80: 430–431.

McPhee SJ, Lingappa VR, Ganong WF, Lange JD (1995) Pathophysiology of Disease. An introduction to clinical medicine. London: Appleton and Lange.

Medicom Zeneca (1992) Workshop Series: Heart Failure. Core module. London: Grange Press.

Meltzer LE, Pinneo R, Kitchell JR (1983) Intensive Coronary Care. A Manual for Nurses, 4th edn. Boston, MA: Brady.

Messerli FH (1994) The ABC's of Antihypertensive Therapy. London: Raven Press.

Metcalfe H (2000a) Recording a 12 lead ECG part 1. Nursing Times 96(19): 43–44.

Metcalfe H (2000b) Recording a 12 lead ECG part 2. Nursing Times 96(21): 45–46.

Metheny N (1996) Fluid and Electrolyte Balance: nursing considerations, 3rd edn. Philadelphia, PA: Lippincott.

Millam D (1988) Managing complications of IV therapy. Nursing 18(3): 34–42.

Miller J (1989) Intravenous therapy in fluid and electrolyte balance. Professional Nurse 4(5): 237–240.

Millner R, Treasure T (1995) Explaining Cardiac Surgery. Patient assessment and care. London: BMJ Publishing Group.

Moore M (1998) Differentiating chest pain. Clinical principles of assessment. Australian Nursing Journal. Clinical Update 5(9): 21–24.

National Institute for Clinical Effectiveness (2000) Guidelines on the use of glycoprotein IIb/IIIa inhibitors in the treatment of acute coronary syndromes. London: NICE.

National Institute for Clinical Effectiveness (2001) Prophylaxis for patients who have experienced a myocardial infarction. Drug treatment, cardiac rehabilitation and dietary manipulation. London: NICE.

O'Connor L (1995) Pain assessment by patients and nurses and nurses' notes on it in early acute myocardial infarction. Intensive and Critical Care Nursing 11: 183–191.

Patterson D, Treasure T (1993) Disorders of the Cardiovascular System. London: Arnold.

Peters J (1998) A review of the factors influencing nonrecurrence of venous leg ulcers. Journal of Clinical Nursing 7(1): 3–9.

Place B, Graham S (2000) Non-invasive vital organ assessment. Nursing Times Plus 96(20): 6–9.

Priebe H, Skarvan K (2000) Cardiovascular Physiology, 2nd edn. London: BMJ Books.

Pyatt JR, Hughes C, Mullins PA, Saltissi S (1999) The effect of an acute chest pain nurse specialist on the delivery time of thrombolysis therapy in AMI. British Journal of Cardiology 6(9): 499–507.

Quinn T (1995) Can nurses safely assess suitability for thrombolytic therapy? A pilot study. Intensive and Critical Care Nursing 11: 126–129.

Quinn T (1999) Thrombolysis in accident and emergency: the exception not the rule. Are we denying patients lifesaving treatment? Accident and Emergency Nursing 7: 39–41.

Rhodes MA (1998) What is the evidence to support nurse led thrombolysis? Clinical Effectiveness in Nursing 2(2): 69–77.

Riley I, Blue L (2001) Assessing and managing chronic heart failure. Professional Nurse 16(5): 1112–1115.

Sheppard M (2001) Positive inotrope therapy. Nursing Times 97(17): 36–37.

Sheppard M, Wright M (2000) Principles and Practice of High Dependency Nursing. London: Ballière Tindall.

Speechley V, Toovey J (1987) Problems in IV therapy. Professional Nurse 2(8): 240–242.

Springhouse (1997) ECG Interpretation Made Incredibly Easy. Springhouse, PA: Springhouse Corporation.

Standing J (1997) Chest pain assessment tools. Journal of Clinical Nursing 6: 85–92.

Stubbing N (1996) Using non-invasive methods to perform vascular assessment. Nursing Standard 10(45): 49–50.

Sutton GC, Chattergee K (1998) Heart Failure: an illustrated text. London: Current Medical Literature.

Swales J, Sutton GC, Chattergee K (1998) Hypertension: an illustrated text. London: Current Medical Literature.

Telion C, Carli P (2001) The management of acute coronary syndromes. British Journal of Intensive Care Autumn: 156–166.

Thelan LA, Urden LD, Lough ME, Stacy KM (1998) Critical Care Nursing. Diagnosis and Management, 3rd edn. New York: Mosby.

Thompson DR, Ersser SJ, Webster RA (1995) The experiences of patients and their partners one month after a heart attack. Journal of Advanced Nursing 22: 707–714.

Thompson DR, Webster RA (2000) The cardiovascular system. In Alexander MF, Fawcett JN, Runciman PJ (eds) Nursing Practice: hospital and home. The adult, 2nd edn. Edinburgh: Churchill Livingstone.

Tierney S, Fennessy F, Bouchier Hayes D (2000) ABC of arterial and vascular disease. Secondary prevention of peripheral vascular disease. British Medical Journal 320: 1262–1265.

Timmis AD, Nathan AW, Sullivan ID (1997) Essential Cardiology, 3rd edn. Oxford: Blackwell Science.

Van de Werf F (1999) Single bolus tenecteplase compared with front loaded alteplase in acute myocardial infarction: the ASSESNT – 2 double-blind randomised trial. The Lancet 354: 716–721.

Walker WF (1996) A Colour Atlas of Peripheral Vascular Disease, 2nd edn. New York: Wolfe Medical Atlases.

Walton S, Underwood SR, Hunter GC (1989) A Colour Atlas of Diagnostic Investigation in Cardiology. New York: Wolfe Medical Atlases.

Welch J (2000) Using assessment to identify and prevent critical illness. Nursing Times Plus 96(20): 3–4.

Woods SL, Sivarajan Froelicher ES, Underhill Motzer S (2000) Cardiac Nursing, 4th edn. Philadelphia, PA: Lippincott.

Chapter two

The respiratory system

Lee Cutler and Phil Murch

Introduction

This chapter presents a review of important aspects of respiratory physiology, assessment, disorders and management of the most common respiratory conditions. To develop and use appropriate knowledge and skills in practice, nurses must be able to understand the respiratory system in context. It is important to understand the role of the respiratory system in meeting the metabolic needs of the cells of the body. These cells are diverse and make up the tissues, organs and systems of the body. Thus inadequate respiratory function will affect a wide range of cells, tissues and organs. Dysfunction of the respiratory system and its effects on other organ systems are examples of disease. Such diseases are the concern of nursing, and nurses have key roles, through their proximity to patients, in the assessment, therapeutic intervention and monitoring of such conditions.

Physiology of the respiratory system

Oxygen at the cellular level

One of the fundamental needs of the cells in the body is to receive oxygen (O_2) and 'fuel' (e.g. glucose, protein and fats), which are used to produce energy and maintain cellular functions. If O_2 is present (aerobic metabolism) during the breakdown of 'fuel', the process is much more efficient and more energy is released.

The process of breaking down 'fuel' (catabolism) to release energy gives off waste products, including water (H_2O), carbon dioxide (CO_2) and a substance called pyruvate. Under normal conditions none of these is toxic and CO_2, pyruvate and water are eliminated. In the absence of O_2 (anaerobic metabolism) the breakdown of 'fuel' is less efficient and, instead of pyruvate, lactic acid is produced and a 'metabolic acidosis' results. If there is poor circulation, as may be the case in conditions that result in a lack of oxygen supply to tissues, the acid accumulates and begins to disrupt further the cellular environment and functioning.

If CO_2 is not removed, because of respiratory dysfunction, it builds up. CO_2 also converts to acid in body fluids and, if not removed by efficient respiration and circulation, may also contribute to a 'respiratory acidosis'. A downward spiral of cellular, organ and multi-organ dysfunction and death can soon ensue if O_2 is not supplied to the tissues of the body and CO_2 is not eliminated. As the illness severity of patients in acute hospital settings increases, the fundamental needs of the cell for oxygen and 'fuel' are an evermore important focus of healthcare professionals involved in direct care. Therefore an understanding of the process of O_2 intake delivery is essential.

The process of taking O_2 in from the atmosphere and delivering it to tissues can be broken down into several sequential stages. If dysfunction occurs at any of these stages, tissue oxygenation and CO_2 elimination are impaired. These stages are presented in Figure 2.1.

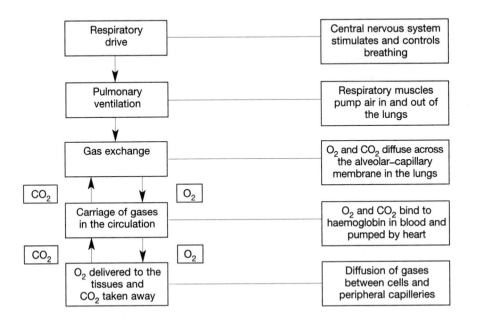

Figure 2.1 Oxygen delivery and carbon dioxide elimination.

Each stage of the process will be discussed before consideration of what happens when there is dysfunction in the system and the implications for collaborative management and nursing care.

Respiratory drive

Breathing essentially involves the pumping of air in and out of the lungs so that gas exchange (of O_2 and CO_2) can take place. A system of 'controllers' regulates this pulmonary ventilation. Breathing rate, depth and pattern can be affected anywhere in the respiratory control system. 'Effectors' and 'sensors' are depicted in Figure 2.2. Some knowledge of these is useful for the clinician caring for individuals with actual or potential respiratory dysfunction.

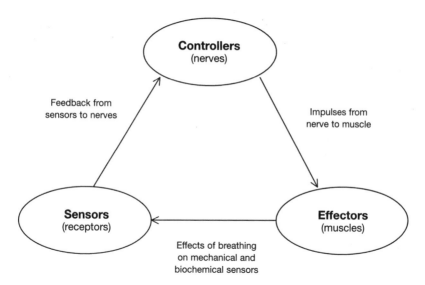

Figure 2.2 The triad that influences respiratory drive.

Controllers

Ventilation is controlled by several areas within the central nervous system (CNS) so that breathing is regular, co-ordinated and of adequate depth and rate. Four groups of cells within the brain stem – the pneumotaxic centre, the apneustic centre, the ventral respiratory group and the dorsal respiratory group – exhibit significant control over respiratory rate, rhythm and depth.

Normal breathing is referred to as eupnoea ('good breathing'). However, other patterns of abnormal breathing will be seen in clinical practice and are presented on page 51.

Beyond these automatic regulatory mechanisms breathing is significantly affected by some voluntary control, i.e. the cerebral cortex allows voluntary breathing to override the automatic control of the brain stem. This may be seen in anxiety states, during pain or when different patterns of breathing are required, such as when talking, singing, etc.

Action point 1

Why is it important to assess your patient's respiratory function?

When assessing breathing it is important to establish the extent to which fast breathing is compensatory (e.g. breathing fast due to hypoxia – controlled by the respiratory centre) or due to voluntary override of automatic breathing caused by anxiety or significant pain.

The experience of acute illness, hospitalization, and therapeutic interventions and care by clinical staff contributes significantly to the patient's anxiety. The fact that clinicians are measuring vital signs on a relatively frequent basis reinforces the patient's perception of being seriously ill.

Breathing rate, depth and pattern can be affected by dysfunction anywhere in the triad/feedback system. Figure 2.3 gives graphical representations of normal breathing (eupnoea) as well as other abnormal or compensatory mechanisms of breathing that might be seen in clinical practice.

Effectors

The effectors of breathing are the respiratory muscles that work under CNS control to cause co-ordinated inspiration and expiration.

The principal respiratory muscle causing inspiration is the diaphragm, which does approximately 80% of the work of breathing at rest. The diaphragm is a sheet of muscle that separates the thoracic and abdominal cavities, and is dome shaped when relaxed. Contraction of the muscle causes it to flatten, pulling downwards, and thus increasing the vertical diameter of the thorax and pulling air in. This is much the same action as the downward drawing of the plunger of a syringe, and draws in air in much the same way by creating a lower pressure on the inside of the syringe (a vacuum) than in the atmosphere outside the body.

A secondary, but still important, group of respiratory muscles is the intercostals. In inspiration, the external intercostal muscles contract, lifting the ribcage upwards and outwards. This increases the lateral and anterior–posterior diameter, creating a vacuum and, like the diaphragmatic action,

Graphical representation	Description	Key notes
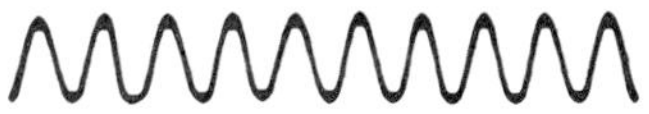	*Eupnoea* Regular rhythm with a rate of 12–20 per min	This is normal, effortless breathing as seen at rest in the individual without pulmonary or respiratory drive problems
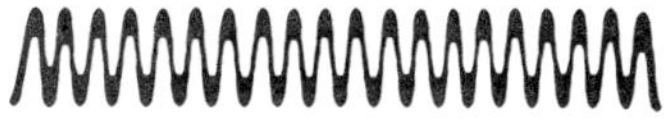	*Tachypnoea* Rapid shallow breathing > 20 per min	This may be seen in the individual who has pulmonary disorders affecting gas exchange, or in states of anxiety, fear and pain
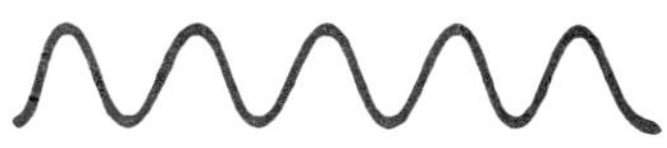	*Bradypnoea* Slow breathing < 12 per min	This may be normal in sleep or abnormal in the individual who is comatose/semi-comatose (e.g. overdose of opiate or sedative drugs, head injury, intracranial bleed, hypothermia)
	Apnoea Absence of breathing	Always abnormal – may precede or follow immediately after cardiac arrest
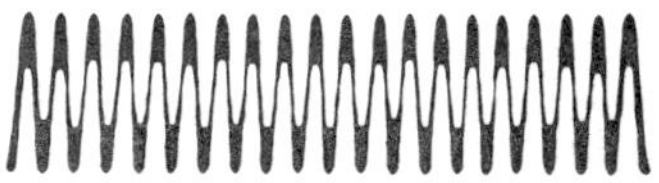	*Hyperpnoea* Increased depth of regular respiration with a normal to increased rate	Normal in exercise, but also seen in anxiety and pain Deep sighing breaths with no pauses and a rate > 20 may be seen in metabolic acidosis (e.g. renal failure, diabetic ketoacidosis) and is called *Kussmaul's* breathing.
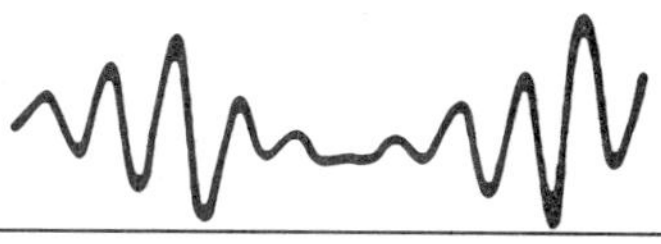	*Cheyne–Stokes* Alternation between hyperpnoea and apnoea	Damage or dysfunction in the brain. Often seen in the terminal stages of advanced disease (e.g. immediately before death in advanced cancer)
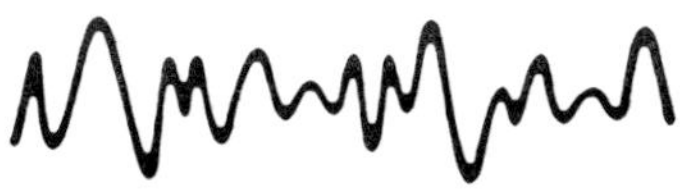	*Ataxic* Irregular breathing with random rapid and shallow breaths	This may be associated with lesions (tumours, traumatic damage, haemorrhage) in the medulla and pons within the brain stem. May involve periods of apnoea and is then called *cluster* or *Biot's* breathing.
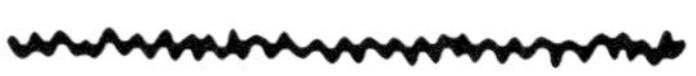	*Neurogenic hyperventilation* Rapid shallow breathing associated with coma and occurring over a prolonged period	Lesions in the pons and midbrain (head injury, raised intracranial pressure, intracranial bleeding)

Figure 2.3 Normal breathing (eupnoea) and abnormal and compensatory mechanisms.

sucking air into the lungs. Other muscles that also help the intercostals are the pectoralis minor and the sternocleidomastoid muscle These latter groups are used increasingly as breathing requires more effort.

Expiration occurs when the inspiratory muscles relax. The elastic recoil of the lung and chest wall means that, at rest in health, expiration is mostly a passive manoeuvre involving little muscular assistance. However, when needed – on exertion or in disease – the muscles of expiration are the abdominal muscles and internal intercostals. Contraction of the abdominal muscles causes a pushing up of the diaphragm against the lungs, forcing air out by reducing the vertical diameter of the thorax and creating a higher pressure in the lungs than in the atmosphere outside the body. Contraction of the internal intercostals pulls the ribs inwards and downwards, reducing the anteroposterior diameter of the thorax and the lateral diameter and thus forcing air out.

If you notice someone actively exhaling, this indicates an increase in the work of breathing – this is clinically significant and often indicates deterioration of the pulmonary condition or that the patient has had increased demand for oxygen through activity or pyrexia.

In conditions that are characterized by significant narrowing of the airways (e.g. asthma, chronic bronchitis, emphysema) it is common to see use of, and increased size of, accessory muscles of inspiration (e.g. the sternocleidomastoid muscle) and expiration (e.g. the abdominal muscles).

Integration of controllers and effectors

For the respiratory muscles (effectors) actually to cause the respiratory 'pump' to work, they need to be functioning and stimulated by nerves that are themselves intact and functioning. This means that dysfunction of the nervous and muscular systems can result in inadequate pulmonary ventilation and respiratory failure. Acute and chronic conditions may contribute to inadequate respiratory 'pumping'. Some examples are given below.

System	Example
Central nervous	Coma from head injury or drug overdose Spinal injury severing nerves that supply the diaphragm
Muscular	Muscular weakness, acutely from electrolyte imbalances, or chronically from muscular dystrophy

---

Sensors

The sensors provide feedback to the CNS, thus influencing the stimulus to breathe and hence the way the muscles (effectors) affect the 'ventilatory pump'. A summary of the key factors, effects and mechanisms in this feedback system is given in Table 2.1.

In health, a rise in Pa_{CO_2} is a significant stimulus to breathe. It is more important and stimulating than the pH of arterial blood and the Pa_{O_2}. However, in chronic disease states that are associated with such a degree of

Table 2.1 Key factors, effects and mechanisms in sensory feedback

Factor	Effect	Mechanism
Pa_{CO_2} (normal 4.5–6 kPa)	Elevated Pa_{CO_2} stimulates increased rate and depth of breathing resulting in 'blowing off' of the CO_2	CO_2 passes from the blood into the cerebrospinal fluid (CSF) around the brain, causing it to become more acidic. This is picked up by receptors in the respiratory centre
	Reduced Pa_{CO_2} causes a reduction in ventilation. However, this is limited, since to breathe too little would reduce the blood oxygen levels	CSF becomes more alkaline and breathing is suppressed to some extent. This is the opposite of the mechanism described above
Reduced arterial pH (acidaemia) (normal 7.35–7.45)	Increased rate and depth of breathing – much the same as when CO_2 rises	Acid blood does affect the pH of the CSF but is also detected by receptors in the carotid blood vessels and the aorta
Reduced Pa_{O_2} (hypoxaemia) (normal 10–12 kPa)	Increased breathing in order to take in more O_2	Like changes in blood pH – a low blood O_2 is detected by receptors in the carotid blood vessels and the aorta
Arterial blood pressure (BP)	An acute rise in BP causes slowing of breathing	This is called the 'respiratory pressor reflex'
	An acute fall in BP causes a reflex increase in respiratory rate and depth	The high/low pressure is detected by the aortic and carotid baroreceptors (pressure receptors)
Stretch of lungs	Initiation of respiration when lungs are deflated and receptors are not stretched	Hering–Breuer inspiratory reflex
	Initiation of expiration when lungs are fully inflated and receptors are stretched	Hering–Breuer expiratory reflex
Other miscellaneous factors	Pain – sudden pain causes an initial apnoea but prolonged pain causes an increase in depth and rate of respirations	
	Stimulation of larynx or pharynx – this causes a temporary apnoea as a protective mechanism against inhalation of foreign bodies or noxious substances	

respiratory dysfunction that $PaCO_2$ is continuously elevated, receptors that are usually sensitive to these levels become desensitized. Such disease states include chronic obstructive pulmonary disease (COPD). The result is that low PaO_2 takes over as the primary stimulus to breathe.

This is termed 'hypoxic drive' – because hypoxaemia (low blood O_2) is the main stimulus to breathe. It is important to note that not all those with COPD will have hypoxic drive – it is only in the most severe cases that this occurs. None the less, the possibility of causing apnoea through giving too much O_2 remains a prevalent fear among medical and nursing staff. This issue will be revisited later in the chapter.

Pulmonary ventilation

Before gas exchange can take place between the alveoli and the pulmonary capillaries, effective pulmonary ventilation must take place. Some of the key factors that determine this have been described above. These are essentially the controllers, effectors and sensors that help drive the system. However, for the effectors to cause pulmonary ventilation via the 'respiratory pump', the mechanics of breathing have to be functioning normally. Significant respiratory dysfunction seen in clinical areas affects the flow of air in the whole or part of the lungs. Pulmonary ventilation and its clinical relevance for the nurse will be examined in this section.

The process of moving gas into the lungs has been considered above. The air that enters the lungs does so because the pressure inside the lungs is less than that in the atmosphere. As the pressure between the atmosphere and the lungs equals out, air flow slows down. With the elastic recoil of the lungs and chest wall, and when the muscles of expiration contract, the lungs are 'squeezed'. This causes a rise in intrathoracic pressure above that of the atmosphere, and air is exhaled (Figure 2.4).

This pressure gradient is one factor that significantly affects gas movement. The others are resistance and compliance.

Resistance

Resistance is the force exerted on air as it passes through the airways. The force restricts air movement and is greatest when air is passing quickly through long, narrow airways. It is least when air is passing slowly through short, wide airways. Resistance is created as air swirls around turbulently in the airways.

A common respiratory condition characterized by high airway resistance is asthma. The effects of high resistance in asthma mean that great effort ('work of breathing') is required to move air along the airways. It is

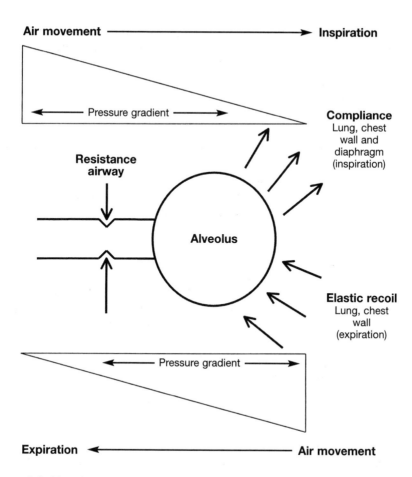

Figure 2.4 Air movement.

especially difficult to breathe out, as air becomes trapped within the lungs and the muscles of expiration (not usually used to a great extent) become tired. Any air that does move tends to cause vibrations and musical sounds when the chest is auscultated (listened to with a stethoscope). These sounds are called wheezes. However, as the resistance increases further and the respiratory muscles tire, less air is moved and the wheezing stops – this is an ominous sign that the patient may soon stop breathing.

Compliance

Compliance is the degree to which the alveolar air sacs, the lungs as a whole and the thorax can stretch and accept the air that is being inspired. High compliance means the lungs are quite elastic and can stretch but also recoil at the beginning of expiration. Poor compliance means the lungs are stiff and that the 'work of breathing' is high on inspiration. Similarly, stiff lungs that have low elastic recoil do not deflate passively to the same degree as in health and the work of breathing is high in expiration.

Poor compliance is associated with numerous conditions. Some of these conditions affect the lung tissue, e.g. fibrosing alveolitis is a chronic condition where there is scarring and fibrosis of lung tissue. Scar tissue is stiff and inelastic. The lung may be stiff in specific regions because of infection and collapse or tumour. Other conditions affect the chest wall making it stiff, e.g. pain or hypothermia and the associated muscle rigidity; bony deformities such as kyphosis (curvature of the spine) or rib fractures. Another way lung compliance may be reduced is through abdominal distension or tension.

Clinical application

High resistance and poor compliance mean that the lung will not easily accept air despite a pressure gradient between the lung and the atmosphere outside the body. The work of breathing is high and respiratory effort may result in poor pulmonary ventilation.

Measures to reduce resistance and improve compliance are important aspects of respiratory therapy.

Example 1: Compliance
Lung compliance may be reduced through abdominal distension. This may be due to peritonitis, the management of which is complex. However, it may be distended because of constipation and/or the swallowing of air, which is common in breathless individuals who are acutely ill. The insertion and aspiration of a nasogastric tube, adequate hydration and aperients to alleviate constipation may be simple measures that reduce the extent to which the diaphragm is splinted (immobilized) by its underlying stomach and bowel contents.

Example 2: Resistance
Resistance may be increased by the presence of pulmonary secretions in the major airways in the lungs. Effective clearance of secretions is dependent on many factors, including adequate hydration, analgesia (e.g. following abdominal surgery) and acceptance by the patient that to cough up sputum is not bad manners but necessary if prevention of pneumonia and recovery are to be achieved. Clearing pulmonary secretions may significantly reduce airway resistance, reduce the work of breathing and enhance pulmonary ventilation.

Table 2.2 gives examples of the clinical conditions that might affect these factors.

Table 2.2 Clinical conditions affecting air movement

Factors in air movement	Clinical conditions
Resistance	Acute bronchospasm (e.g. in asthma) Airway oedema (e.g. in anaphylaxis) Airway obstruction (e.g. inhaled foreign body) Breathing through an artificial airway (e.g. tracheostomy, Guedel airway) Pulmonary secretions (e.g. bronchitis, pneumonia)
Compliance	Lung infection and inflammation (e.g. pneumonia) Pulmonary oedema (e.g. in acute heart failure) Stiff muscles (pain, fitting, hypothermia) Chest wall/thoracic abnormalities (e.g. kyphosis, scoliosis) Diaphragmatic splinting (abdominal distension) Chronic lung disease (e.g. chronic bronchitis)
Ability to create a pressure gradient	Muscle wasting (e.g. chronic disease, after mechanical ventilation) Muscle fatigue (e.g. acute prolonged dyspnoea) Neurological conditions (e.g. multiple sclerosis) Muscle weakness (e.g. electrolyte imbalance, malnutrition)

Lung volumes

The tidal movement of air carries O_2 (21% in air) into the lungs to be exchanged at the alveolar level from the alveoli into the capillaries. It also carries CO_2, a cellular by-product of metabolism, out, after it has been exchanged in the lungs from the capillaries to the alveoli. The amount of air that moves in and out of the lungs is important to ensure that gas exchange takes place. The relationship of ventilation to perfusion (the other important factor in gas exchange) will be discussed later in this section; however, it is first important to examine the different pulmonary volumes in the normal and abnormal respiratory cycle and explain their relevance to clinical practice.

The total lung capacity is around 5700–6200 ml (Figure 2.5). This can be divided into smaller volumes, which are affected by disease, activity and respiratory phase. The normal inspiratory and expiratory volumes are around 500 ml (or 0.7 ml/kg of body weight). This is referred to as the tidal volume (TV). After normal tidal expiration, the lungs are not empty and even more air can be exhaled. A forceful expiration of as much air as possible is called the expiratory reserve volume (ERV) and is around 1000–1200 ml in an adult. Similarly, it is possible to inhale forcefully a volume of air above the normal tidal volume. This is called the inspiratory reserve volume (IRV) and is around 3300 ml. Even after a forced expiration, air will remain in the lungs. This is called the reserve volume (RV) and is around 1200 ml.

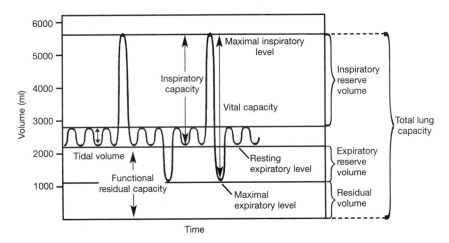

Figure 2.5 Lung volumes.

Respiratory failure or dysfunctions in the acute or chronic situation are often the result of altered lung volumes, which may be caused by a number of factors. These include failure of respiratory controllers, effectors and sensors. Alternatively it may be due to problems within the lung that cause air spaces (alveoli) to be filled with fluid (e.g. pulmonary oedema in acute heart failure), immune cells and pus (e.g. in pneumonia) or compressed (e.g. by air in a pneumothorax or a tumour as in lung cancer). Many treatments are aimed at maximizing lung volumes and this is the basis for much, if not all, respiratory physiotherapy. A more detailed discussion of respiratory therapy will follow later in the chapter. However, an example of how lung volumes, gas exchange and respiratory therapy apply to the clinical situation is presented below.

Clinical application

When a lung is compressed or is under-ventilated for a prolonged period (e.g. several hours) the volume of air left in the lungs after expiration becomes reduced. This volume is called the functional residual capacity (FRC), and it serves two purposes. First, it takes part in gas exchange – so if it is reduced there may be impaired oxygenation and CO_2 retention. Second, a semi-inflated lung (with a normal FRC) takes much less effort to inflate on inspiration than one that is almost deflated (reduced FRC). Thus an individual with a reduced FRC may have impaired gas exchange and increased 'work of breathing'. This may manifest as an increased respiratory rate (tachypnoea), use of accessory muscles, and a tendency to become fatigued and retain pulmonary secretions. In the worst cases, this may result in respiratory failure, exhaustion and secretion retention, and/or pneumonia.

Consider the process of having major abdominal surgery. It involves a prolonged period of under-inflation of the lung. This is so that the lungs and diaphragm are not forced downwards, obscuring the surgeon's field of view. It is not uncommon for postoperative patients to need supplemental oxygen via a facemask for some time. This is because they have a reduced FRC from the use of anaesthetic gases and minimal volume ventilation. It is also made worse by the fact that inhaled anaesthetic gases are very easily absorbed in the lungs, causing absorption collapse (or 'atelectasis') of the alveoli, especially in the most distal parts of the lungs.

In the worst cases, usually elderly people or those with chronic lung disease, postoperative patients may need to have air forced into their lungs to re-expand them – returning to the FRC. This may mean being taken to an intensive care unit (ICU) and receiving mechanical ventilation or receiving continuous positive airway pressure (CPAP) via a facemask with an airtight seal. CPAP will be discussed in more depth later in the chapter.

Action point 2

Spend some time with a respiratory physiotherapist and undertake the following:

- Find out what methods are employed with a range of patients to maximize lung volumes (acutely ill, chronically ill, medical patients, surgical patients).
- Consider what you can do as a nurse on an ongoing basis with these patients to facilitate the achievement of maximum lung volumes.
- Reflect on the indications for the approaches used by physiotherapists and try to identify occasions when the physiotherapist could be called to help a patient with lung volume problems.
- Ensure you understand the physiological basis for maximizing pulmonary ventilation and lung volumes, reading a range of books and articles if necessary.

Gas exchange within the lungs

The random movement of gas molecules within compartments (e.g. the lungs) and across membranes that divide compartments (e.g. the alveolar capillary membrane) is called diffusion. It is generally the case that the particles move from an area of high concentration to an area of low concentration, until there is an even number of molecules within all areas of the compartment or on either side of a permeable membrane.

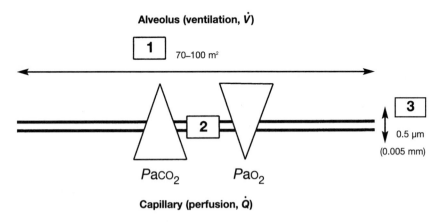

Figure 2.6 The factors that determine gas exchange. (1) The surface area available for gas exchange. (2) The difference in gas concentrations on either side of the alveolar–capillary membrane. (3) The distance the gas has to travel between alveolus and capillary.

There are three factors that affect gas exchange (diffusion) across the alveolar–capillary membrane within the lungs (Figure 2.6), and it is important for nurses to know about these:

1. The surface area available for gas exchange.
2. The difference in gas concentrations across the alveolar–capillary membrane.
3. The distance the gas has to diffuse.

Understanding these is the key to understanding many respiratory disorders and therapies – some of which will be discussed later in the chapter.

Surface area available for gas exchange

For gas exchange to take place across the alveolar-capillary membrane, the surface area of lung – with blood on one side and ventilated lung on the other – has to be adequate. The surface area of healthy lungs is between 70 and 100 m^2 – around the size of a tennis court. When this is reduced, less gas exchange takes place.

When lung volumes are decreased during collapse or shallow breathing, for example, there is said to be 'shunting' of blood from the right side of the heart to the left, without it taking part in gas exchange. This is because areas of deflated lung are still perfused with blood – but the perfusion is wasted because of 'shunting'.

When ventilated areas of lung are not well perfused, e.g. when there are blood clots in pulmonary blood vessels (i.e. pulmonary embolism or PE), the lung ventilation is wasted, i.e. the oxygen in the alveoli cannot diffuse from the alveoli into blood vessels that are clotted off. This wasted ventilation is called 'dead space'.

When there are significant differences between the amount of ventilation (abbreviated to $\dot{V}$) and perfusion (abbreviated to $\dot{Q}$) there is said to be a $\dot{V}{:}\dot{Q}$ mismatch. The two types of $\dot{V}{:}\dot{Q}$ mismatch are as described above: 'shunting' and 'dead space'.

When a patient experiences a blood clot travelling into the lung (a PE), the scan used to detect such a problem compares ventilation and perfusion and is called a $\dot{V}{:}\dot{Q}$ scan. A scan may be carried out in the more minor cases, but a large PE causes critical illness or, in serious cases, death; thus the diagnosis is made clinically by doctors because the patient is unable to tolerate a $\dot{V}{:}\dot{Q}$ scan or the scan is too late. PE is a relatively rare but serious postoperative complication.

Differences in gas concentrations

A further factor important in gas exchange is the difference in gas pressures across the alveolar–capillary membrane. Diffusion occurs most readily when there is a significant difference in the concentration of O_2 and CO_2, e.g. between the capillary and the alveolus. In this scenario, the gas moves from a high concentration to a low concentration.

When someone under-ventilates their lungs, the O_2 reserves in the lungs get used up as the O_2 moves into the capillary. This results in less of a difference between the two sides of the membrane and reduced gas exchange.

A frequent intervention is to give supplemental O_2 to those with respiratory problems, and this is done to increase the concentration of O_2 in the alveoli. This in turn increases the difference in concentrations of O_2 on either side of the alveolar–capillary membrane. This means that O_2 will move more readily from the alveolus (high concentration) to the capillary (low concentration).

Distance the gas has to diffuse

This third factor relates to the thickness of the alveolar–capillary membrane. The thicker the membrane, the further the gas has to travel in a very short space of time as blood travels past the alveolus. In healthy lung tissue, the alveolar–capillary membrane is around 0.5 μm or 0.005 mm. If the alveolus becomes fluid-filled, as in pulmonary oedema from heart failure, the layer of fluid inside the alveolus adds to the distance gas has to travel. Not only does it have to travel through the wall of the alveolus and blood vessel, but also the fluid that has flooded into the alveolus. A further example of when this distance is increased is when the alveolar wall becomes thickened with fibrous tissue, as in chronic bronchitis or fibrosing alveolitis.

Carriage of gases in the circulation

The previous sections have described a series of processes that are essential if O_2 is to be delivered to the cells that need it for metabolism, and CO_2 is to be eliminated as a waste product of that metabolism.

The processes of driving breathing, ventilating the lungs and facilitating gas to exchange across the alveolar–capillary membrane are what might be thought of as the respiratory elements of 'feeding' (O_2) and allowing 'elimination' from metabolism (CO_2). The next processes in this series are the carriage of gases in the blood and the cardiac pumping of that blood to organs and tissues via the circulatory system. (The circulatory system is given fuller consideration in Chapter 1.) However, since the respiratory system and circulatory system are integrated and because the effectiveness of the respiratory system is, in part, measured by blood gases and O_2 saturation of haemoglobin, the carriage of gases in blood is given some consideration here.

There are two ways that O_2 and CO_2 are carried in the blood. First, they are dissolved in the plasma. Plasma is the straw/yellow-coloured fluid part of the blood in which the cells are bathed. Gases dissolve in this fluid in much the same way they dissolve in other fluids. For example, lemonade or other fizzy drinks contain dissolved CO_2, which is released to a great extent when you take the top off a bottle.

The other way that gases are carried is by binding to haemoglobin, a protein found in red blood cells (erythrocytes). When there is a normal amount of haemoglobin in blood (around 15 g/dl), 100 ml of oxygenated, arterial blood will carry just over 20 ml of O_2. Around 20 ml of this is carried bound to haemoglobin and around 0.3 ml is carried as dissolved gas in the plasma. When the blood is deoxygenated after it has delivered its O_2 to the tissues, these figures will be around 20–25% lower. More CO_2 than O_2 is carried in the plasma and less is carried bound to haemoglobin. It is not until there is severe respiratory failure that levels of CO_2 begin to rise in the blood because of a failure to eliminate it. Therefore, the main focus of clinical assessment and this section will be on carriage of O_2.

In clinical practice, the amount of O_2 carried on haemoglobin is measured using a pulse oximeter. This is a device that is usually attached to the patient's finger or ear lobe by a clip and shines red light through the blood. It measures the angle at which the light bounces off the haemoglobin and from this it calculates the extent to which the haemoglobin is 'saturated' with O_2. The normal range is above 95%.

The amount of a gas dissolved in the plasma or contained in air is referred to as the partial pressure and is usually abbreviated to P. It is often measured in millimetres of mercury (mmHg) but more commonly in the UK in kilopascals (kPa). The partial pressure of arterial (oxygenated blood) is usually abbreviated to PaO_2, where the 'a' is a shorthand reference to arterial.

The PaO_2 is measured from a blood sample inserted into a blood gas machine (as is the $PaCO_2$). Normal levels for PaO_2 are around 10–13 kPa and for $PaCO_2$ around 4.2–6 kPa).

Action point 3

Why measure PaO_2?

Blood gases require a needle to be inserted into an artery, which can be quite painful for the patient. And since the overwhelming majority of O_2 is carried on haemoglobin – and this can be measured non-invasively and painlessly with a pulse oximeter – is it really necessary or important to measure arterial blood gases (PaO_2 and $PaCO_2$)?

The answer, in some instances, is yes. When individuals have advanced respiratory failure they may begin to retain CO_2. If this builds up it can make the blood acid (acidaemia), adversely affecting cellular functioning in the body. In addition, high CO_2 levels (hypercapnia) can cause respiratory depression and coma. Individuals who have a severe respiratory disorder will usually receive a high concentration of supplemental O_2 and this may keep the O_2 saturations within normal levels. However, pulse oximetry does not measure CO_2 levels and clinicians may be reassured that the patient is satisfactory because their saturations are normal when they are actually retaining CO_2. Checking blood gases would give $PaCO_2$ measurements.

Another reason to measure blood gases is that saturations are affected by how much O_2 is being used at the cell level and how healthy the haemoglobin is, as well as the amount replenished in the lungs. However, the dissolved gases in the arterial blood (PaO_2 and $PaCO_2$) are affected only by the gas exchange in the lungs and therefore are a good measure of respiratory dysfunction or failure.

Another way of thinking about this is that the O_2 that crosses from the lungs to the blood is measured as PaO_2. What happens to it after that, i.e. binding to haemoglobin (saturation), carriage to the tissues (circulation) and use by cells in tissues of the body (metabolism), all affect the saturation reading on pulse oximetry. Therefore PaO_2 isolates the gas exchange from the bigger picture and, because of this, is worth checking in many situations.

Oxygen–haemoglobin binding

The PaO_2 is a good measure of gas exchange. It is the amount of gas dissolved in the plasma, and can be thought of as the loading force that drives the binding of O_2 to haemoglobin. However, despite the presence of a high PaO_2 in plasma surrounding red blood cells – i.e. a high loading force – there are several factors that can affect the binding and thus the carriage of O_2 to the tissues that need it.

If the blood is acid, the body temperature is high or the haemoglobin is already heavily loaded with CO_2 (which it also carries), it will not pick up and carry as much O_2. These factors can adversely affect tissue oxygenation and should be managed in the seriously ill patient to optimize the binding of O_2 to haemoglobin.

A measure as simple as reducing pyrexia has a double effect on oxygenation. First, reducing body temperature to the normal range allows more oxygen to bind with haemoglobin. Second, hot tissues burn more energy and O_2 so they may cause an O_2 debt in the system, which failing lungs may not meet.

If the blood is alkaline, the body temperature is low or the amount of CO_2 bound to haemoglobin is low, more O_2 will be picked up and carried. The problem in this case is that although it carries more O_2, it will not release it, in the tissues. Rather, it stays bound to the haemoglobin and is recirculated back to the lungs and heart.

An important part of the nurse's role in the acute care setting is to monitor and control some of the factors that determine oxygen–haemoglobin binding and O_2 demands. These will be considered in greater depth later in this chapter and will be discussed within the context of a more comprehensive respiratory therapy model.

Conditions causing respiratory dysfunction and failure

In essence, the concept of failure is that the organ or system is unable to meet the needs of the body. The respiratory system is important in ensuring O_2 delivery to cells and elimination of CO_2 from them. When the respiratory system is unable to meet one or both of these metabolic demands, failure is said to exist. However, before failure, there is usually a phase of compensation when there is increased breathing in an attempt to overcome the gas exchange problems. The phase of reduced gas exchange and attempted compensation is the 'dysfunction' that precedes failure (Figure 2.7).

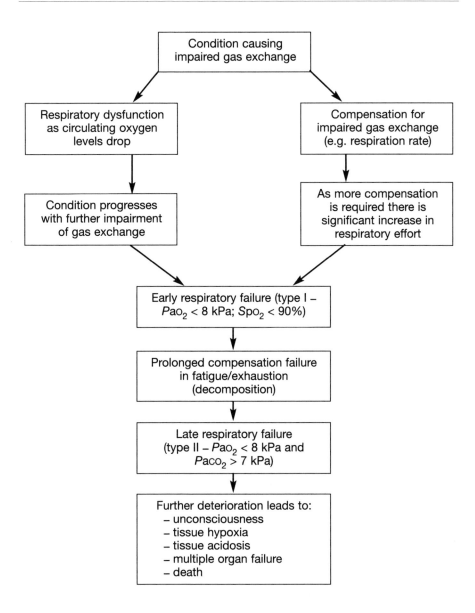

Figure 2.7 Respiratory function and failure. Spo_2, saturation oxygen level in the plasma.

Some common conditions that cause respiratory dysfunction and failure are considered next, while the respiratory assessment important in identifying and monitoring patients with respiratory problems is considered later in the chapter.

Common disorders of the respiratory system

Asthma

Asthma is a chronic hyper-reactive lung disease. Individuals who suffer from asthma are subject to intermittent bouts of widespread, reversible airway obstruction. This is a result of:

- narrowing of the airways leading to the lungs, caused by muscle contraction
- glands under the lining of the airways producing more mucus or phlegm than usual
- swelling of the inner linings of the airways.

There are three main signs of asthma:

1. repeated sudden shortness of breath
2. wheezing, which can be heard especially when breathing out
3. cough, usually a dry cough with the feeling of a 'tight chest'.

An asthma attack where symptoms worsen considerably is usually transient and reversible. Many things can make asthma symptoms worse, the most common being allergic reaction or viral infection.

Asthma can be described as mild, moderate or severe. Mild asthma, meaning occasional bouts of wheezing or breathlessness, is present most of the time, but it does not interfere with everyday activities at work or in the home. Moderate and severe asthma interfere with daily activities. The amount of mucus produced by the glands that line the airways may build up to form plugs, which block the flow of air in that part of the lungs. This in turn increases the work of breathing and in certain cases causes hypoxia.

Asthma trigger factors

Certain trigger factors can be responsible for irritating the airways and provoking an asthma attack. They include the following:

- Allergy: often to pollen, house dust mites, or microscopic moulds in the air.
- Infection: colds or other virus infections.
- Emotions: crying and laughing both affect breathing patterns and may trigger asthma in some people.
- Environment: tobacco smoke, pollution or chemicals encountered at work, school or in the home.

- Exercise: airways enlarge to meet the need for more air when we exercise. Narrowing of the airways after exercise can sometimes be excessive, provoking an asthma attack.

Action point 4

After reading the earlier section on key concepts in respiratory physiology and the brief overview of asthma presented above, consider how gas exchange in individuals with asthma might be affected.

Chronic obstructive pulmonary disease

This is the umbrella name applied to all diseases where air flow into the lungs is permanently restricted, i.e. airways are permanently reduced in size (or narrowed) compared with a normal airway.

COPD results from a combination of chronic bronchitis and emphysema. These illnesses develop over several years. Long-standing irritation leaves the airways permanently swollen and narrowed (bronchitis). Irritation also causes increased production of mucus. This can block airways that are already narrowed. In almost all cases, the cause of the illness is cigarette smoking – 99% of people who have COPD will have smoked or are still smoking.

Over time, many individuals with COPD become reliant on lower levels of O_2 and may have high accompanying levels of CO_2. These low levels of O_2 stimulate spontaneous respiration. This is known as hypoxic drive. If inappropriately high concentrations of O_2 are given to a patient who usually has a high CO_2 level and relies on low O_2 levels to stimulate breathing, respiratory depression may result. This may worsen respiratory function and lead to a further increase in CO_2 levels. However, it should be pointed out that such occurrences are rare and it is usually more important to give O_2 than to tolerate low O_2 levels for fear of respiratory depression.

The management of the patient with hypoxic drive is outlined in the key considerations when nursing the patient with altered respiratory function

Chronic bronchitis

Chronic bronchitis is chronic inflammation of the airways following years of irritant exposure. In most cases, the long-term exposure is to pollutants such as tobacco smoke, although industrial pollution also contributes. Chronic bronchitis is said to exist when there is a productive cough for 6 months in any one year or 3 months in each of two consecutive years.

Over several years, the airways are damaged. The pollutants cause irritation and coughing, which stimulate extra mucus production. The mucus blocks the airways. Further damage to the lung occurs due to a breakdown of airway tissue, which causes yet more narrowing. Damage to the airways can lead to scarring, otherwise known as fibrosis. The combination of damage to the airways and excessive production of mucus reduces physical defences against infection and predisposes the sufferer to recurrent pulmonary infections.

Emphysema

Emphysema is usually found in association with chronic bronchitis. The air spaces at the end of the airways (the alveoli) in the lungs become over-inflated and damaged. Over time, the air sac walls are broken down by enzyme activity. Also, as the airways are narrowed by mucus, air becomes trapped in these air sacs. With no way of escape, air is compressed when breathing out, which stretches and distends the air sac walls. Emphysema causes shortness of breath, which is usually worse in winter.

Nothing can be done to repair the lungs and therefore treatment is aimed at preventing further damage. Stopping smoking is essential. Reducing mucus production in the bronchial tubes reduces blockage of the airways and can improve symptoms.

Action point 5

After reading the earlier section on key concepts in respiratory physiology and the brief overview of COPD presented above, consider how gas exchange in individuals with COPD might be affected.

Pulmonary congestion/heart failure

Breathlessness can be caused by heart problems, as well as lung problems. Chronic heart failure may accompany chronic lung conditions such as COPD or may occur as a result of a myocardial infarction (MI, heart attack). The failing heart is unable to clear blood adequately from the lungs as it passes through to become oxygenated, resulting in pulmonary congestion.

In the elderly individual, a degree of heart failure may accompany many acute or chronic pulmonary disorders as they place an extra workload on the heart. It is important to consider this, as the management of the patient may differ considerably, depending on whether heart or respiratory failure exists alone or in combination.

Fuller consideration of heart failure can be found in Chapter 1.

Pneumonia

Pneumonia can be defined as an acute inflammation of the functional tissue (bronchioles, alveoli and interstitial tissue) of the lung as a result of infection by micro-organisms. Pneumonia can be categorized according to:

- whether the infection originated primarily in the lung (primary pneumonia) or was a secondary complication of a viral illness, such as chickenpox
- where the infection was acquired (hospital, community, while on a mechanical ventilator)
- whether the pneumonia is caused by common micro-organisms (bacteria, viruses, fungi) presenting in a typical picture or whether the micro-organisms are less common (e.g. *Legionella* spp.) and present as an atypical picture
- whether the way the infection and inflammation affect the lungs is restricted to a lobe (lobar pneumonia) or is more diffuse in nature (bronchopneumonia).

This section will not go into great detail about these categories of pneumonia but will present some of the key concepts related to this type of pulmonary disorder.

The development of pneumonia requires the following:

- exposure to a virulent pathogen, or
- large exposure to a pathogen, and/or
- an immunocompromised host.

As the lung is infected, the process (the pathophysiology) is responsible for the significant, sometimes life-threatening, problems that follow.

Bronchopneumonia

It is most common that the disease process causes widespread patchy areas of collapse, consolidation and production of purulent (pus-containing) sputum. This type of pneumonia is most common in debilitated individuals and postoperatively, and is called bronchopneumonia.

Lobar pneumonia

When the infecting organism is *Streptococcus pneumoniae* ('pneumococcus'), the pneumonia can be quite localized, affecting one or more lobes and causing solidification (consolidation) of the lobe(s). This type of pneumonia may also affect younger and previously healthy individuals, causing a sudden severe illness. The patient has a very high fever and often little sputum initially as the infected area is a solid mass rather than a number of exuding open lung areas.

The points discussed here regarding respiratory disorders are only the most basic and fundamental ones. For a deeper understanding the reader is referred to textbooks that focus on disease and internal medicine.

Respiratory assessment

This section gives a brief overview of the 'why', 'when', 'who', 'where', 'what' and 'how' of respiratory assessment.

Why and when to assess

Assessment is the means of gaining much useful information about the patient. Without this information it is difficult to prioritize care and decide on appropriate interventions, or to evaluate their effectiveness. Similarly, without assessment it is difficult to understand the patient's experience of illness and perceptions of care, which are important prerequisites to excellent nursing care.

The gathering of information about a patient and their respiratory problems should be a continuous process and should begin as early as possible in an episode of care. Initial assessment will give a baseline against which future assessment findings and patient trends can be compared. Historical information (from the patient's past), on the other hand, can give important details about why the patient may have respiratory problems and how the problems have impacted on his life over previous weeks, months or years. These historical facts may also help in the future management and planning of care, e.g. the extent to which the patient has been rehabilitated to their previous state of health or needs additional follow-up support or therapy.

Continuous assessment is a way of determining trends in a patient's progress. This is the means by which deterioration can be identified and necessary intervention commenced, and also the way in which improvements can be identified. It is as important for the patient to know about these as it is for the clinical professionals, because without this knowledge the patient may not appreciate the severity of his illness, may not comply with care or treatment plans or may lose hope despite improvement in his condition. Table 2.3 provides a summary of important reasons for respiratory assessment.

Table 2.3 Rationale for respiratory assessment

Respiratory assessment allows the nurse to make the following clinical judgements:

- Whether the patient has a chronic, acute or acute-on-chronic respiratory disorder
- The extent to which the disorder impacts on the patient's life when at home
- Whether the patient is critically ill and requires immediate medical attention
- Whether the patient is deteriorating or improving
- Whether the patient is able to care for personal needs, such as hygiene, nutrition and elimination, independently, or what level of help is needed
- The patient's insight into the disorder and the treatment they are receiving
- The awareness of the family about their loved one's problems and treatment

Who should assess

Nurses are in a key position to pick up on early respiratory dysfunction before respiratory failure ensues. This is because the trends in patient mood, activity tolerance and general appearance, which are early signs of illness, are best detected by those close to the patient and who know them well. This puts the nurse in a position of some advantage over the doctor, who generally relies on 'snapshot' views of the patient and on being called by the nurse when something is wrong.

Early intervention is likely to lead to a much better chance of recovery than if the patient deteriorates into respiratory failure before there is intervention. For this reason the nurse's assessment skills and vigilance need to be well developed and exercised.

Assessment, both initially and as an ongoing activity, is a multidisciplinary responsibility. The optimum team not only assesses, but also shares, this information within the team.

Where to assess

The patient may share sometimes embarrassing, and often confidential, information during an admission or more in-depth review assessment. Because of this, the optimum location for assessment is one that affords the individual privacy. However, this is often not a secluded, sound-proof cubicle, but a bed close to other patients in the middle of a busy hospital ward.

The assessment may not always be a discrete or isolated activity, but may be an ongoing activity as part of daily interactions with the patient.

What to assess and how

> **Action point 6**
>
> During the clinical assessment process several important questions
> should be present in the nurse's mind:
> - What is the nature of the problem?
> - How hard is the patient working to breathe?
> - Are there signs that the patient is failing to meet the O_2 needs of
>   the body or is retaining CO_2?

Since the role of the respiratory system is to help supply life-sustaining O_2 to
tissues of the body, thus maintaining vital organ function, at times nurses
may be called on to assess or care for patients who are in a life-threatening
state. The first judgements that should be made when assessing a patient are:

- 'To what extent do I need to assess?'
- 'How urgent is the need for further treatment or medical intervention?'

These are particularly relevant when the patient is first admitted to hospital. It could be that a very limited assessment is needed to find out that what
is really most important is not a thorough health history interview, but rather
an urgent review by a doctor and an increase in the level of treatment. The
nurse may not be conscious of systematically assessing but rather is aware of
salient clinical signs that indicate the nature and severity of the problem.
Nurses often remark that there is something wrong with the patient, without
being able to articulate clearly what the specific problem is.

The nature of an assessment may therefore vary according to the particular situation and how severely ill the patient is. The nature of the problem
may be classified as critical and in need of urgent intervention or it may be
non-critical and in need of further assessment by the nurse. The initial assessment process is presented in Table 2.4.

> **Action point 7**
>
> Are there signs of respiratory failure and decompensation indicating
> that the nature of the problem is because of any or all of:
> - airway
> - ventilation
> - gas exchange?

A comprehensive assessment involves an interview with the patient and/or
relatives to gather information about the patient's health history. Table 2.5

Table 2.4 The initial assessment process (Thelan et al. 1998)

Airway problem	Ventilation problem	Gas exchange problem
• Noisy breathing • Recession above the clavicle and between the ribs on inspiration • Flaring nostrils • Use of accessory muscles • See-saw motion of chest and abdomen	• Absence of breath exchange at mouth/nose • Minimal chest wall movement • Decreased breath sounds (listen with stethoscope)	• Cyanosis • Low saturation of plasma O_2 (SpO_2) • Tachypnoea • Confusion • Agitation

lists of some important information that can be gained from such an interview. The relevance of many of the points will be obvious to the reader, such as tobacco use and its links with chronic lung disease. However, it is beyond the scope of this book to discuss their relevance and the reader is referred to texts that consider in more depth the links between aspects of lifestyle and respiratory disease.

Table 2.5 Information to be gained from a patient interview

Current complaints by the patient
- Main complaints/symptoms (e.g. cough, dyspnoea, fatigue)
- Duration and nature of symptoms (e.g. cough productive of sputum for one week)
- Effect of symptoms on daily life and care needs as a result (e.g. too breathless to walk to shops, therefore daughter does shopping)
- Related factors (e.g. what makes symptoms better or worse?)
- Treatments – past and present (e.g. prescriptions from GP or medicine bought over the counter at chemist)
- Patient and family's perception/understanding of the symptoms/illness and their cause (e.g. inconvenience of having to be admitted to hospital or extremely worried that the problem is life threatening)

Patient's health history
- Previous illness and operations (e.g. has had a 'bad chest' for 20 years)
- Factors that might be linked to respiratory disorder (tobacco use, work environment, allergies to pollen)
- Family history (e.g. mother died of emphysema)

What to assess in a health history interview

The health history interview offers the chance for the nurse not just to listen to what the patient is saying, but also to notice important signs, perhaps through 'looking', 'listening' and 'feeling' as the interview progresses. For example, the patient may not be able to talk in sentences without pausing to breathe – an important sign of severe dyspnoea. A wheeze may be audible as the patient exhales, or as the nurse touches the patient's hand she may notice that the skin is cool and pale or warm and flushed. A clinical assessment of the patient thus begins during the interview and can also be followed up with a more detailed survey of the patient.

How hard is the patient working to breathe?

Reviewing Figure 2.7, which outlines the process of respiratory dysfunction and failure, it can be seen that prior to failure there is some dysfunction and compensation as the individual increases the effort he puts into breathing – the 'work of breathing'. Such signs as an increase in respiratory rate and use of accessory muscles will be seen long before a reduction in oxygen saturations. Although pulse oximetry is a useful and easy-to-use method of assessing oxygenation, it will not indicate that the patient is having to work very hard to maintain normal saturations. Increased work of breathing is an important sign of compensation and may exist when some of the clinical findings listed below are noted:

- restlessness
- agitation
- unco-operative behaviour
- increased respiratory rate
- concentration on breathing
- increased blood pressure
- increased heart rate
- sweating
- use of accessory muscles (shoulder shrugging, tensing of stenocleidomastoid muscles in neck)
- mouth breathing

Signs of increased work of breathing

The work of breathing can be reduced in some instances by helping the patient to change position or by administering bronchodilator drugs. These strategies will be discussed more fully in the final section of this chapter.

Action point 8

Are there signs that the patient is failing to meet the oxygen needs of the body or is retaining CO_2?

As respiratory dysfunction progresses to failure and blood O_2 levels begin to drop, important signs can be identified and should be reported to senior nurses and doctors urgently. Similarly, the retention of CO_2 late in the failure process may also be noticeable and should be reported. Table 2.6 gives an overview of how low O_2 and high CO_2 may manifest themselves in patients.

Table 2.6 How respiratory failure manifests itself (adapted from Thelan et al. 1998)

System affected	Hypoxaemia ($\downarrow O_2$)	Hypercapnia ($\uparrow CO_2$)
Central nervous	Restlessness Agitation Irritability Confusion Personality changes Impaired judgement Memory loss Sleep disturbance Bizarre behaviour Decreased consciousness	Headache Drowsiness Decreased consciousness Blurred vision Confusion Seizures Sleep disturbance
Cardiovascular	Tachycardia Bounding pulse Hypertension (systolic) Wide pulse pressure Dysrhythmias Palpitations Chest pain	Same as hypoxaemia Skin flushing
Pulmonary	Tachypnoea Hyperventilation Dyspnoea Accessory	Same as hypoxaemia
Renal	Decreased urinary output Oedema	Same as hypoxaemia
Gastrointestinal	Decreased bowel sounds Abdominal distension Anorexia Nausea and vomiting Constipation Gastrointestinal bleeding	Same as hypoxaemia
Skin	Pallor Cyanosis Cool skin Clammy skin	Flushing Clammy skin

The care and management of the patient with altered respiratory function

Nurses have a pivotal role in managing the patient's respiratory function, either autonomously or in collaboration with other members of the multidisciplinary team. Timely and appropriate management of the patient's respiratory function can have a tremendous impact on the experience of illness and the eventual outcome for patients and their families and friends.

The nurse–patient relationship is integral in this. Developing a rapport with your patient, coupled with good communication, is essential in order to gain the patient's confidence, minimize anxiety, gain compliance with treatment regimens and promote trust.

Caring for the patient with altered respiratory function, whatever the cause, represents a significant challenge for all nurses. If shortness of breath is used as a simple example, this has the potential to lead the patient into a vicious cycle of events that can have extremely serious consequences (Figure 2.8). As nurses with developing skills and knowledge in this area, we should be able to intervene in such cycles and protect the patient from further deterioration. However, it is also important to recognize that in certain instances, despite best efforts, sometimes such cycles are unbreakable.

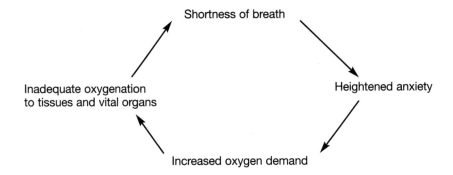

Figure 2.8 The vicious cycle of breathlessness and increased oxygen demands.

The nursing role in the care and management of the patient with altered respiratory function

As nurses, we need to meet this challenge and strengthen our skills in caring for these patients. Many of the nursing roles and activities that make up the patient's respiratory care can be drawn from Figure 2.9, which summarizes the aims that underpin respiratory therapy. The key nursing roles and activities that develop from these statements will be examined in more detail.

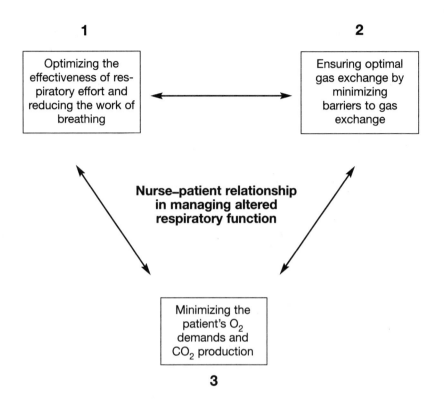

Figure 2.9 The aims of respiratory therapy.

Action point 9

- What do you perceive to be the key nursing roles and activities that centre on managing a patient with respiratory dysfunction?
- Consider where these roles might lie within the boxes of Figure 2.9 and whether they lend themselves best to box 1, 2 or 3, or a combination of all three.

Clinical application

1. 'Optimizing the effectiveness of respiratory effort and reducing the work of breathing' can be achieved by encouraging and helping the patient to cough and expectorate sputum, for example. This is effective by ensuring that airways are clear, thus allowing air movement with less work by the patient. Other examples include giving prescribed bronchodilators or passing a nasogastric tube to relieve gastric gas and the splinting effect this has on the diaphragm.

2. 'Ensuring optimal gas exchange and minimizing barriers to gas exchange' can again be achieved by airway clearance. Sputum retention and reduced lung ventilation mean reduced surface area available for gas exchange. Surface area reduction is one of the three major factors in reduced gas exchange. Other examples may include ensuring that the patient does not become overloaded with fluid, which may pool in the lungs and act as a gas exchange barrier

3. 'Minimizing the patient's O_2 demands and CO_2 production' can be achieved by reducing the amount of work a patient has to do to ventilate his lungs effectively (point 1 above). The more work an individual has to do, the more oxygen the respiratory muscles use and the more CO_2 they produce. Other examples include reducing body temperature when an individual is pyrexial. For each 1°C above normal, the metabolic rate increases by around 10%, burning more O_2 and producing more CO_2.

With significant clinical experience and the development of expertise, it becomes apparent to the practitioner that the basic things are the ones that are most important. Vigilance in ensuring that these are features of care will go a long way to promoting the patient's recovery from respiratory dysfunction. Factors such as adequate nutrition and hydration, a balance of activity and rest, giving adequate O_2 and monitoring responses to these as well as pharmacological therapies are the important basics. However, there is a prerequisite to all of these, which is unique to nursing – the nurse–patient relationship.

Key intervention 1. *Aim to build close and therapeutic relationships with your patient*

This is the basis for all the following interventions and for all nursing care. The relationship nurses have with patients and the way nurses use their knowledge within these relationships is what makes nursing unique and puts nurses in a special, and often optimum, position to help those experiencing illness.

Without, and even with, these relationships, compliance with simple aspects of care such as keeping an oxygen mask on can be major obstacles. The patient's understanding of the importance of such compliance is paramount, but again is difficult to achieve unless the patient trusts the nurses and believes what they say. So many things come from the nurse–patient relationship and it is often such a challenge to build that this brief mention does not do justice to its fundamental importance. This is the basis for teaching the individual and family, gaining their consent, meeting their social, psychological, spiritual and cultural needs, and much more. The reader is advised to read broadly on this subject, and to reflect and engage in diverse clinical experiences around this element of nursing.

Action point 10

- Choose a patient with respiratory dysfunction newly admitted to your clinical area.
- Be conscious of your interactions with the individual ('observe yourself') as well as other members of the nursing team. Ask yourself what attitudes (e.g. the need for honesty and friendliness) and behaviours (introducing humour into conversations) have positive and negative effects on the individual and the nurse–patient relationship.
- Undertake this over a period of days and reflect on the extent to which what you think of as 'positive relationships' affect patient trust in the nurses, compliance with care, mood and progress towards recovery.

Key intervention 2. Help the individual to achieve the optimum position

Safe and appropriate positioning of the patient can do much to improve comfort, ease the work of breathing, improve the uptake of O_2/nebulized medication and improve the patient's overall oxygenation. This also helps safeguard against developing a chest infection.

Positioning significantly influences lung function and inspiratory and expiratory lung volumes. The optimal position to ensure that maximal lung volumes are involved in gaseous exchange during spontaneous respiration is standing.

Think of athletes who have just completed a race. More often than not they remain standing, leant slightly forwards while breathing rapidly and sometimes through pursed lips. There is rationale for this: the fast respiratory rate is an attempt to draw more oxygen in to meet the needs of the body during the race, while simultaneously allowing for efficient removal of waste gas, CO_2. Body position ensures that inspired air gets to all areas of the lung. Breathing through pursed lips or sighing through pursed lips is an attempt to hold airways open irrespective of the respiratory cycle in order to improve oxygenation. This principle can be carried over to CPAP, a breathing circuit that can help with spontaneous respiration in certain instances.

Consider the breathless asthmatic patient. In certain instances the only position they may feel comfortable in is sitting out of bed, partially leant over a table. When you notice positional changes to standing, or near standing, accompanied with breathing through pursed lips, you know that the patient is mimicking an athlete and trying to maximize ventilation and oxygenation.

The following positions are the next-best positions to adopt in order to maximize oxygenation:

- sitting upright in a chair
- sitting upright in bed
- side lying in bed.

Lying in bed in a slumped sitting position represents poor positioning as it leads to diminished airflow to the bases of the lungs and the upper abdominal contents compress against the bases of the lungs. This phenomenon also inhibits the movement of the diaphragm and this is sometimes referred to as diaphragmatic splinting. In conditions where there is marked abdominal distension, this effect is more profound, and in many cases can cause significant collapse of the lung bases, thus in turn reducing the amount of airways (surface area) available for gaseous exchange.

Side-lying positions are preferable to a slumped supine position; this is because the abdominal contents move downwards, allowing the uppermost lung more freedom to expand and drain any secretions that may be present. The lung that is nearest to the bed does not expand as fully as the uppermost lung, which is stretched, but this 'dependent' lung does experience the greatest amount of tidal flow (in and out) of air and enjoys better perfusion (blood flow), as blood flow is influenced by gravity and favours the 'dependent' lung.

These basic principles of positioning, and its effects on lung ventilation, gas exchange and secretion drainage, underpin physical therapy in clinical practice. It explains why physiotherapists often request alternate side lying for their patients who are in bed with respiratory problems. It also explains why physiotherapists try to establish whether patients who are difficult to position in bed, or who slump in the bed, can stand or sit out in a chair.

Correct positioning of the patient will help to:

- improve spontaneous ventilation and increase lung volumes available for gaseous exchange, thus improving oxygenation
- drain secretions
- decrease the work of breathing
- minimize the risks of chest infection.

Key intervention 3. *Monitor the rate and the rhythm of respirations*

Monitoring and recording the patient's respiratory rate are among the most important observations the nurse can make. In certain instances they can be a reliable predictor of impeding critical illness. A normal resting respiratory rate is 10–20 breaths per minute. Respiratory rates of less than 8 per minute or greater than 30 per minute are clinically significant and should not be ignored. Equally important is observing the rhythm of respirations, as this can also provide valuable information about the patient's clinical condition. Respiratory patterns were discussed earlier.

Accurate recording of the respiratory rate on the observation chart serves as a record of when certain key changes took place and provides valuable clues about the patient's care. For example, did the high respiratory rate coincide with a change in treatment, such as a reduction in the frequency of a nebulizer or a reduction in a diuretic or inspired O_2 concentration?

When monitoring the rate and rhythm of your patient's respirations it is well worth considering the following points in patients who have a raised respiratory rate:

- Establish the current respiratory rate and compare it with the trend over the past 24 hours. Has this rate climbed recently or has it been progressively climbing over a prolonged period of time?
- Is this change linked to any other recent developments, such as a sudden climb in temperature, sudden decrease in level of consciousness or reduced oxygen saturation? It could be that an elevated respiratory rate is a consequence of a worsening chest infection. The change in respiratory rate could herald something that warrants urgent medical attention, such as a pneumothorax (collapsed lung with air in the pleural space).
- Is anxiety/restlessness an issue? This can be a manifestation of hypoxaemia (low blood O_2) or it could increase the patient's O_2 demands and go on to make them hypoxaemic. If the patient does not become calmer after reassurance and careful explanation of these experiences, a medical review will be of value as the patient may require sedation. However, in certain instances sedation may compromise an already compromised respiratory function, hence the rationale behind having medical approval prior to administering sedative drugs.
- If your patient is breathless with a high respiratory rate, carefully stage nursing interventions, e.g. bathing, sheet changes, positioning, as these may increase O_2 demand and worsen the breathlessness. Establish whether certain interventions cam be minimized or performed together, e.g. sheet change and pressure area check in conjunction with physiotherapy. This avoids repeatedly revisiting the patient and increasing O_2 demands.
- It may be that during such periods physical activity is limited and the associated risks need to be considered such as deep vein thrombosis (DVT) prophylaxis.

In patients who have a reduced respiratory rate, it is worth considering the following points:

- Establish the current respiratory rate and compare it with the trend of the past 24 hours. Has this rate dropped recently or has it been progressively lowering over a prolonged period of time?

- See if a link can be made between the low respiratory rate and the patient's history. In certain instances, such as drug overdose, reduced respiratory rate may be a consequence of this. If this is the case, the nurse should ascertain from the medical staff agreed criteria for when to contact them in the event of any further deterioration.
- Consider the impact of sedation or analgesics; these drugs can have profound effects on the respiratory system. Opiate analgesics such as morphine/diamorphine cause respiratory depression. Reduced respiratory rate may well be a consequence of opiate overdose
- Is this change linked to any other recent developments, such as a sudden climb in temperature, sudden decrease in level of consciousness or reduced O_2 saturation? It could be that this change in respiratory rate is a consequence of a worsening infection.

The rate and rhythm of respiration can be heavily influenced both positively and negatively by pharmacological agents. Monitoring the rate and rhythm of your patient's respiration will help to detect any change in their clinical condition. It is a vitally important observation and in certain instances may be indicative of pending critical illness. However, it is important to place this observation in the context of the previous trend in respiratory rate and the type of patient you are looking after.

Changes in your patient's respiratory rate may have a direct influence on the care you give, e.g. the breathless patient requiring staggered or carefully managed nursing interventions to avoid exhaustion.

Key intervention 4. *Administer prescribed pharmacological agents and monitor for their effects and complications*

The role of pharmacological agents and of the pharmacy service also form a large part of the respiratory care a patient receives. Administration of the appropriate pharmacological agents has a tremendous impact on improving the patient's respiratory function as well as influencing outcome. It is vital that nurses have a good understanding of the relevant pharmacological agents used to improve respiratory function. Detailed description of all the associated respiratory pharmacology is beyond the realms of this chapter. However, Table 2.7 summarizes some of the key pharmacological agents used in improving respiratory function and the main clinical considerations.

It is important to emphasize that all inhaled drugs are most effective if they are inhaled as deeply as possible while the patient is in a position that facilitates maximal lung ventilation, e.g. sitting upright.

Table 2.7 Pharmacological agents used to improve respiratory function

Drug	Mode of action	Key clinical considerations
Oxygen	Increases alveolar O_2 concentration and thereby increases the amount of O_2 crossing into the pulmonary capillaries. This treats hypoxaemia	Administration is controlled by flow meter and the type of delivery device being used The amount of O_2 required for any patient is whatever amount will stop them being hypoxemic and keep their O_2 saturations > 95% (> 90% in some chronic lung diseases)
Bronchodilators Beta-2 agonists Short acting, e.g. salbutamol, terbutaline; long acting, e.g. salmeterol, formoterol	Beta-2 receptor stimulation, reverses airway obstruction in bronchospasm by relaxing bronchial smooth muscle.	Short-acting beta-2 agonists administered by inhaler or nebulizer are effective within 5 min and have a short duration of action (4–6 h). Useful in acute asthma attacks Long-acting beta-2 agonists are useful for night-time use These drugs are effectively stimulants and can also cause restlessness, agitation, insomnia, tremors, tachycardia and other unpleasant side effects especially in high doses (refer to the *British National Formulary*, BNF)
Antimuscarinics, e.g. ipratropium bromide	Muscarinic receptor blockade reverses airway obstruction in bronchospasm by relaxation of bronchial smooth muscle	Antimuscarinic bronchodilators are probably of most use in the treatment of COPD but may also be used in chronic asthma
Phosphodiesterase inhibitor, e.g. aminophylline, theophylline	Inhibition of phosphodiesterase reverses airway obstruction in bronchospasm by relaxation of bronchial smooth muscle	Theophylline is administered orally. Aminophylline may be administered orally or by slow Intravenous injection or infusion Plasma level monitoring of these two drugs is important to keep the plasma level of the drug within the therapeutic range These drugs are stimulants, similar in a way to salbutamol and can cause similar side effects, especially insomnia, tachycardia and tremors (refer to the BNF)

Table 2.7 Pharmacological agents used to improve respiratory function (contd)

Drug	Mode of action	Key clinical considerations
Corticosteroids, e.g. beclomethasone, prednisolone, hydrocortisone	Reduces airway inflammation, thereby reducing oedema and secretion of mucus into the airway	This group of drugs do not give immediate relief of broncho-spasm. Symptom control with corticosteroids may take 3–7 days Must be used regularly when administered by inhaler Can also be administered orally and parenterally This group of drugs has many short- and long-term side effects, including alterations in metabolism, fluid and electrolyte balance, immune functioning and tissue healing (refer to the BNF)
Respiratory stimulants, e.g doxapram	Stimulates peripheral chemoreceptors and central respiratory centres in the medulla, causing the patient's respiratory centre to increase respiratory effort	May be of use in COPD patients when ventilatory support is contraindicated If given to patients who are suffering from respiratory fatigue it may merely hasten their ensuing failure and worsen their respiratory muscle fatigue Administered by slow intravenous injection or infusion
Antibiotics, e.g. amoxicillin, erythromycin, cefuroxime	Examples of infecting organisms: *Streptococcus pneumoniae*, *Haemophilus influenzae*, *Staphylococcus aureus*, mycoplasma, etc. Antibiotics have bactericidal and/or bacteriostatic properties	Choice of antibiotic depends on factors such as sensitivity of known or likely infecting organism, side effects of the drug, route of administration of the drug, allergies, etc. The many groups of antibiotics have numerous side effects (refer to the BNF)

Action point 11

Select a range of patients who are being treated for respiratory dysfunction. Identify what drugs they are receiving and read around those drugs. Get to know the drugs well and consider what implications their actions, interactions, side effects and potential complications have for the care you deliver and, most importantly, for the patient and their experience of illness and therapy.

Key intervention 5. Monitor the amount of O_2 your patient requires and how this impacts on O_2 saturation when pulse oximetry monitoring is used

The amount of inspired O_2 patients require can also provide you with valuable information on their respiratory status. Normal healthy respiratory function sees us generating a satisfactory O_2 saturation of 95–98% in atmospheric air, which contains 21% O_2. If you adopt this as a baseline, then it can sometimes help you gauge the significance of altered respiratory function.

If your patient is generating poor O_2 saturations (85–90%) on 60% O_2, you now know the O_2 requirement is three times greater than normal and with poor O_2 saturation; O_2 is failing to diffuse across the alveolus into the pulmonary circulation. With any form of O_2 therapy, the nurse should ensure that the inspired air is adequately humidified, so that the extra flow of O_2 does not make the airways too dry and the sputum does not become overly viscous, thus making it difficult for the patient to expectorate.

Giving O_2 to patients with COPD

Certain patients, particularly those with long-standing COPD, can go on to develop hypoxic drive (discussed earlier in this chapter). This can lead to dilemmas and confusion about how best to manage the O_2 therapy of these patients, especially when they become acutely ill.

Oxygen therapy and managing the patient with known hypoxic drive

One commonly asked question is:

- 'What happens if I am worried about my patient's oxygenation and he has known hypoxic drive?'

In this situation it is very important to avoid giving unnecessarily high levels of O_2, but it is equally important to safeguard your patient against hypoxia.

Oxygen should not be withheld in the presence of high $P\text{CO}_2$ levels nor withdrawn if the patient worsens.

Management strategy

Initially, the aim should be to achieve an O_2 saturation > 92% (this may vary according to the doctor's preference), with monitoring of arterial blood gases. If the $P\text{CO}_2$ rises to > 10 kPa, then the O_2 should be reduced and the desired parameters for acceptable saturation amended to 2–3% below the previous scale.

Inadequate reversal of hypoxia, e.g. saturation < 85%, can be suggestive of a worsening clinical condition, such as pulmonary embolism, pulmonary oedema or pneumothorax, and in this case specialist help should be sought (Tuxen 1997).

The practicalities of delivering appropriate amounts of O_2 in the clinical situation require some knowledge of the different delivery devices and in what situations they should be used. Table 2.8 summarizes some of the key points about the various O_2 delivery devices available.

Table 2.8 Oxygen delivery devices

Equipment	Objective	l/min	$F\text{IO}_2$ (%)	Advantages/Disadvantages
Nasal cannula	Provides O_2 through a low-flow oxygen delivery system	1 2 3 4 5 6	24 28 32 36 40 44	Can be used with mouth breathers Convenient Comfortable Good low flow Allows for talking and eating Oxygen content delivered to the patient difficult to assess accurately because it depends on the patient's respiratory pattern May cause sinus pain >2 l/min requires added humidity or it will have a drying effect on the nasal mucous membranes Nasal passages must be patent

Table 2.8 Oxygen delivery devices (contd)

Equipment	Objective	l/min	F_{IO_2} (%)	Advantages/Disadvantages
Simple facemask	Provides O_2 through a mask and a low-flow oxygen delivery system	5 6 8	50 50 60	Simple set-up; good for emergency situations Can get uncomfortable Poor patient tolerance O_2 content delivered difficult to assess accurately because it depends on the patient's respiratory pattern Cannot provide enough humidity for prolonged use Must be removed for meals Tight-fitting mask can cause pressure sores
Non-rebreathing mask	Provides higher O_2 concentrations	6 8 10–15	55–60 60–80 80–90	Delivers the highest possible oxygen concentration (55–90%) possible from a low-flow system Good for short-term therapy and transport Requires a tight seal May irritate skin
Air-entrainment (Venturi) mask	Provides a high flow of O_2 with a precise F_{IO_2} in a selected range	4–8	Determined by colour coding (varies according to manufacturer)	Accurate O_2 level Simple set-up; good for emergency situations Can only have F_{IO_2} in selected range Hot and confining Must fit snugly
Facemask with high flow and wide-bore tubing	Can provide a high flow and O_2 concentration, as well as humidification		Usually determined Air/ oxygen mixing device	With O_2 analyser gives an accurate and high concentration of O_2 Can give a high flow for patients with a high minute volume and high inspiratory flow rates Can be humidified Requires a tight-fitting mask Can feel warm and confining for patient

F_{IO_2}, fraction of inspired oxygen.

Key intervention 6. Aim to achieve a balance between activity and rest

It is of paramount importance to help and encourage the individual who is at risk of respiratory deterioration to change position frequently and to be as mobile as possible. This helps to recruit and expand areas of lung that have collapsed or are compressed in particular positions. Activity stimulates deeper breathing and the expectoration of sputum.

Part of this regimen of activity and mobilization may well include hourly deep-breathing and coughing exercises, especially in the postoperative patient, where the key aim is to prevent complications such as pneumonia.

A deep-breathing exercise that the physiotherapist may instruct patients to undertake, especially in the postoperative period, is the sustained maximal inspiration (SMI) manoeuvre. This involves asking the patient to take as large a breath as possible and holding at the end of inspiration for 3–5 seconds. This is far more effective than merely taking deep breaths without holding, and helps to maintain the maximum surface area for gas exchange and prevent lung collapse and sequential complications such as pneumonia.

Coughing is another useful manoeuvre, not least because before coughing one generally takes a deep breath. Coughing helps to clear airways, reducing airway obstructions and the work of breathing that such obstruction may bring.

The emphasis placed on activity must be proportional to the individual's tolerance and the severity of respiratory distress. Activity uses more O_2 than rest and generates more CO_2 as a by-product. Some patients may be in such critical conditions that they cannot tolerate any activity, even coughing. Others may be able to transfer from bed to bedside chair or walk short distances. A key consideration in the nurse's mind should be 'what demands will this activity place on the individual in terms of extra O_2 for the cells?'. It should be remembered that the more muscle involved, the higher the demands will be. Walking across a hallway to the toilet may seem a small expenditure of energy to us, but may be too much for some patients – especially if O_2 therapy has to be discontinued to do this.

Adequate rest is necessary for healing, as is sleep, and these are part of a whole range of requirements for recovery.

Key intervention 7. Aim to promote the conditions for healing to take place

A vast range of physiological factors can contribute to healing and the recovery of the individual from acute respiratory dysfunction or the maintenance of maximum achievable health in those with chronic pulmonary disease. These will be given some consideration here, but a fuller discussion is beyond the scope of this chapter and the reader is referred to other texts and articles on the topics (see Further reading).

Aside from elements such as O_2, cells also need nutritional 'fuel' to sustain their normal functions and recover from insult or injury. Adequate nutrition can have many beneficial effects in all disease states; in respiratory disease, it can help to:

- protect the pulmonary system from infection or help to fight off an existing infection through boosting the immune system
- replace energy stores that are used up during the exertion that is a result of increased work of breathing in respiratory dysfunction
- deliver the nutrients required by cells to replace dead or damaged cells and tissue
- help maintain a normal electrolyte balance essential for normal respiratory muscle functioning
- keep a healthy mucous lining in the lungs to trap invading bacteria when coupled with adequate hydration, as well as allowing expectoration of sputum through reducing its viscosity.

Many of these effects are not guaranteed even if the individual has an adequate and well-balanced nutritional intake. Substances such as steroid hormones are produced during times of stress, wakefulness and physiological exertion. While steroids can be beneficial in their anti-inflammatory effects in conditions such as acute asthma, they also reduce immunity, delay tissue healing and cause muscle breakdown. Reducing the amount of circulating steroids through measures that promote rest and sleep, limit physical exertion, and relieve anxiety and pain is an important element of nursing. Promoting sleep also has a very positive effect, in that tissue repair and regeneration is promoted through the release of growth hormone and the inhibition of steroid production. On the other hand, controlling pain not only reduces steroid production but may also allow greater lung expansion, mobility, deep breathing and coughing – especially if the pain was abdominal or thoracic in locality.

These key nursing interventions are the fundamentals that are likely to have a great influence on patient outcomes and experiences. However, on occasions, there is a need for advanced therapeutic regimens, which, in addition to maintaining these key interventions, might be considered advanced respiratory support.

Advanced respiratory support

There are varying degrees of advanced respiratory support. These primarily include high flow oxygen therapy, continuous positive airway pressure (CPAP) and bi-level positive airway pressure (BIPAP). It may be that some patients are treated by being stepped up and down through all of these methods and other patients are treated with just one method. The treatments selected will be determined on individual patient need and by the clinicians attending to the patient at the time.

It is vitally important that nurses recognise the value of optimizing and treating the patient with altered respiratory function at the earliest opportunity in order to avoid critical illness. We should also recognize points in time when a patient's respiratory support should be accelerated and when it should be limited, or when unsure, know where to access further opinion. Systems such as CPAP are considered as advanced respiratory support. They are more commonplace in intensive care units and high dependency units, but are increasingly common in acute ward areas supported by critical care outreach teams. These will be described briefly here, more for completeness rather than an attempt to give the reader a working knowledge. For this you are referred to texts on critical care nursing.

High flow oxygen therapy

This is a technique whereby a specialized oxygen flow converting device is connected to a piped oxygen supply, which gives the patient flow rates of oxygen at a higher rate of flow than conventional delivery devices. This increased flow rate of oxygen can have the beneficial effect of improving oxygen uptake in poorly ventilated areas of the lungs. This in turn can improve the patient's overall oxygenation in certain instances.

Continuous positive airway pressure

CPAP is a method of providing positive airway pressure throughout all phases of the respiratory cycle (inspiration and expiration), through a specially designed respiratory circuit. The circuit has the ability to administer a higher flow rate of gas than conventional delivery systems; this also has the beneficial effect of improving oxygen uptake in poorly ventilated areas of the lungs.

CPAP also involves breathing out against a resistance which is generated by a specially designed valve known as a positive end expiratory pressure (PEEP) valve. This has the additional effect of improving the functional residual capacity of the lung (which is the functional volume left in the lungs at the end of expiration). This increases the surface area of the alveoli available for gas exchange and prevents alveolar collapse. This in turn increases the potential for improved oxygenation.

Reconsider for a moment the athlete completing a race. As mentioned earlier note, how the athlete breathes out through pursed lips. This is a mimicking of the PEEP effect which is an attempt to hold the alveoli open, allowing for increased oxygenation.

Mask bi-level positive airway pressure (BIPAP)

BIPAP is delivered via a machine and a respiratory circuit designed specifically for this purpose. BIPAP differs from CPAP, as BIPAP gives the patient additional assistance on inspiration to a pre-determined pressure level, while also providing the PEEP effect.

BIPAP is often linked with the term 'non-invasive ventilation' (NIV). NIV refers to the technique of improving alveolar ventilation without an endotracheal tube. The term bi-level refers to the two elements of positive pressure used, the first being the positive pressure from an enhanced spontaneous inspiratory breath and the second level referring to the positive pressure from the PEEP effect.

Think of BIPAP as a way of optimizing respiratory function by giving the patient enhanced inspiration while allowing the patient to breathe out against a resistance, in order to help maximize oxygenation.

Artificial mechanical ventilation

This represents the highest level of respiratory support and is used in a variety of different clinical conditions. Artificial mechanical ventilation involves using a ventilator to support the respiratory system. This is often used as support for patients in respiratory failure. Artificial mechanical ventilation without other interventions, e.g. physiotherapy, sputum clearance, antibiotics and appropriate use of pharmacologic agents, will not improve respiratory function; it may merely serve to improve blood gases and take over the work of breathing for the patient. This technique will only be seen in intensive care units.

Summary

This chapter has focused on the respiratory system and attempted to relate theory and practice in four key areas. These are the fundamental physiological concepts that are required to understand respiratory disorders and their treatment. It has also considered respiratory dysfunction and failure, and examined some of the common respiratory disorders that may be seen in clinical practice in the acute care area. Respiratory assessment and therapy have also been examined, with the aim of giving the beginning nurse a view of the most important key concepts, as well as some of the detail.

Timely and appropriate management of the patient's respiratory function can have a tremendous impact on the patient's condition and eventual outcome. Following studies by McQuillan et al. (1998) and McGloin and Adams (1997), who discovered suboptimal standards of care for the seriously ill in acute ward areas, there is a much greater appreciation of the value of treating and optimizing the patient's condition at the earliest possible opportunity. This will reduce the likelihood of the patient going on to develop a critical illness that may require a prolonged hospital stay and the associated risks involved. This may not always be possible, but it should remain a guiding principle of care. The authors believe that the nurse–patient relationship is a prerequisite for such care.

References and further reading

Bassett C, Makin L (2000) Caring for the Seriously Ill Patient. London: Edward Arnold.

Benner P, Wrubel J (1989) The Primacy of Caring: stress and coping in health and illness. Menlo Park, CA: Addison Wesley

McGloin H, Adams S (1997) The quality of pre-ICU care influences the outcomes of patients admitted from the ward. Clinical Intensive Care 8: 104.

McQuillan P et al. (1998) Confidential enquiry into quality of care before admission to intensive care. British Medical Journal 316: 1853–1858.

Thelan LA et al. (1998) Critical Care Nursing: Diagnosis and management 3rd edn. St Louis, MI: Mosby.

Thibodeau G, Patton K (1999) Anatomy and Physiology, 4th edn. St Louis, MI: Mosby

Tuxen DV (1997) Acute respiratory failure in chronic obstructive airways disease. In Oh TE (ed) Intensive Care Manual, 4th edn. Oxford: Butterworth-Heinmann.

CHAPTER THREE

The digestive system

MARGARET R KAY

Introduction

To function effectively, the human body requires fuel. This is derived from ingested food and fluids, which supply the dietary nutrients needed to meet the body's metabolic demands, and depends on a healthy digestive system.

This chapter is designed to equip the nurse with the knowledge needed to inform the care required by the patient with a disease of the digestive system. The importance of food and nutrition is introduced, followed by a review of the dysfunction of specific organs, and the treatment and nursing considerations required for the patient with disorders of the upper and lower digestive tract.

After reading this chapter, the nurse should be able to identify nutritional need and recognize the symptoms associated with each condition discussed, which will enable her to provide relevant and effective nursing care for patients with a dysfunctioning digestive system.

Nutrition

Action point 1

What does nutrition mean to you? And why is it important to ensure good nutrition for your patients?

The science of nutrition is the study of all processes for growth, maintenance and repair of body tissues that depend on the digestion of food. From this we can deduce that a healthy digestive system and the ability or opportunity to take in food that comprises a healthy diet are necessary for maintaining good nutritional status.

Food facts

Food is necessary for life, since it provides the body with the essential nutrients to enable health and wellbeing. The food we eat falls into five essential classes, which, along with water, make up the diet. They can be grouped as energy giving, body building or protective (Figure 3.1).

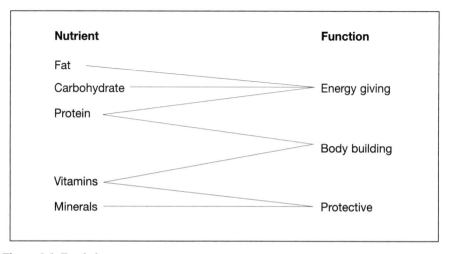

Figure 3.1 Food classes.

Dietary fibre, both soluble and insoluble, is also important since it absorbs water, stimulates the muscular movement of the digestive tract, provides bulk and produces gas, which aerates faeces. This results in easier, more frequent defecation and the prevention of constipation.

Action point 2

Reflect on these five classs of nutrient and identify the food sources from which each can be derived.

The nutrients enter the digestive system, which acts like a human food processor. It comprises a group of organs and structures that wreck mechanically and change chemically the complex structure of food and drink into small, simple molecules that can be absorbed, circulated, used or stored.

Knowledge of the system is essential for the nurse who is responsible for a full assessment of digestive function and the implementation of relevant care.

The digestive system – a basic overview

Alternative names for this system are the alimentary tract or gastrointestinal (GI) system (gut), although the latter is technically incorrect as it refers only to the stomach and the intestines. In fact, the digestive system stretches from the mouth to the anus (Figure 3.2).

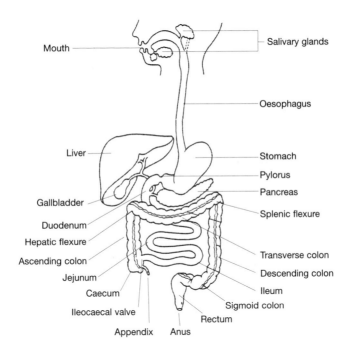

Figure 3.2 The digestive system. Reproduced from Elcoat (1986) by kind permission of Baillière Tindall.

The digestive system is basically made up of a tube of varying diameters, approximately 5–7 metres long in the adult. The organs that make up the system are divided into main and accessory structures which complement each other with regard to their digestive function (Table 3.1).

Table 3.1 Organs of digestion

Main	Accessory
Mouth	Teeth and tongue
Pharynx	Salivary glands
Oesophagus	Liver
Stomach	Gallbladder
Small intestine	Pancreas
Large intestine	Appendix

Histology of the digestive tube

Despite possessing specific functions, the main organs of digestion are constructed from the same basic arrangement of four main tissue layers (Figure 3.3). Any disease or damage to these tissues will impact on the process of digestion and absorption of nutrients.

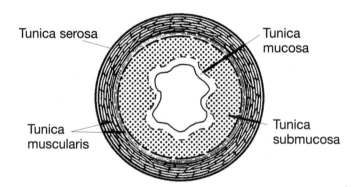

Figure 3.3 Simple cross-section of the digestive tube.

Tunica serosa

This is the outermost layer of strong connective and adipose tissue containing large nerves and blood vessels. Within the abdomen this is known as the peritoneum; outside the abdomen, i.e the mouth and oesophagus, it is called the adventitia.

Tunica muscularis

The tunica muscularis is composed of two layers of juxtaposed muscle fibres: an innermost circular layer and an outer longitudinal layer. The stomach has an additional oblique layer. Parasympathetic nerve bodies and fibres (myenteric nerve plexus) lie between the muscle layers that exert control primarily over the motility of the tract.

Tunica submucosa

This is a thick connective tissue layer containing blood vessels, small glands and nerves (submucosal nerve plexus). It is particularly important for control of secretion throughout the digestive tract.

Tunica mucosa

This is the innermost layer, and comprises the mucous epithelium that lines the lumen of the tract, loose connective tissue rich in blood and lymphatic vessels, and a thin layer of muscle that enables the mucosa to fold.

The peritoneum

This is the largest serous membrane of the body and is comprised of two layers: the parietal layer, which lines the abdominal cavity; and the visceral layer, which covers the abdominal and pelvic organs. The stomach and parts of the intestines are almost completely surrounded by a double fold of peritoneum and connective tissue – the mesenteries, which attach these structures to the posterior abdominal wall and provide a route for blood vessels and nerves. Other organs of the digestive tract, e.g. the duodenum and descending colon, lie against the abdominal wall and have no mesenteries. These are described as retroperitoneal, because only the anterior surface is covered with peritoneum. Any leakage into the peritoneal cavity from within the digestive tract will cause inflammation of the peritoneal layers and result in a serious and potentially fatal condition – peritonitis.

Functions of the digestive system

The digestive system performs a number of intricate tasks that render food less complex and more acceptable to the system. This occurs through five essential activities.

Ingestion

Taking food and fluid into the digestive system, usually via the mouth in the healthy individual.

Movement or propulsion

The transfer of food from the mouth to the anus. This includes the voluntary act of swallowing and peristalsis, the involuntary neuromuscular activity that uses alternate waves of contraction and relaxation of organic muscles to advance the substance onwards.

Digestion

The mechanical and chemical breakdown of complex food compounds.

Absorption

The movement of the end products of digestion from the lumen of the diges-tive tube, via the mucosal cells, to blood or lymph for distribution to body cells.

Defecation/Elimination

The excretion of unabsorbed and indigestible substances in the form of faeces.

Elaborate neural and hormonal mechanisms ensure that food taken into the digestive system is moved to sites for enzyme activity, which reduces complex foods into small molecular units that can be absorbed easily (Table 3.2).

Action point 3

Think about your experiences in practice and consider circumstances that can affect any of the normal processes of digestion in patients you have cared for.

Table 3.2 Summary of the process of mechanical and chemical digestion

Organ(s)	Chemical(s) and secretions	Action	Result
Mouth, teeth, tongue, salivary glands	Salivary amylase Mucus	Tearing, chewing, lubricated by mucus, mixing, rolling, breakdown of starch initiated	Bolus ready for swallowing Polysaccharides reduced to disaccha-ride (maltose)
Pharynx, oesophagus	Salivary amylase Mucus	Bolus received and propelled into oesophagus by pharyngeal muscles Polysaccharide breakdown contin-ued by salivary amylase	Oesophageal peristal-sis is stimulated moving bolus forward to the stomach

Table 3.2 Summary of the process of mechanical and chemical digestion (contd)

Organ(s)	Chemical(s) and secretions	Action	Result
Stomach	Gastrin, pepsinogen, hydrochloric acid (HCl), pepsin, mucus, intrinsic factor	Receives, stores and mixes the bolus with gastric juice containing chemicals and the hormone gastrin. Begins protein digestion when inactive enzyme pepsinogen is activated by HCl to enzyme pepsin	Bolus is reduced to a semi-liquid substance, chyme. Proteins reduced to peptides. Stomach contents ready to move into duodenum
Duodenum, jejunum and ileum (small intestine)	Intestinal juice containing bicarbonate, bile, and enzymes enterokinase and cholecystokinin (CCK), maltase, sucrase and lactase, and the hormone secretin	Carbohydrate and protein digestion continues. Fat digestion begins with the chemical action of the enzymes	Digestion is completed. The complex food ingested is now simplified to glucose, amino acids, fatty acids and glycerol and is able to be absorbed into the blood via the villi in the small intestine. Once absorbed the nutrients are metabolized (see Chapter 6)
Colon, rectum and anus	Mucus containing gut flora (bacteria)	No digestive function. Stores and concentrates undigested cellulose, absorbs salt and water, synthesizes vitamin D and B complexes. Expels faeces via rectum and anus	Forms and eliminates faeces from the body by defecation, a reflex act that responds to distension in the rectum

The impact of malnutrition

All body systems are dependent on nutritional supply and elimination of waste, a service provided by the digestive system. People with digestive dysfunction are a particularly vulnerable group because reduced appetite, inadequate diet and nutrient malabsorption will impede these normal functions. This will contribute not only to loss of weight and lean body mass but, over time, can have wide-reaching systemic consequences (Tables 3.3 and 3.4).

These serious and potentially life-threatening problems must be avoided at all costs. It is the responsibility of all healthcare professionals to prevent or correct undernourishment, and a team approach to nutritional care was advocated over 25 years ago to help achieve this. The purpose was to develop evidence-based standards and guidelines for nutritional assessment. Lennard Jones (1992) endorsed this position and advanced the argument for nutritional assessment for all hospital patients, a recommendation supported by dieticians and the British Association for Parenteral and Enteral Nutrition. (BAPEN).

Table 3.3 Effect of protein–energy malnutrition on body systems

Cardiovascular	Wasting and weakened myocardium, and reduced contraction and conduction, resulting in reduced cardiac output and increased risk of cardiac failure. Reduced arterial and venous pressure and increased risk of thromboembolism
Respiratory	Weakened/atrophied respiratory muscles result in reduced respiratory response to hypoxia Retention of pulmonary secretions, increasing the risk of infection and pneumonia
Digestive	Atrophy of gut mucosa, and reduced hormone and enzyme secretion, resulting in impaired integrity of gut structure and function
Musculoskeletal	Reduced skeletal muscle mass and muscle wasting, resulting in fatigue, muscle weakness and reduced mobility Reduced osteoclast activity resulting in bone loss. In elderly people increased risk of fractures
Endocrine	Rapid depletion of liver glycogen stores and decreased secretion of hormones, i.e. insulin, cortisol, growth hormone, triiodothyronine, resulting in reduced metabolic rate, lethargy and tiredness
Renal	Impaired ability to concentrate filtrate leads to increased urine output, resulting in increased risk of dehydration Reduced ability to excrete sodium ions resulting in an increased risk of circulatory overload if fluid volume increases

Table 3.3 Effect of protein–energy malnutrition on body systems (contd)

Skin	Augumented atrophy and desquamation increase fragility of skin, which can be damaged easily. In severe cases, local tissue oedema can occur. Combined effects increase the risk of skin breakdown, pressure sore formation and impair wound healing
Immune	Both humoral and cellular immunity are impaired, leading to reduced production of lymphocytes and complement, resulting in increased risk of infection and delayed wound healing

Table 3.4 Characteristics of vitamin deficiency

A	Deterioration of poor light vision, dry conjunctiva, dry scaly skin
D	Proximal muscle weakness, bone pain, bone deformity and fractures in severe cases
E	Shortened life span of erythrocytes and leucocytes, possible lack of control of limb movements and unsteady gait
C	Lethargy, fatigue, weakness, dry skin, small haemorrhages into joints and muscle, purpura of lower limbs, gum disease (gingivitis) and loss of teeth, impaired wound healing
B_1 (thiamine)	Cardiac failure, tachycardia, oedema, anorexia, nausea, vomiting, weakened calf muscle
B_2 (riboflavine)	Inflammation of the mouth (stomatitis), cracks at corners of the mouth, swollen red lips
B_6 (pyridoxine)	Irritability, insomnia, weakness, mental confusion, depression, stomatitis, glossitis, dermatitis (perineum, scrotum)
Niacin	Dry skin, hyperpigmented on exposed areas, dermatitis, peripheral neuropathy, dementia, apathy, atrophic changes to the tongue, diarrhoea

Nutritional assessment objectives and process

Nutritional assessment is a decisive factor when planning care for patients with disorders of the digestive system. The nurse can be instrumental in detecting the presence or risk of malnutrition.

Objectives

- To establish the degree of risk of the patient becoming undernourished.
- To enable care to be planned that recognizes the need for nutritional support.
- To liaise with relevant members of the multidisciplinary team.

Process

This process has been made easier by the development of risk assessment tools that provide a useful framework and guidelines for nurses to follow. No standard assessment tool exists. Bond (1997) provides a comprehensive summary of several published tools and many hospitals have developed their own. What is evident is that each uses a combination of subjective and objective measures to identify malnutrition and calculate the degree of risk. Achieving validity of these tools is difficult, because malnutrition is complex and nutritional needs vary between individuals. The Malnutrition Advisory Group (MAG 2000) has attempted to address this by developing a standard tool and advocates its use nationwide to enable national comparisons to be made.

Methods for nutritional assessment

Subjective methods

Obtaining subjective data is integral to the overall assessment of the patient. By using skilled clinical observation and effective questioning, the nurse will be able to estimate the patient's nutritional status.

Action point 4

Reflecting on the systemic consequences of malnutrition, what would lead you to suspect that a patient is undernourished?

Did you include:

- clothes too big?
- pale, rough, dry patchy skin?
- dry, swollen, cracked lips?
- red, swollen, bleeding gums?

- dull, dry, brittle, sparse hair?
- pale, dry, dull eyes?
- brittle, ridged, peeling nails?
- oedematous legs and ankles?
- general weakness and lethargy?

Specific questions relevant to the digestive system should centre around what is the norm for the individual and reflect weight loss, appetite, eating patterns, eating and swallowing difficulties, nausea, vomiting, diarrhoea, constipation, and past history and current diagnosis of GI disease.

Objective methods

Body weight

This is a basic objective mechanism that, when correctly interpreted, provides information about body fat stores and lean body mass. One drawback of this method is that some patients are too ill to be weighed.

Body mass index (BMI)

This uses weight as a nutritional index by using 'power' indices where height is expressed as a power function of weight, i.e. BMI = weight (kg) divided by height (m) squared.

Interpreting BMI

< 20 = long-term health hazard
20–24.9 = desirable
25–39.9 = overweight
30–39.9 = obese
> 40 = morbid obesity

Disadvantages of this method:

- muscular patients may be classified as obese
- does not take into account shortening of spinal column with age
- may be affected by retention or loss of body fluid.

Weight loss over time

The percentage of weight loss over time is calculated as follows: usual weight minus actual weight multiplied by 100, divided by usual weight.

Indication of significant weight loss

> 1–2% in one week
> 5% in one month
> 10% in six months

It is simple to calculate body weight, BMI and weight loss over time, and these data can be combined with the subjective information. This will constitute an initial screening, which will identify people who are, or have an increased risk of becoming, undernourished. This will lead to a more comprehensive assessment that involves measurement of:

- muscle bulk, subcutaneous fat, skin-fold thickness and hand grip strength
- biochemical measurements to identify concentrations of serum albumin and retinol-binding protein, and total lymphocyte count.

These last measures provide informative data, but the nurse should be aware that they can reflect the patient's clinical condition rather than nutritional status; therefore a combination of all data is essential to obtain a complete overview of nutritional deficit.

Action point 5

Check out the nutritional assessment tool used as your clinical base and identify the types of data collected. How is the level of risk calculated: quantitatively, qualitatively or a mixture of both?

Providing nutritional support

When planning nutritional care, the goal for nursing is to ensure that the patient will acquire the required daily nutrients (Table 3.6) and not become undernourished, or that existing malnourishment will be reversed.

Whenever possible, nutritional support should be introduced before malnutrition has developed.

Table 3.6 Normal adult daily protein–energy and fluid requirements

Nitrogen	8–12 g
Calories	1500–2000 kcal
Fluid	2000–2500 ml

Action point 6

What is the primary consideration when selecting the best method of nutritional support?

The cardinal rule is 'if the gut works, use it', since this maintains normal structural integrity and prevents translocation of gut bacteria to other organs of the body.

Ability to take food via the normal oral route is the first consideration. Where no deficit exists and the patient can eat and drink independently, the nurse is charged with the responsibility for providing the patient with a well-balanced diet. This should be based on the 'healthy plate' principle, advocated by the Health Education Authority (Figure 3.4).

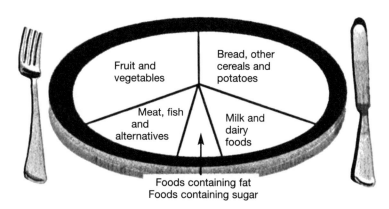

Figure 3.4 The healthy plate.

Additional sweet or savoury liquid supplements (e.g. Fortisip, Ensure, Fresubin) can be provided for patients with increased nutritional need or swallowing difficulty.

When eating is not possible

When the digestive system dysfunctions, oral intake may be impossible or insufficient either to meet metabolic demand or to be managed by the digestive system. This increases the patient's chances of becoming undernourished.

In these circumstances, artificial, specialized nutritional support is required, where nutrients are delivered directly into the body by tube. Two options are available: enteral and parenteral nutrition. The route selected depends on two essential factors:

• the health, state and functional ability of the gut
• the length of time nutritional support is required (Figure 3.5).

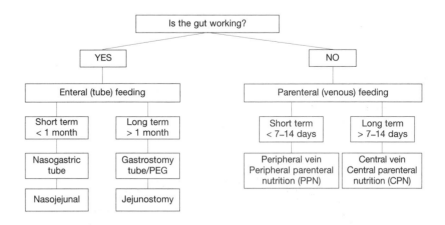

Figure 3.5 Is the gut working? PEG, percutaneous endoscopic gastronomy.

Enteral is the preferred alternative to oral intake when the gut is functional. The mouth is bypassed and nutrients are delivered directly into the stomach or small intestine (Figure 3.6).

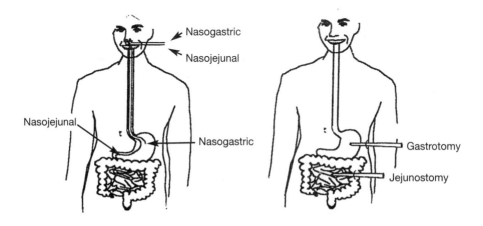

Figure 3.6 (a) Sites used for nasoenteral tubes; (b) sites used for enterostomy tubes.

Nursing management of enteral feeding

- Before administering feed directly into the stomach check the position of the tube by:
    - aspirating gastric content and testing for acidity with blue litmus, which turns pink on contact with aspirate
    - injecting a small amount of air down the tube into the stomach and listening with a stethoscope for bubbling
- Flush the tube with either sterile or cooled boiled water before and after feeding: nasoenteral tube 15–20 ml, enterostomy tube 30–50 ml
- Use an enteral feeding pump to ensure that the feed is delivered at the correct rate
- Feed in a semi-recumbant position with the patient's head raised at least 30° to prevent aspiration, nausea, vomiting and abdominal distension.
- Change the administration set daily
- Follow principles of good hygiene to prevent contamination of the feed
- Record volume administered on the fluid balance chart
- Observe for diarrhoea or constipation
- Provide mouth care 2-hourly

Parenteral refers to any route into the body other than the digestive tract. In this case, the digestive system is bypassed and a highly concentrated solution of essential nutrients is infused into the circulatory system via a central vein, a technique known as total parenteral nutrition (TPN) (Figure 3.7).

Nursing management of parenteral nutrition

- Never administer feeds directly from the refrigerator
- Verify the patient's details on the label of the feed
- Inspect the solution for cracking or separating – if present, do not use
- Apply a strict aseptic technique when changing the bag, manipulating the administration set or dressing the catheter exit site
- Change the administration set every 24 h
- Administer via a volumetric pump to ensure the correct flow rate. Never try to 'catch up'; this could precipitate metabolic disturbance
- Do not use the feeding line for delivering any other substance, e.g. blood or drugs
- Flush the line with 0.9% saline if a blockage occurs
- Measure temperature, pulse and respirations 4-hourly to detect infection or respiratory problems associated with a direct central catheter
- Check capillary blood glucose to detect hyper- or hypoglycaemia 6-hourly for first 24 h after initial commencement of PN, and then daily
- Keep an accurate record of feed delivery, i.e. date, start time, stop time, volume infused and reference number of feed
- Maintain accurate record of fluid balance
- Provide mouth care 2-hourly

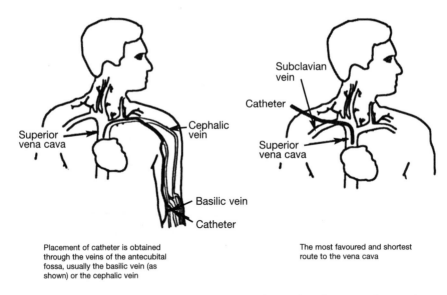

Placement of catheter is obtained through the veins of the antecubital fossa, usually the basilic vein (as shown) or the cephalic vein

The most favoured and shortest route to the vena cava

Figure 3.7 Sites used for central venous access. (a) Peripherally inserted central catheter (PICC); (b) direct central venous cather.

The dysfunctional digestive system

Diseases of the digestive tract are common and a frequent cause of primary healthcare consultation and hospital admission. Almost everyone will demonstrate symptoms of GI 'upset' at some time in their life, and this could be caused by a condition that is acute, chronic, benign or malignant. These will manifest as one or more symptoms that may affect the functions of the tract (Table 3.6).

Table 3.6 Main symptoms of diseases of the digestive system

- Dysphagia
- Heartburn and regurgitation
- Pain – retrosternal, abdominal, perineal
- Nausea and vomiting
- Weight loss and anorexia
- Altered bowel habit – diarrhoea, constipation
- Rectal bleeding
- Jaundice

These generic symptoms, which indicate that a problem exists, underlie the actual cause of the disease and can be associated with a number of disorders. The exact disease or condition will be determined by physical examination and diagnostic investigations (Table 3.7).

Table 3.7 Towards a diagnosis – clinical investigations for disease of the digestive system

Laboratory investigations	Haematology – full blood count (FBC) for indicators of infection, leucocyte count, for anaemia, haemoglobin Prothrombin time (jaundiced patients) to estimate clotting time Biochemistry – urea and electrolytes (U&Es), liver function tests (LFTs) Microbiology – faecal and vomit analysis for presence of pathogens
Gastric secretion tests	Analysis of gastric contents and measurement of volume over a specific period of time to determine gastric acid secretion
Imaging	Abdominal x-ray Contrast (barium) radiography, i.e. barium swallow/meal or enema – a liquid containing the contrast medium barium is introduced into the upper or lower digestive tract This outlines the structure and identifies any abnormality Ultrasonography, computer tomography (CT), magnetic resonance imaging (MRI) Specialist techniques that enable more detailed studies of specific structures or the entire abdomen
Endoscopy	Direct visualization techniques to view the digestive tract using a flexible endoscope Upper digestive tract to view the oesophagus (oesophagoscopy), stomach (gastroscopy) and duodenum (oesophagogastroduodenoscopy) Lower tract colonoscopy to view the entire colon and occasionally terminal ileum, sigmoidoscopy to view rectum and sigmoid colon Rigid endoscopy, sigmoidoscopy and proctoscopy to view the rectum and up to the sigmoid flexure of the large bowel

Nursing considerations

The nurse must ensure that the patient receives a full explanation of why the investigation is being carried out. If any specimens have to be collected, the nurse should do so in the correct manner and dispatch them to the laboratory as quickly as possible. For some investigations (i.e. barium studies and endoscopy), the patient will require specific preparation, i.e. nil by mouth for 8–10 hours before upper digestive tract investigation, and bowel cleansing and dietary modification for lower tract investigations. Nil by mouth is also required for 6–8 hours before abdominal CT and MRI scan. The nurse should consult local protocols to ensure that the patient is properly and safely prepared.

Care and management of patients with selected diseases of the digestive tract

Clearly, there are many conditions that can affect the normal structure and function of this extensive body system and it lies beyond the scope of this chapter to explore them all. Beginning with the oesophagus, certain of the inflammatory, obstructive and malignant disorders of the upper and lower digestive tract that the nurse in general practice may encounter have been selected for inclusion. For more detailed and comprehensive information the reader is advised to consult a specific text from the further reading list.

Where surgical options are discussed, it is anticipated that the reader will apply the general principles of safe perioperative care to each case, and only specific aspects of relevant care are included.

Disorders of the oesophagus

The oesophagus or 'gullet' is the tube that acts like a conduit to convey food from the mouth to the stomach by muscular action – peristalsis. At the lower end of the oesophagus is the lower oesophageal sphincter, a muscular structure which opens in response to swallowing and allows food into the stomach. Closure of the sphincter prevents backflow of stomach content into the gullet, therefore protecting the oesophagus from the acid content of gastric juice. However, this valve can dysfunction and give rise to a common disorder of the oesophagus – gastro-oesophageal reflux disease (GORD).

Gastro-oesophageal reflux disease

This common problem, frequently referred to as 'heartburn', accounts for up to 10% of medical consultations (British Society of Gastroenterology 1996). It is caused by the retrograde passage of gastric content into the oesophagus. In most cases, it is short-lived, presents as uncomfortable symptoms and does no actual damage to the oesophagus. Repeated or persistent exposure results in inflammation of the mucosa, a condition known as reflux oesophagitis. This seemingly benign condition has the potential to cause chronic bleeding, resulting in anaemia, and it can cause narrowing of the oesophagus as a result of scar formation. More seriously, it can lead to the pre-cancerous condition, Barrett's oesophagus, where the mucosal cells of the oesophagus change into similar tissue to the gastric mucosa, which renders it vulnerable to cancer. Therefore it is essential that repeated frequent episodes of reflux are investigated and treated.

Causes

- Incompetent gastro-oesophageal valve.
- Hiatus hernia, which causes misalignment between the two parts of the gastro-oesophageal valve, therefore reducing its strength and allowing reflux of gastric juice into the oesophagus.
- Reduction in lower oesophageal sphincter (LOS) pressure caused by smoking, heavy consumption of alcohol, chocolate, and fatty and spicy foods.

Symptoms

- A retrosternal burning sensation that commonly occurrs after meals and may radiate to the throat.
- Occasional regurgitation and a bitter acid taste in the mouth.
- Lying down or bending may initiate pain.

Diagnostic investigations

X-ray
Barium swallow and meal may indicate presence of sliding hiatus or stricture.

Oesophagoscopy (endoscopy)
Direct visualization to determine the extent of inflammation and biopsy if necessary.

Monitoring of pH
Twenty-four-hour measurement of acid levels in the oesophagus, which involves nasogastric intubation. A special tip at the end of the tube measures the acidity at frequent intervals.

Management and treatment

This centres on symptom relief and lifestyle modification and in most cases is managed successfully in primary care. Hospital admission will be necessary if complications arise or surgery is required.

Action point 7

Reflect on the above and identify how nursing care will be implemented for a patient hospitalized as a result of reflux oesophagitis.

A thorough assessment of need is required to inform a plan of care. This will include the following.

Symptom relief

Administer medication that will include a combination of antacids, acid suppressants and motility stimulants, and monitor effect.

Drug therapy

> **Antacids**, e.g. aluminium hydroxide, to neutralize gastric acid
> **Alginate antacid combinations**, e.g. Gaviscon, to increase the pH of gastric content and form a floating raft in the stomach that acts as a physical barrier to reflux
> **Proton pump inhibitors**, e.g. omeprazole, to suppress gastric acid. Can produce rapid relief from heartburn and healing
> **H$_2$-receptor antagonists**, e.g. ranitidine, to reduce stomach acid production
> **Motility stimulants** (prokinetic drugs), e.g. metoclopromide and cisapride, to improve gastric emptying and tighten the lower oesophageal sphincter

Health education

Explain how lifestyle modification alone may resolve the problem. This should include the following:

- Avoid ingesting substances that are known to weaken the lower oesophageal sphincter.
- If appropriate, lose weight and stop smoking.
- Remain upright for 2 h after eating.
- Eat small meals more often. This will avoid overfilling the stomach.
- Do not wear clothing that is tight around the waist.
- Do not eat or drink just before going to bed and elevate the head of the bed at least 15 cm to reduce reflux when sleeping.
- Reinforce the importance of continuing with medication.

Nutritional support

Ensure that a nutritious non-irritant oral diet is provided. Liaise with the dietician to provide liquid supplements if necessary. Monitor intake of food and fluids.

Prepare for diagnostic investigations

- Explain the process and preparation required.
- Provide support during and following investigations.

Prepare for surgery (if appropriate) and provide safe perioperative care

- Explain the surgical procedure.
- Teach deep-breathing techniques to enable satisfactory postoperative respiration.
- Provide appropriate nutritional support pre- and postoperatively.

Common surgical procedure to treat persistent reflux

Nissen fundoplication involves wrapping the fundus of the stomach around the lower end of the oesophagus to which it is sutured. This effectively increases lower oesophageal sphincter pressure and prevents reflux. These days this procedure is often performed via a laparoscope, which makes it minimally invasive with a short recovery time.

Carcinoma of the oesophagus

This is a common cancer in the populations of Asia, the Far East and some parts of Africa. The incidence in the western population is significantly lower, but there is evidence to show that it is increasing by 7% per year, a more rapid increase than in any other malignant tumour in the western world. It is a disturbing condition because the patient's prognosis is poor, and the 5-year survival rate is low. This can be attributed to the rapid growth of the tumour, early invasion of local structures and late presentation of extreme symptoms.

This cancer is more common in older men than women, with a male to female ratio of 3:2 and median age of onset of 60 years.

Pathology

The disease develops as a result of cell changes in the lining of the oesophagus and presents as two histological types:

- squamous cell carcinoma, which is most common and arises in the upper two-thirds of the oesophagus
- adenocarcinoma, less common but on the increase; it is found at the lower end of the oesophagus, close to the oesophagogastric junction.

Causes

Like many cancers the actual cause is unknown, but a number of contributory factors that increase the risk are evident (Table 3.8).

Symptoms

The early symptoms are insidious and tend to creep up, and there is often a delay in seeking medical advice. As the tumour grows, the lumen of the oesophagus narrows, which results in the most common symptom – difficulty swallowing (dysphagia). Initially, this occurs with solid food, but progresses to liquids as the tumour obstructs the oesophagus. There is pain between the shoulder blades associated with ingesting food, and regurgitation of unaltered food a few minutes after swallowing. The person avoids ingesting food to prevent these uncomfortable and distressing symptoms, which results in rapid weight loss and fatigue. At this point the person may visit the doctor, although in some cases people do not seek medical help until they develop the late symptoms of persistent heartburn, vomiting and vomiting blood (haematemesis). Some patients ignore the symptoms and are admitted to hospital with aspiration pneumonia caused by overspill of food into the trachea; they will also be severely undernourished and dehydrated.

Table 3.8 Contributory factors to carcinoma of the oesophagus

- Smoking
- Alcohol
- Heavily salted and smoked fish in diet
- Iron deficiency
- Pre-cancerous changes in Barrett's oesophagus

Towards a diagnosis

Clinical examination and a careful history will precede the common investigations used for diagnosis.

- Barium swallow – may demonstrate stricture at the tumour site.
- Oesophagoscopy and biopsy – confirms the diagnosis.
- Bronchoscopy – to detect malignant spread to the trachea.
- CT and MRI – to assess the extent of disease and inform best treatment option.

Treatment

Because it is usually diagnosed late, less than 10% of patients have a curable tumour. However, whether palliative or curative, treatment of some kind is available. This may be surgery, radiotherapy, chemotherapy or a combination of any of these. More recently, laser and photodynamic therapy have been introduced. The treatment used depends largely on the site and stage of tumour growth and whether it has spread beyond the oesophagus.

The surgical option

The best chance of a cure is surgery, which carries a 5-year survival rate of between 50 and 80%, if the disease is confined to the oesophageal mucosa or submucosa alone (Ellis and Cunningham 1994).

The surgery is major, complex and not without risk of serious complications. It involves mobilizing the stomach and resection of the diseased oesophagus. In the standard Ivor Lewis procedure, an abdominal and thoracic incision is made, the stomach is mobilized, pulled into the chest cavity and joined to the remaining portion of the oesophagus by gastro-oesophageal anastomosis (Figure 3.8a). Alternatively, a section of colon is transposed to the thorax to connect the resected margins (Figure 3.8b).

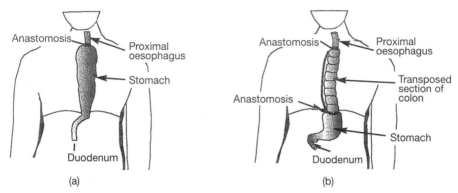

Figure 3.8 Surgery for carcinoma of the oesophagus. (a) After gastric 'pull-up'; (b) after colonic translocation.

Nursing considerations

Patients undergoing this operation will be anxious and concerned. They will need careful and considerate attention to prepare them for surgery. This will involve the following:

- Comprehensive nutritional assessment and the provision of appropriate nutritional support. Preoperative parenteral nutrition may be required if the patient is undernourished. This can be maintained postoperatively; however, in some cases a jejunostomy feeding tube is inserted during surgery to provide postoperative nutrition.
- Preparation for being nursed in a high-dependency unit (HDU) or intensive care unit (ICU) postoperatively and for the presence of intravenous (IV) lines, nasogastric tube and a chest drainage tube.
- Encourage the patient to practise deep-breathing exercises taught by the physiotherapist.
- Collaborate with the dietician and patient to plan and implement a postoperative nutritional regimen, which considers the altered anatomy and capacity of the gut.
- Support and prepare the patient and family for the possibility of an inoperable tumour.

Postoperative care is managed in the HDU or ICU for several days, where, along with standard postoperative observation, specific attention is paid to:

- maintaining intravenous fluids and jejunostomy feed
- monitoring urine output
- pain management via either epidural analgesia or patient-controlled analgesic system
- observation of chest drain for obstruction
- nasogastric drainage and aspirate
- wound management
- teaching and encouraging deep-breathing exercises instigated by the physiotherapist
- oral hygiene.

Frequency of observations will be established by local hospital protocols and identified in care pathways. Oral fluids will be commenced on the advice of medical staff.

Adjuvant therapy

Radiotherapy can be used to shrink the tumour in preparation for surgery. Chemotherapy is only of value for chemosensitive tumours and is usually employed in combination with radiotherapy.

The side effects and complications of these treatments often exacerbate the situation for a debilitated, malnourished person. The nurse acts in a supporting and comforting role to ensure that distressing symptoms are relieved and the patient's dignity is maintained.

The palliative option

If surgery is not possible, palliation is the sole form of treatment to relieve dysphagia and prevent nutritional deficit and dehydration. The nurse must prepare the patient for endoscopic procedures to dilate the oesophagus, the insertion of self-expanding metal stents (tubes), or endoscopic laser treatment that will ablate but not cure the tumour. Radiotherapy can be used to shrink the tumour and maintain some oesophageal patency.

Whichever course of action is taken, it is important that the patient receives appropriate nutritional support. Some debate exists about the best way to achieve this and opinion is split about the value of introducing gastrostomy feeding while total dysphagia is developing. It is essential that each patient is treated as an individual and cared for in a supportive and informative environment where the nurse represents their needs and wishes.

Disorders of the stomach and duodenum

The stomach is a J-shaped pouch which is continuous with the oesophagus and connects with the first part of the small intestine, the duodenum. It acts as a short-term reservoir for food, which is liquefied by mechanical churning. The gastric musosa contains several types of secretory cell that work together to secrete gastric juice containing hydrochloric acid, which activates the protein-digesting enzyme pepsin. The mucosa is protected from the acid and enzyme by a coat of mucus secreted by epithelial cells. The body creates a fine balance between these destructive and protective forces, by producing just enough acid and enzyme to digest the food but not enough to overwhelm the protective layer. However, there are occasions when this delicate balance is disturbed, mainly due to disruption of the mucous layer. This can result in a peptic ulcer.

What is a peptic ulcer?

A peptic ulcer is a common disorder that arises from disruption or weakening of the mucosal barrier, which allows the acid and pepsin literally to eat away the delicate tissues below. The result of the body digesting itself in this way is a crater-like hole, an ulcer, which can occur in the oesophagus, but is more commonly found in the stomach (gastric ulcer) or duodenum (duodenal ulcer). The incidence of gastric and duodenal ulcers is higher in males than in females. Some age-related variance exists: the age of onset for gastric ulcers is 50+ years, while for duodenal ulcers it is 25–50 years.

For years it was believed that the causes of peptic ulcer were emotional stress, tobacco smoking and alcohol consumption. While these are still regarded as influential factors, they are no longer believed to cause ulceration, but they do worsen the symptoms and affect the healing potential of an existing ulcer. The development of a peptic ulcer caused by mucosal incompetence is now attributed to two primary causes: *Helicobacter pylori* and non-steroidal anti-inflammatory drugs (NSAIDs).

Helicobacter pylori

This bacterium, discovered in 1982 by two Australian doctors, has been identified as the dominant cause of peptic ulcer. It is found in 80% of people with gastric ulcer and 90% with duodenal ulcer. The bacterium has the ability to burrow into the gastroduodenal mucosa and protect itself from the acid environment of the stomach. This invasion disrupts the protective mucous layer and exposes the mucosa to the corrosive action of gastric juice.

Non-steroidal anti-inflammatory drugs (e.g. aspirin, ibuprofen)

Most of these drugs are believed to inhibit the production of mucosal prostaglandin, a chemical that inhibits gastric acid and enhances mucosal defence. Taking NSAIDs on a regular basis therefore increases the vulnerability of the mucosa to corrosive damage.

Symptoms

The most common symptom is a gnawing and burning pain, similar to 'heartburn', in the central upper abdomen. In gastric ulcer, pain is exacerbated by eating, but there is no consistent pattern of pain. In duodenal ulcer, the pain is more consistent and occurs 2–4 hours after eating, but is often relieved by food. Pain that awakens the patient at night is highly suggestive of duodenal ulcer.

Less common symptoms are bloating, belching, nausea and vomiting, which are associated with obstruction of the pylorus caused by oedema and scarring following healing of recurrent ulceration.

In some cases people have very minor symptoms or none at all.

Diagnosis and treatment

Barium meal is an option, but these days the gold standard diagnostic technique is gastroscopy and biopsy to detect the presence and site of the ulcer and a tissue biopsy to test for *H. pylori*.

The goal of treatment is to:

- relieve symptoms and treat the ulcer with drug therapy, as in reflux oesophagitis, with additional stomach lining protectors, e.g. bismuth subsalicylate
- eradicate the cause of the ulcer, which will include:
    stopping NSAIDs
    treating *H. pylori* (if present) – regimens vary, but will include a combination of antibiotics and as above
- prevent recurrence and complications.

Nursing considerations

The widespread availability of endoscopy and the discovery of *H. pylori* have revolutionized the management of uncomplicated peptic ulcers. Treatment is mainly on an outpatient basis, with the patient seen by the nurse in the clinic or endoscopy suite.

The nurse's role in these circumstances is to ensure that the patient is fully conversant with the process of endoscopy and understands the treatment

Gastrojejunostomy and vagotomy

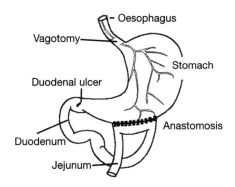

The jejunum is anastomosed to the stomach. Provides a second outlet for gastric contents. Vagus nerve is split to reduce gastric secretions

Polya gastrectomy (Bilroth II)

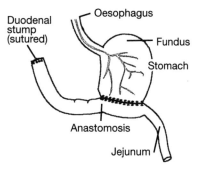

Diseased section resected. Duodenal stump is closed and stomach anastomosed to jejunum

Truncal vagotomy and pyloroplasty

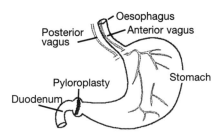

Pylorus is incised longitudinally and closed transversely to allow muscle relaxation. A wider outlet is established. Vagotomy reduces gastric secretions and emptying

Highly selective vagotomy

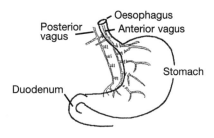

Branches of the vagus nerve that supply the pyloric sphincter are kept intact. The remaining nerves are divided. Results in a reduction in gastric secretions but motility is unaffected

Total gastrectomy with jejunal pouch

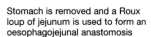

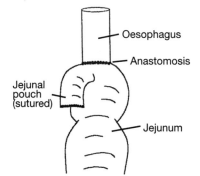

Stomach is removed and a Roux loup of jejunum is used to form an oesophagojejunal anastomosis

Figure 3.9 Some surgical procedures used to treat peptic ulcers and gastric carcinoma. Reproduced from C Torrance and E Serginson: Surgical Nursing, 1997, by kind permission of Baillière Tindall.

regimen and potential side effects of drugs prescribed. If *H. pylori* is the underlying cause of the ulcer, the patient must be made aware of the importance of completing the full treatment regimen to eradicate the bacterium, or the chances of recurrence will be high. The patient who smokes should be advised to stop, since to continue will maintain high acid levels, which will make ulcer healing more difficult.

In cases where the ulcer does not respond to drug therapy, surgery can be undertaken. The procedure – a highly selective vagotomy (Figure 3.9) – involves severing some of the branches of the vagus nerve that innervate the parietal cells of the gastric mucosa, with subsequent reduction in gastric secretions.

Unfortunately not all ulcers will be diagnosed, and in some cases the patient will not comply with the treatment regimen. In these cases the ulcer will become chronic and serious complications can arise (Table 3.9).

Action point 8 – case scenario

Jim Hill is admitted to the surgical ward with a bleeding peptic ulcer. He is shocked and vomiting a copious amount of fresh blood. He is very anxious and afraid that he will die. He is scheduled for endoscopic therapy to arrest the bleeding.
• What nursing actions will be carried out to ensure this patient is safe and comfortable before the endoscopy?

The goal of caring for a shocked patient is to restore normal function as soon as possible and prevent complications. This is achieved by close observation and the application of technical and communication skills. It includes the following.

• Monitor vital signs every 15–30 min.
• Maintain intravenous infusion of fluids or blood.
• Administer prescribed percentage of oxygen.
• Administer prescribed analgesic to control or relieve pain.
• Pass nasogastric tube and maintain on free drainage or low suction. Aspirate 1- to 2-hourly.
• Observe colour and amount of gastric drainage.
• Observe for melaena stools.
• Monitor urine output (patient will be catheterized). Less than 30 ml/h indicates renal insufficiency.
• Nil by mouth and provide mouth care.
• Give information about the endoscopy process.
• Continuously inform the patient about progress and enable the expression of fears and anxieties.

Table 3.9 Acute complications of peptic ulcers and treatment options

Complication	Symptoms	Treatment options
Haemorrhage – the most common cause of death from peptic ulceration. It is caused by the erosion of a blood vessel at the site of the ulcer. In most cases, bleeding will stop spontaneously, but approximately 20% of cases will rebleed (Butler 1997) and require treatment to arrest bleeding and prevent death from exsanguination	• Haematemesis – initially dark brown due to the action of gastric juice and may contain small solid particles often referred to as 'coffee grounds'. Continued bleeding becomes bright red and may contain clots • Hypovolaemic shock induced by loss of circulating volume, demonstrated as weakness, dizziness, fainting, pallor, hypotension, tachycardia • Melaena – passage of black, tarry, foul-smelling faeces	Endoscopic treatment: • Injection therapy – adrenaline causes haemostasis by vasoconstriction or sclerosants create vascular thrombosis and secondary surrounding fibrosis • Thermal techniques – produce local heat at bleeding point to cause coagulation and contraction Surgery – undersewing the blood vessel in duodenal ulcer or gastric resection (Figure 3.9)
Perforation – the ulcer burrows through the stomach or duodenal wall, releasing the contents into the peritoneal cavity. This is a surgical emergency requiring immediate treatment	• Abdominal pain – sudden onset and very severe. Increased by movement • Rigid abdomen indicative of peritonitis • Vomiting • Indications of clinical shock	• Emergency surgery to oversew the ulcer, resect the affected part or provide a second outlet for gastric contents and divide the vagus nerve to reduce gastric secretions (Figure 3.9)
Pyloric obstruction – occurs when the ulcer is at the pylorus or duodenum constriction of the pylorus, caused by oedema or inflammation in acute ulceration or by scar tissue from healed recurrent ulcers. Results in retention of gastric contents	• Nausea and vomiting – the stomach fills with retained food that must be expelled to obtain relief • Epigastric pain after eating • Constipation – dehydration and absence of waste in colon • Weight loss – nutrients unable to access small intestine for absorption	• Decompression – aspiration of stomach contents via a nasogastric tube • Stomach washouts with warm water • Endoscopic pyloric balloon dilatation – useful in prolonged obstruction • Surgery – to either refashion the pylorus or remove stenosed gastric or duodenal tissue and reduce stimulation of gastric juice (Figure 3.9) • Total parenteral feeding if malnourished

The surgical option

The surgical management of peptic ulcers is mainly reserved for the treatment of complications, particularly perforation and outlet obstruction or when endoscopic haemostasis fails. A range of procedures is used and many surgeons have their own preferred approach, which will also depend on the site of ulceration and the specific complication.

The nursing objective is to manage the patient's perioperative care, to prevent complications and to maximize comfort, commensurate with the care of a patient undergoing major abdominal surgery.

Postoperatively, specific attention is paid to:

- preventing dehydration and malnutrition:
    - maintain intravenous infusion
    - commence sips/30 ml of water hourly 24–36 h postoperatively
    - increase oral fluids when bowel sounds return
    - gradually build up to a normal diet
    - liaise with the dietician to provide liquid supplements as required
    - observe for abdominal distension and pain associated with food intake
- gastric decompression and prevention of vomiting:
    - maintain nasogastric tube on free drainage
    - aspirate 1- to 2-hourly
    - do not move or reposition nasogastric tube unless discussed with the surgeon (could disrupt anastomosis)
- record amount and type of aspirate
- daily nasal toilet around exit site of tube
- 2-hourly mouth care:
    - remove nasogastric tube when bowel sounds return and aspirate is diminished (on advice of the doctor).

Gastric (stomach) carcinoma

Pathogenesis

This cancer arises from malignant changes in gastric mucosal cells, which eventually displace the normal cells and form a 'lump' of tissue that ceases to carry out its normal physiological functions. There is decreased production of protective mucus, which exposes the lump to the corrosive forces of gastric juice, which creates a malignant ulcer. Eventually the tumour spreads beyond the mucosa, invades the muscle layer and may break through the stomach wall to invade surrounding tissues.

Incidence and symptoms

The past 50 years has seen a changing trend in gastric carcinoma, with a gradual decline in the incidence of cancer in the distal part of the stomach and
an increase in cases where the cardia-oesophageal and gastro-oesophageal
junctions are affected (National Cancer Institute 2000). This has been attributed to the increasing prevalence of Barrett's oesophagus. Gastric cancer is
regarded as the fourth most common cancer in Europe and the second most
common worldwide. The disease presents more commonly in males than
females and is rare in people under the age of 40, the peak incidence occurring between the ages of 70 and 80 years.

Just as in oesophageal cancer, the prognosis is poor. The 5-year survival
rate is low, epitomized by the UK mortality from this disease of 10 000 deaths
per year. This is attributed to the fact that initial symptoms are frequently
minor and vague, and mimic dyspepsia and heartburn. It is often not until
the late symptoms of weight loss, poor appetite, tiredness, nausea, vomiting,
hoarse voice, and epigastric or abdominal pain manifest that medical advice
is sought, by which time the tumour has metastasized. In severe cases, the
diagnosis will be made when the person is admitted to hospital with gastric
haemorrhage, perforation, outlet obstruction or signs of advanced disease,
i.e. palpable epigastric mass, jaundice, ascites and enlarged liver. This is
unfortunate, because studies in Japan have reported 5-year survival rates
greater than 90% when the tumour is detected and treated early. These findings led to the instigation of asymptomatic screening programmes in Japan
and some South American countries where the cancer is particularly
prevalent.

Diagnosis and treatment

Barium meal is an option and this will reveal the presence of either a
space-occupying lesion or an ulcer with a rolled edge. The primary diagnostic investigation is either gastroscopy or oesophagogastroscopy,
because these enable the mucosa to be examined directly and tissue biop-
sies to be obtained to determine the stage of the cancer according to the
TNM (tumour, node, metastases) classification of tumours. Ultrasound,
CT or MRI will be undertaken to confirm metastases. The combined
results will inform the doctor about the best treatment option to offer to
the patient.

Surgery is required either to cure or to palliate the condition. Curative
surgery involves either partial or total gastrectomy, depending on the site
of the tumour (see Figure 3.9). The overall 5-year survival rate from this
approach is approximately 20% and following palliative surgery only 5%
(Cushieri et al. 1996). Adjuvant chemotherapy and radiotherapy can be

used and, although these can downgrade tumours and assist in the treatment of metastases, they do not improve survival rates.

Nursing considerations

Following the diagnosis the patient will be anxious and concerned about the treatment and prognosis of the disease. The nurse must be available to listen to the patient, answer questions honestly, and provide information about surgery or other planned treatment.

Nutritional support is essential and TPN may be required to provide a calorific boost prior to surgery and maintain nutrition for a short time afterwards. The nurse must provide support and monitor the delivery of TPN carefully, so that any complications are detected early.

The immediate postoperative care for a patient following gastric resection mirrors that provided for patients following surgery for peptic ulcers. In some cases of total gastrectomy, a thoracotomy may be necessary and the care reflects that of the patient undergoing oesophagectomy.

The impact of gastric resection

In the long term, it is estimated that 30% of patients undergoing gastric resection will have significant problems associated with the changed size and restructuring of the gastric pouch. These include weight loss, iron deficiency anaemia and the unpleasant experience of dumping syndrome soon after eating.

Cause and symptoms of dumping syndrome

Following gastric resection, gastroenterostomy or vagotomy, normal pyloric control is lost. Undiluted hyperosmolar food and fluid will pass suddenly into the jejunum. This results in a rapid fluid shift and temporary reduction in circulating volume. The patient will be pale, sweating, nauseous, dizzy, faint, feel palpitations and have a feeling of epigastric fullness.

The nurse should give advice about how to manage these problems. This includes eating small, high-protein, low-carbohydrate meals often to offset the symptoms of dumping syndrome. If it does occur, the patient should lie down for 10–15 minutes after eating. It is important to emphasize that these symptoms should pass within a year of surgery, but if they become too troublesome the patient should consult a doctor, who may prescribe an anticholinergic drug to slow down GI activity. Exceptional tiredness could indicate anaemia, so the patient should be advised to report it to the GP immediately. Following total gastrectomy the patient will require parenteral vitamin B_{12} at 3-monthly intervals to prevent pernicious anaemia, which would otherwise arise due to the loss of the intrinsic factor normally secreted by cells in the gastric mucosa. Additionally, patients whose surgery was palliative should be informed about cancer support services and pain management facilities to improve their quality of life.

The small and large intestine (colon)

These are the structures of the lower part of the digestive tract, commonly known as the bowel. The small intestine is a long, coiled tube, which is divided into three anatomical regions: the duodenum, jejunum and ileum. It is here that the process of digestion is completed and nutrients are absorbed through the specially adapted mucosa into the blood. Dysfunction of these structures will impede the movement, digestion and absorption of nutrients and consequently threaten the patient's nutritional status.

The large intestine is approximately 1.5 m long and extends from the ileocaecal valve to the anus. It includes the colon, which is divided into ascending, transverse, descending and sigmoid regions. The main functions of this structure are conservation of water and electrolytes, and the formation and storage of faeces until evacuation. Bacterial activity in the colon contributes to the production of gas and decomposes bilirubin to urobilinogen, which gives the characteristic brown colour to faeces. Vitamin K and some B vitamins are synthesized by this bacterial action. Disorders of this structure will affect the elimination of faecal waste, which can be accelerated, resulting in diarrhoea, or slowed, resulting in constipation. Disease of the ascending colon can reduce the normal absorption of water and electrolytes and contribute to dehydration.

A major cause of intestinal disruption is inflammation, which can occur anywhere in the small and large intestines and will affect movement, secretion and absorption.

Inflammatory bowel disease (IBD)

This umbrella term can describe any condition that invokes the inflammatory response in bowel tissue, but, by convention, it is reserved to denote two chronic, relapsing and remitting disorders – ulcerative colitis (UC) and Crohn's disease (CD).

Globally, the incidence of IBD is high in Scandinavia, the UK, North America, Australia and much of north-west Europe (Hungin and Rubin 2000), with UC being more prevalent than CD.

These are serious diseases of the digestive tract that cause misery, pain, embarrassment and distress to those unfortunate enough to be affected. While recognized as distinctly separate diseases that possess unique pathological differences (Table 3.10), they do share some similar features:

- Their cause is unknown, although several theories exist, including immunological, genetic and dietary factors. An association with tobacco smoking has emerged, in that CD occurs more often in smokers and UC in non-smokers.
- Typically presents in people between the ages of 15 and 30 years, but can be younger or older.
- Affects both sexes equally.
- Symptoms include abdominal pain, diarrhoea, urgency, rectal bleeding (more common in UC), weight loss, fatigue, anaemia, low-grade infection (more common in CD).
- Both carry a risk of developing colorectal cancer. This is higher in UC than CD.
- Extracolonic manifestations emerge as inflammatory conditions of the skin, joints, kidney, liver and eyes.

Table 3.10 Pathological differences between ulcerative colitis and Crohn's disease

Ulcerative colitis	Crohn's disease
Begins at the rectum and extends proximally to involve part of or the entire colon	Affects any part of the digestive tract from mouth to anus, more commonly confined to terminal ileum and colon
Inflammation usually confined to mucosa. Crypt abscesses form and become necrotic and ulcerated	Affects full thickness of structure involved, i.e. transmural, with bowel-wall thickening and 'skip lesions'
Craggy, irregular, continuous ulcers	Patchy linear and transverse mucosal ulcers, with intervening mucosal oedema, create cobblestone appearance
No granulomata	Granulomata occur, mainly in the submucosal layer
Fistula formation is rare	Fistula may occur to the skin, bladder or vagina
Stricture is rare	Stricture is common
Proctitis common, no perianal involvement	Perianal disease occurs

Getting the diagnosis right

The patient may have been experiencing unpleasant symptoms for some time. The most common symptom is diarrhoea, which can be attributed to a number of causes. It is critical that the correct diagnosis is made because despite the symptomatic similarity and same investigations used to diagnose UC and CD (Table 3.11), treatment strategies, particularly surgery, and potential complications differ.

> **Action point 9**
>
> What specific details will be required from the history of the patient's illness?

Did you include:

- frequency of defecation and presence of blood and mucus in the stool?
- presence of abdominal pain, particularly after eating?
- nutritional assessment, which will indicate weight loss, nutritional deficit and signs of fatigue?

Table 3.11 Investigative techniques used to diagnose inflammatory bowel diseases

Disease	Investigation	Site investigated
Crohn's disease affecting the colon, or ulcerative colitis	Barium enema	Whole colon
	Colonoscopy (avoided during active disease, because of the risk of perforation)	Whole colon
	Sigmoidoscopy	Anus, rectum and sigmoid colon
	White cell labelling scan	Any areas of inflammation or infection
Crohn's disease	Barium meal and follow-through	Stomach and small intestine
Crohn's disease (small bowel)	Abdominal ultrasound	Small intestine and abdominal organs

- duration of symptoms?
- indications of extracolonic inflammation, e.g arthritis, uveitis?

Nursing considerations

Colonoscopy and barium enema require specific physical preparation to clear the bowel of faeces. The nurse should provide the patient with clear written and verbal information about the preparation and possible after-effects of these investigations.

- Stop solid food intake the day before the procedure. Clear fluids only, i.e. fruit juice, black tea or coffee, can be taken up to the time of the investigation.
- Give instructions about how to use the bowel-cleansing solution, e.g. Klean-prep, Picolax.
- Advise about the possible after-effect of constipation following a barium enema.
- Advise about the possibility of feeling bloated or experiencing mild abdominal pain after colonoscopy.
- Any rectal bleeding must be immediately reported to the GP, or nurse if in hospital.

The procedures are uncomfortable, invasive and embarrassing, so the nurse must ensure that the patient's dignity is maintained throughout. Following diagnosis, the nurse should provide the patient with a full explanation of how best to manage the condition. This should include useful literature and details of the National Association for Colitis and Crohn's Disease (NACC) so that the patient can obtain additional support and information from this self-help group.

Therapeutic management

The primary aims of treatment are to achieve and maintain remission of symptoms. Uncomplicated cases of either CD or UC will be successfully managed with drug therapy, which includes the following:

- Aminosalicylates, e.g. sulphasalazine, mesalazine – widely used but generally more effective in UC than CD.
- Corticosteroids, e.g. prednisolone, hydrocortisone – used for more severe cases and constitute the first line of treatment in acute exacerbation.
- Immunomodulatory agents, e.g. azathioprine, cyclosporin – used in severe cases that have failed to respond to steroid therapy. More effective in CD than UC.

- Antibiotics, e.g. metronidazole – used in CD, but long-term use is contraindicated because of side effects.

In most cases, diagnosis and treatment will occur on an outpatient basis, where the condition will be regularly monitored. An inflammatory bowel or GI nurse specialist will enhance the quality of these visits by providing clinic attendees with a comprehensive service that complements medical treatment and maintains continuity of care between hospital and community.

Circumstances where hospitalization will be required

Unfortunately, when a severe attack of either UC or CD does not respond to conventional drug therapy, hospital admission is necessary. The purpose of this is to:

- rest the gut by restricting oral intake
- reduce the inflammation by administering intravenous steroids and rectal steroids for patients with UC
- correct fluid and electrolyte imbalance with intravenous fluids
- treat infection associated with CD with intravenous antibiotics
- maintain nutritional status: parenteral nutrition will be required for malnourished and severely debilitated patients.

The patient in these circumstances is weak, debilitated, dehydrated, lethargic and anorexic, and often has a high temperature. Nursing interventions are essential to support the usual activities of living and maintain the planned therapeutic regimen.

Action point 10

What nursing actions will be required to ensure that the patient receives the appropriate care?

- Safe administration of prescribed medication.
- Four-hourly measurements of vital signs to detect significant changes that could indicate bowel perforation or peritonitis.
- Administration of intravenous fluids as prescribed, to prevent dehydration.
- Easy access to the toilet, to maintain dignity and privacy.
- Observation of faecal output, i.e. frequency, colour, consistency, presence of blood and mucus.
- Nutritional support: parenteral nutrition may be instigated to enable the gut to rest. When oral intake is commenced, consult with the dietician to provide a well-balanced diet consisting of the patient's preferred foods.

- Monitor urine output for diminished or excessive amount.
- Record fluid balance and report significant negative or positive balance.
- Weigh daily to evaluate weight loss or gain.
- Assist with general hygiene and mouth care, to maintain comfort and self-esteem.
- Assist with perianal hygiene after defecation and provide barrier cream if required.
- Conduct accurate pain assessment, administer prescribed analgesics and evaluate the effect.
- Encourage the patient to rest throughout the day.
- Provide accurate information about progress and treatment, and enable the patient to ask questions and express anxiety and concerns.
- Prepare for surgery, if necessary, in conjunction with the colorectal/stoma care nurse specialist.

When is surgery necessary?

In both UC and CD, surgery is avoided for as long as possible. It is generally undertaken when conservative treatment has failed, the patient's condition has deteriorated and pre-malignant changes have been identified at annual screening or in response to an emergency.

While the conservative management of patients is similar, the reasons for surgery, the surgical options and the outcomes differ between the two conditions. Therefore to avoid confusion these will be considered separately.

Surgery to treat Crohn's disease

Crohn's disease is incurable by either medical or surgical means. The main objectives of surgery are to control symptoms, maintain the continuity of the bowel and restore health by alleviating complications such as:

- abscess
- fistulae
- haemorrhage
- obstruction
- perforation with peritonitis
- anorectal disease
- toxic colitis or megacolon.

Surgery is dictated by the problem that exists, and can be elective or emergency. In both instances, a number of surgical procedures can be undertaken. Surgeons have their own preferences, but the overriding intention will always be to conserve as much bowel as possible (Table 3.12). The reason for this is the danger of recurrence, because further surgery will mean loss of more bowel, with the likely consequences of diarrhoea, malabsorption, electrolyte imbalance and nutritional deficiency.

Table 3.12 Surgical procedures used for Crohn's disease, and patient outcome

Procedure	Description	Outcome
Small bowel resection	The most common operation on the small bowel to relieve obstruction. The terminal ileum and caecum are resected. Ileocolic anastomosis maintains continuity of bowel. If the bowel is dilated or toxic, a stoma may be fashioned	Diarrhoea may be experienced. Decreased absorption of fat and vitamin B_{12} due to loss of terminal ileum
Stricturoplasty	Longitudinal excision of the stricture that is closed transversely. The technique was developed to treat bowel strictures but conserve bowel and prevent nutritional deficit	Narrowed area of bowel is widened without loss of any intestine. Patient can eat and nutritional status will be improved
Segmental resection of colon	Diseased segment of colon is excised and anastomosed. There is a high incidence of recurrence that requires further resection	Retains continuity of bowel and avoids stoma formation in the short term
Subtotal colectomy with ileostomy	Removal of colon with preservation of rectal stump	Ileostomy and rectal conservation. This enables ileorectal anastomosis later if the rectum is healthy
Panproctocolectomy	Removal of the entire colon and rectum. Avoided if possible	Permanent ileostomy

Surgery to treat ulcerative colitis

Just as in CD, surgery is indicated to treat similar complications in patients with UC. However, the major difference here is that surgical removal of the large bowel and rectum will cure UC and eradicate the risk of colon cancer, which is increased in patients who have had active disease for 10 years or more. Curative surgery eliminates the miserable and restraining symptoms of the disease, but it involves removal of the rectum and entire colon (proctocolectomy) and results in a permanent ileostomy or the formation of an ileoanal pouch, which retains bowel continuity and faecal continence (Figure 3.10).

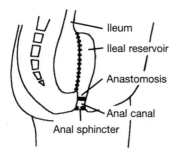

Entire large bowel is removed up to anorectal junction. Anal sphincter muscles are left intact. Pouch is constructed from ileum to form a reservoir and joined to anal stump

Figure 3.10 Ileal pouch and anal anastomosis. Reproduced from C Torrance and E Serginson: Surgical Nursing, 1997, by kind permission of Baillière Tindall.

This latter development is encouraging patients to elect for surgery much earlier. It is a lengthy process and generally requires the patient to undergo two or three operations, over several months, which will involve the formation of a temporary loop ileostomy. However, patients are prepared for this temporary inconvenience because, when completed, the pouch hides the fact that the colon is gone and there is an element of control over defecation, which is not possible with a permanent ileostomy.

Nursing considerations

A rectal drain is inserted into the pouch during surgery to remove collections of old blood. The drain is flushed twice daily with 30 ml of saline to prevent blockage. It is removed when bile-stained drainage is noted, usually around the fourth or fifth postoperative day.

The nurse must observe for any potential complications that arise, which include:

- rectal leakage
- inflammation of the pouch
- diarrhoea
- perianal soreness
- night-time defecation.

Persistence of these problems or the development of anal cancer will result in excision of the pouch and a permanent ileostomy. The patient will be supported through these episodes and personal needs discussed in relation to the management. The nurse can provide information about self-help groups, such as the Kangaroo Club, based at John Radcliffe Hospital, Oxford, from whom the patient can acquire additional information and long-term support.

The colorectal/stoma care nurse specialist is invaluable to provide support for patients requiring surgery to treat IBD. Specific information about the surgery is essential, and details of aftercare and potential complications must be explained. Careful preparation for a stoma and subsequent stoma care must be undertaken.

The specific principles of nursing care for patients requiring colorectal surgery and stoma care are included at the end of this section on colorectal disorders.

Colorectal cancer

Colorectal cancer is a collective term used to describe adenocarcinomas found in the large bowel and rectum. Ninety-eight per cent of these cancers are of this same histological type and can be present anywhere along the entire length of the colon or in the rectum. The greatest incidence, over 60%, occurs in the sigmoid region and rectum.

This cancer poses a significant health threat in the western world and the incidence is increasing. In the UK, it is the second most common cancer after lung cancer and the morbidity and mortality rates are alarming. Approximately 28 000 new cases are diagnosed each year and in 1998 there were 14 732 deaths from this disease (Kocher and Saunders 1999). These statistics are being attributed to the increasing elderly population, since colorectal cancer is age related. It is less common under the age of 40 years and peaks at 60–70 years.

Symptoms

The symptoms are few and quite vague in most cases, and will vary according to the site of the tumour (Table 3.13). As the tumour develops, the severity of the symptoms will increase and give rise to obstruction or perforation of the bowel, and weight loss will be noticed.

Towards a diagnosis

Early diagnosis is the key to successful treatment and increases the chance of 5-year survival. One or more of the diagnostic tests available will be conducted:

• Faecal occult blood test (FOBT): used to detect hidden blood in the faeces.
• Digital rectal examination (DRE): the doctor inserts a gloved finger into the rectum to feel for abnormalities.

Table 3.13 Symptomatic presentation by tumour site

Caecum and ascending colon	Transverse and descending colon	Rectum
Faecal occult blood	Colicky abdominal pain	Pain
Anaemia	Constipation followed by diarrhoea	Tenesmus (ineffectual and painful straining at stool)
Fatigue	Melaena	Early morning bloody diarrhoea
Palpable mass	Obstruction	Rectal bleeding

- Rigid sigmoidoscopy: direct viewing of the sigmoid colon using a rigid, lighted instrument – a sigmoidoscope.
- Colonoscopy: an examination of the rectum and entire colon using a flexible colonoscope. Biopsy can be taken during this examination to 'stage' the tumour and determine the extent of pathology, according to the 'Dukes' classification.
- Double contrast barium enema: a series of x-rays that illustrate the diseased area.

Patients considered to be at high risk of colorectal cancer, i.e. IBD or genetic predisposition, are offered annual screening, usually by colonoscopy. Screening of the wider population in the UK is currently under scrutiny, but to date no national screening programme exists. In America, annual FOBT is recommended as part of any routine physical examination for people over the age of 40 and flexible sigmoidoscopy every 3–5 years from 50 years of age.

Treatment

Surgery is the primary treatment. This involves the removal of the tumour and a section of healthy colon or rectum and adjacent lymph nodes. Pre- and postoperative radiation and chemotherapy may also be used. The surgical approach is determined by the location of the tumour, and whenever possible bowel continuity is maintained (Table 3.14). Unfortunately in some cases this is not always possible and either a temporary or a permanent stoma is required.

Intestinal obstruction

Either the small or large bowel can become totally or partially obstructed, which will stop or reduce the free passage of intestinal contents. The bowel distal to the obstruction collapses and the accumulating air and fluid in the

Table 3.14 Surgical procedures used to treat colorectal cancer

Location of tumour	Procedure	Description	Outcome
Caecum or ascending colon	Right hemicolectomy	Removal of part of the terminal ileum, caecum and ascending colon. Ileum is joined to transverse colon	Continuity of bowel maintained. No stoma
Transverse colon	Transverse colectomy or right or left hemicolectomy	Depends on the location of the tumour along the transverse colon. Diseased area excised and end-to-end anastomosis is formed	Continuity of bowel is maintained. No stoma
Descending colon	Left hemicolectomy	Diseased area removed and end-to-end colonic anastomosis	If the tumour is at the proximal descending colon, continuity is maintained. If it occurs at the distal or sigmoid region, a temporary defunctioning colostomy or ileostomy (surgeon's preference) may be required
Sigmoid colon	Sigmoid colectomy	Removal of the diseased part of the sigmoid colon Anastomosis with descending colon	Bowel continuity is maintained but a temporary defunctioning colostomy may be required
Rectosigmoid junction or proximal rectum	Anterior resection	Diseased areas of the rectum and sigmoid colon are excised. An anastomosis between the sigmoid colon and distal rectum	Bowel continuity is maintained Temporary defunctioning colostomy or ileostomy is required

Table 3.14 Surgical procedures used to treat colorectal cancer (contd)

Location of tumour	Procedure	Description	Outcome
Distal rectum and anus	Abdominoperineal excision of rectum (AP resection)	Rectum and anus are removed using an abdominal and perineal approach	Bowel continuity interrupted. A permanent descending colostomy is fashioned
Sigmoid or rectal perforation	Hartman's procedure	The diseased area is resected. The rectal stump is either sewn and left *in situ* or exteriorized as a mucous fistula. Colostomy is formed from descending colon	Bowel continuity is not maintained. Colostomy (can be temporary or permanent) with or without mucous fistula

proximal bowel cause it to distend. Bacteria proliferate in the obstructed bowel and the wall becomes oedematous. As the distension increases, the blood supply is stretched, leading to ischaemia and necrosis with subsequent perforation.

The obstruction can be caused by functional impairment, such as handling of the intestine during surgery which leads to paralytic ileus, or from irritation to the peritoneum as in peritionitis. The most common causes, however, are mechanical, and include:

- adhesions resulting from previous surgery, abdominal sepsis or inflammatory disease
- hernia (strangulated or not)
- tumours (carcinoma, lymphoma)
- faecal impaction
- bolus obstruction, e.g. swallowed foreign object, gallstone
- twisted bowel (volvulus)
- stricture.

Symptoms

Most obstruction occurs in the small bowel and is sudden and dramatic. Large bowel obstruction is less common and takes a more chronic course. The severity of the symptoms will depend on whether the bowel is completely or partially obstructed and the region of bowel affected (Table 3.15).

> **Action point 11**
>
> Reflecting on the above, what do you think the presenting symptoms of bowel obstruction will be?

The inability of the gut to absorb vital water and electrolytes, and persistent vomiting, gives rise to the physical signs of dehydration and electrolyte imbalance. Conservative treatment is employed to prevent hypovolaemia and subsequent shock, which could prove fatal.

Table 3.15 Cardinal symptoms of mechanical bowel obstruction

Symptom	Small bowel	Large bowel
Vomiting	High obstruction, i.e duodenum to jejunum, severe vomiting of acidic juices. Low obstruction, i.e. jejunum to ileum, less severe vomiting of alkaline juices and faecal fluid	Little or no vomiting until the bowel is fully distended. Then vomiting is severe
Pain	Intense, intermittent, 'colicky' central abdominal pain with complete or incomplete obstruction. Constant pain in strangulation or infarction	Mild suprapubic discomfort
Abdominal distension	Limited and relieved by vomiting	Can become extreme in low colonic obstruction
Absolute constipation	No faeces or flatus passed	Distal segment of large bowel empties. Nothing else can enter, therefore no faecal material or flatus is passed

Specific management and nursing care

- Administer prescribed analgesic and antiemetic.
- Allow nil by mouth to prevent build-up of intestinal contents.
- Insert a nasogastric tube to decompress the gut and prevent vomiting.
- Aspirate the nasogastric tube 1- to 2-hourly and maintain on free drainage.

- Record amount and type of aspirate and drainage.
- Maintain intravenous infusion as per regimen to restore fluid and electrolyte balance.
- Record 4-hourly temperature, pulse, respirations. If there are indications of shock, check every 30 min to 1 h until an acceptable limit is reached.
- Observe urine output (the patient will be catheterized).
- Maintain a fluid balance chart.
- Provide support to meet personal hygiene needs, including daily nasal toilet around nasogastric tube and 2-hourly mouth care.
- Change position 2-hourly to reduce the risk of pressure sores.
- Large bowel obstruction caused by faecal impaction may be relieved by enema.

Is surgery an option?

Surgery will be undertaken to relieve the obstruction if:

- the underlying cause needs surgical treatment, e.g. carcinoma, hernia
- the patient does not improve with conservative treatment, e.g. adhesion obstruction
- there are signs of strangulation or peritonitis (Cushieri et al. 1996).

Principles of nursing management for the patient undergoing colorectal surgery

Assessment of need is the starting point for any nursing care plan and how this is achieved is dictated by circumstances. The need for colorectal surgery can be planned or emergency; the significant difference between the two is that for planned or elective surgery there is more time to prepare the patient than in the emergency situation. However, the same principles of safe perioperative care apply.

In an emergency situation, the patient will be admitted with acute symptoms and the problem could be referred to as an 'acute abdomen'. The priority is for surgery to be undertaken as soon as possible, therefore leaving little time for a comprehensive preoperative assessment, detailed investigations or patient education.

The main objectives are pain relief, preventing dehydration and safe preparation for surgery. This can be achieved by carrying out the same nursing actions required for the conservative treatment of the patient with an acute intestinal obstruction, with the following additions:

- Explain the reason for surgery and check that the patient fully understands.
- Answer questions honestly and openly.

Action point 12 – case scenario

On admission, Mrs Jones aged 65 years is experiencing acute abdominal pain and vomiting. Her skin is pale, cool and clammy, and her mouth is very dry. Her blood pressure is 90/50 mmHg and her pulse is 95 beats/minute. She is anxious and afraid and does not understand what is happening to her. Surgery is required to relieve an acute intestinal obstruction.

- What are the nursing priorities for the preoperative care of Mrs Jones?

Postoperative care is managed in the same way as for the patient recovering from elective surgery, with the added consideration that more information may be required to enable the patient's individual needs to be met.

When surgery is planned

Although time is available to prepare someone for elective surgery, we must not assume that the patient will be any less anxious than one admitted as an emergency. The bonus here is that, since the advent of preoperative assessment clinics, patients undergoing elective colorectal surgery will have time to acquire and use the information provided. The colorectal/stoma care nurse specialist will be involved from the outset and will provide continuous support throughout the perioperative period and beyond.

Assessment of need is identified on admission to inform the plan of care. Care plans differ between organizations; they may be based on integrated pathways of care or core care plans, or reflect a model of nursing, such as Roper et al. (1996), but all will include the general principles of perioperative care that are relevant for all patients. The information provided here refers to specific requirements for pre- and postoperative care required by the patient undergoing elective colorectal surgery.

Preparing the bowel for surgery

A clean bowel is essential to prevent spillage of faecal material into the abdominal cavity during surgery, which will cause serious infective complications.

It is essential that the patient understands what to do and what to expect from this process. Various approaches are taken, but these days they are much less aggressive than in the past, mirroring the preparation required for barium enema or colonoscopy. The purging substances used cause fluid loss and potential dehydration, so the patient must be advised to drink at least 3 litres of fluid in 24 hours.

The nurse must check and record the result of each bowel action to establish the cleanliness of the bowel. This can be quite embarrassing for the patient but can be offset by the nurse explaining the importance of a clean bowel.

No solid food is allowed for 24 hours prior to surgery, but the patient can have clear fluids for 4–6 hours before surgery, and will then be allowed nil by mouth in preparation for general anaesthesia.

The nurse must ensure that preoperative antibiotics are given according to the treatment regimen, since these are effective in 'sterilizing' the bowel and preventing postoperative wound infection.

Postoperative care

The patient's physical recovery is paramount in the first days after surgery. Nutritional support, fluid balance, pain management and nasogastric aspiration should be managed as previously described for the patient undergoing surgery to the upper digestive tract.

If the rectum has been removed there will be a perineal wound that is uncomfortable and troublesome. The wound can be entirely sutured or partially sutured and packed, and the nursing management of this wound is determined by the surgeon's approach to perineal closure.

When a stoma is necessary

An unfortunate consequence in some cases of colorectal surgery is a faecal output stoma either to divert faeces away from a healing anastomosis or because the rectum has been excised.

The term 'stoma' literally means 'mouth' or 'opening', which in this case refers to a section of bowel that opens on to the exterior abdomen, through which faeces are evacuated and collected in an appliance attached to the skin.

Two types of faecal stoma are associated with colorectal surgery:

- colostomy – fashioned from any section of the large bowel
- ileostomy – fashioned from ileum.

These stomas can be either temporary or permanent and can be formed in one of four ways: end, loop, double-barrelled or split.

Nursing considerations

The same principles of care apply whichever type of stoma is present. The reason for the operation can influence the patient's feelings about the stoma. For example, in the case of the person with IBD, it may be perceived as a release from the unpleasant and recurring symptoms of the disease. People with colorectal cancer may see it very differently, as they have to cope with the fact that they have cancer while faced with the stoma as a means of a cure. The essential feelings of loss and grief and the prospect of a changed body image can stir up mixed emotions in people as they await surgery (see Chapter 8).

While the support of the specialist stoma care nurse is invaluable, it is essential that the nurse who provides the patient's day-to-day care possesses the knowledge and technical skills to help the patient with stoma care.

Preparing for the stoma

- *Psychological preparation*: facilitated by the stoma care nurse, the patient and family are given the opportunity to express fears and anxieties. The patient's mental attitude to the stoma and ability to cope with this major change to body image and evacuation of faeces are assessed. Verbal information is given, supported by written material, and the patient is offered the opportunity to meet someone who has undergone a similar experience, but this is entirely optional.
- *Ability to manage technical skills*: careful attention to eyesight, manual dexterity and cultural considerations is required to establish whether the patient can manage the practical basis of stoma care.
- *Selecting a site for the stoma*: this is crucial to the success of stoma management. The stoma care nurse will consult with the patient to identify the most appropriate site for the stoma, in relation to the specific stoma raised, abdominal contours and lifestyle practices. The site will be marked in indelible pen and the patient advised not to wash it off.
- *Choosing an appliance*: the patient should be shown the wide variety of appliances available and helped to select one they feel will suit their lifestyle and that they can manage easily. The deciding factors are usually discretion, comfort and security.

After the stoma is fashioned

- *Observations*: immediately postoperatively, the type of stoma must be noted, i.e. colostomy or ileostomy, and the colour assessed for vascular sufficiency. A healthy stoma is deep pink/red and may be slightly oedematous. Any deviation from this should be immediately reported to the doctor and stoma care nurse. Passage of flatus from the stoma will indicate bowel peristalsis and herald the increase of oral fluids. Passage of faeces should be noted, and the type and consistency observed. The condition of the peristomal skin must be closely monitored and any redness or soreness brought to the immediate attention of the stoma care nurse.

- Technical management: this is about changing the appliances, which in the initial postoperative period the nurse will do in the following way:
    - Make the patient comfortable and maintain privacy and dignity.
    - Collect equipment, i.e. bowl of warm water, cloths for washing and drying, stoma measuring guide, appliances, bag for waste.
    - Empty contents of the appliance into a suitable receptacle.
    - Gently remove the appliance from the top, using slight pressure with the fingers on surrounding skin.
    - Dispose of soiled appliance in accordance with hospital policy.
    - Clean the peristomal skin and the stoma with warm water. Avoid soap unless the area is really dirty. If soap is used, rinse well to remove all residue of soap.
    - Dry the skin well and measure the stoma.
    - Fit the appliance of the correct size, which leaves a slight margin of 2–3 mm between the stoma and the peristomal skin. If the stoma is not round, use an appliance that can be cut to shape.
    - Remove the backing from the adhesive plate and fit over the stoma. Rest warm hand on area for a couple of minutes to enhance the adhesion.
    - Inform the patient about each stage of the process to enable self-care at a later time.

NB The nurse will wear gloves and apron when carrying out this procedure.

- *Teaching the patient technical skills*: this should begin in earnest when the patient is free from intravenous lines and wound drain and can move from the bedside to the bathroom. The process requires great sensitivity and skill, since it is a daunting time for patients who are not used to handling their own bowel or coming face to face with faeces. Gentle encouragement is required and a teaching chart is useful to enable the patient to see progress and communicate it to nursing staff involved in the care. Positive reinforcement is necessary to give the patient the confidence and security required in preparation for discharge and the future management of the stoma.
- *Preparing for discharge*: this will begin as soon as the patient is admitted, to enable social circumstances to be prepared. Before discharge, the patient should answer yes to all the items on a simple checklist, which includes the following:
    - Is proficient in appliance management.
    - Knows how to measure stoma.
    - Knows how and where to obtain new supplies.

- Knows how to store and dispose of equipment safely.
- Knows about eating a healthy diet and that no food is restricted.
- Knows about the disadvantages of some food, i.e. create more gas, may cause loose stools.
- Understands the importance of drinking at least 2–3 litres of fluid a day if an ileostomy is formed.
- Knows about access to self-help groups, e.g. British Colostomy Association, Ileostomy and Internal Pouch Support Group.
- Knows how to contact colorectal/stoma care nurse.

For more details on these and other aspects of stoma care, the reader is advised to consult the further reading list at the end of the chapter.

Mouth care

Throughout this chapter frequent reference has been made to the provision of mouth care in a range of circumstances, and it is perhaps one of the most comforting things that even the most junior of nurses can carry out for the patient.

The mouth is the gateway to the digestive system and its health is essential for the normal ingestion of food. A wealth of literature supports the importance of nurse-assisted oral hygiene for dependent and debilitated patients, including those allowed nothing or very little by mouth and who are receiving special nutritional support. The inactivity of oral structures and reduced production of saliva will result in a dry mouth (xerostomia) and a build-up of bacterial plaque that can lead to dental caries. These will increase the risk of or predisposition to inflammation of the oral mucosa (stomatitis) and fungal infections such as candidiasis (thrush). The provision of mouth care, based on best evidence, is essential to prevent these uncomfortable and distressing problems in one area of the digestive tract, when another is the root of the patient's problem.

References and further reading

Allan S (1998) Ileostomy. Professional Nurse (Update) 14(2): 107–112.
Armstrong E (2001) Practical aspects of stoma care. Nursing Times 97(12): 40–42.
Black P (1998) Colostomy. Professional Nurse (Update) 13(12): 851–857.
Bond S (ed) (1997) Eating Matters. Newcastle: Newcastle University.
British Society of Gastroenterology (1996) Guidelines in Gastroenterology 3. Guidelines for oesophageal manometry and pH monitoring. London: British Society of Gastroenterologists.

Bruce L, Finlay MD (eds) (1997) Nursing in Gastroenterology. Edinburgh: Churchill Livingstone.

Bulmer FM (2000) Bowel preparation for rectal and colonic investigation. Nursing Standard 14(20): 32–35.

Butler M (1997) Gastrointestinal bleeding. In Bruce L, Finlay MD (eds) Nursing in Gastroenterology. Edinburgh: Churchill Livingstone.

Campbell T (1999a) Colorectal cancer part 1. Epidemiology, aetiology, screening and diagnosis. Professional Nurse 14(12): 869–874.

Campbell T (1999b) Colorectal cancer part 3. Patient care. Professional Nurse 15(2): 117–121.

Colagiovanni L (1996) Peripheral benefits. Nursing Times. 92(42): 59–62.

Cushieri A, Hennessy TPJ, Greenhalgh RM, Rowley DI, Grace PA (1996) Clinical Surgery. Oxford: Blackwell Science.

Downie G, Mackenzie J, Williams A (1999) Pharmacology and Drugs Management for Nurses, 2nd edn. Edinburgh: Churchill Livingstone.

Elcoat C (1986) Stoma Care Nursing. London: Baillière Tindall.

Ellis P, Cunningham D (1994) Management of carcinomas of the upper gastrointestinal tract. Current issues in cancer. British Medical Journal 308(26): 834–838.

Evans G (2001) A rationale for oral care. Nursing Standard 15(43): 33–36.

Everett SM, Axon ATR (1997) Early gastric cancer in Europe. Gut 41: 142–150.

Finlay T (1997a) Making sense of parenteral nutrition in adult patients. Nursing Times 93(2): 35–36.

Finlay T (1997b) Malignancies of the gastrointestinal tract. In Bruce L, Finlay MD (eds) Nursing in Gastroenterology. Edinburgh: Churchill Livingstone.

Harkness GA, Dincher JR (1999) Medical Surgical Nursing: total patient care, 10th edn. St Louis, MO: Mosby.

Hawkey CJ, Wright NJD (2000) Family Doctor Guide to Indigestion and Ulcers. London: Dorling Kindersley.

Henry L (1997) Parenteral nutrition. Professional Nurse 13(1): 39–42.

Hicks SJ (2001) Gastric cancer: diagnosis, risk factors, treatment and life issues. British Journal of Nursing 10(8): 529–536.

Hudson J, Goldthorpe S (1997) Inflammatory bowel disease. In Bruce L, Finlay MD (eds) Nursing in Gastroenterology. Edinburgh: Churchill Livingstone.

Hungin P, Rubin G (eds) (2000) Gastroenterology in Primary Care: an evidence- based guide to management. Oxford: Blackwell Science.

Jones CV (1998) The importance of oral hygiene in nutritional support. British Journal of Nursing 7(2): 74–83.

Kocher HM, Saunders MP (1999) Complacence or ignorance about rectal bleeding. Colorectal Disease 1(6): 323–333.

Legge A (1999) The bottom line. Health Service Journal October: 16.

Lennard-Jones JE (1992) A Positive Approach to Nutrition as Treatment. London: King's Fund.

Lunn D, Hurrell C, Campbell T (1999) Colorectal cancer part 2. Treatment. Professional Nurse 15(1): 53–57.

Mallett J, Dougherty L (2000) The Royal Marsden Hospital Manual of Clinical Nursing Procedures, 5th edn. Oxford: Blackwell Science.

Malnutrition Advisory Group (2000) Screening Tool for Adults at Risk of Malnutrition. Maidenhead, Berks: BAPEN.

Melville A (2001) Better quality of care for UGI cancer patients. Nursing Times 97(12): 36–37.

Mason I (2001) Inflammatory bowel disease. Nursing Times 97(9): 33–35.

Myers C (ed) (1996) Stoma Care Nursing: a patient centred approach. London: Arnold.

National Cancer Institute (2000). Gastric Cancer. University of Bonn Medical Centre (http://www.meb.uni-bonn.de/cancernet/1000025.html).

Office for National Statistics (1996) Monitor Population and Health Registration of Deaths in 1995, England and Wales. Government Statistical Service DH2 96.

Porrett T, Daniel N (eds) (1999) Essential Coloproctology for Nurses. London: Whurr.

Powell Truck J, Nielsen T, Farwell JA, Lennard-Jones JE (1974) Team approach to long term intravenous feeding in patients with gastrointestinal disorders. The Lancet ii: 825–828.

Pudner R (ed) (2000) Nursing the Surgical Patient. London: Baillière Tindall.

Reilly H (1998a) Enteral feeding an overview of indications and techniques. British Journal of Nursing 7(9): 510–521.

Reilly H (1998b) Parenteral nutrition: an overview. British Journal of Nursing 7(8): 461–467.

Roper N, Logan W, Tierney J (1996) The Roper–Logan–Tierney model. In Walker PH (ed) Blueprint for the Use of Nursing Models. London: NLN Publishing.

Rowlinson A (1999a) Inflammatory bowel disease 1: aetiology and pathogenesis. British Journal of Nursing 8(13): 858–862.

Rowlinson A (1999b) Inflammatory bowel disease 2: medical and surgical treatment. British Journal of Nursing 8(14): 926–930.

Rowlinson R (1999c) Inflammatory bowel disease 3: importance of partnership in care. British Journal of Nursing 8(15): 1013–1017.

Seifrit B (1997) Helicobacter pylori. American Operating Room Nurses' Journal 65(3): 614–620.

Thune I, Lund E (1996) Physical activity and the risk of colorectal cancer in men and women. British Journal of Cancer 73: 1134–1140.

Torrance C, Serginson E (1997) Surgical Nursing, 12th edn. London: Baillière Tindall in association with the RCN.

Tortora GJ, Grabowski SR (2000) Principles of Anatomy and Physiology, 9th edn. New York: John Wiley.

Walsh M (ed) (1997) Watson's Clinical Nursing and Related Sciences, 5th edn. London: Baillière Tindall in association with the RCN.

Wood S (1998) The use of enteral and parenteral feeding. Professional Nurse 14(1): 44–46.

UKCC (1997) UKCC says nurses have a responsibility for the feeding of patients. Press Statement 16/97. London: UKCC.

CHAPTER FOUR

The neurological system

CATHERINE WASKETT AND CHRIS BASSETT

Introduction

The aim of this chapter is to explore the issues surrounding the treatment and care of the neurologically compromised patient in hospital. Many patients in medical or surgical wards are suffering from head injuries, or other neurological problems such as cerebrovascular accident (CVA, stroke), multiple sclerosis or even meningitis. The key to good nursing care, as with all nursing, is related to the assessment of the patient. Accurate observation, detection and the prompt reporting of changes in neurological status can be life saving. This chapter focuses on the injuries and acute illnesses most commonly seen when working in the specialist neurological setting. The chapter does not cover stroke because stroke care is considered as a specialism on its own and is outside the scope of this text. However, much of the information in this chapter is relevant to stroke care.

Anatomy and physiology of the nervous system

To understand fully the care required by the patient with a neurological problem, and of course the rationale for that care, it is important to have some knowledge and awareness of the anatomy and physiology of the nervous system.

The nervous system consists of two main parts: first, the autonomic or automatic part, the function of which is associated with the control of blood pressure and other vital functions, and, second, the central nervous system (CNS). The CNS is made up of the brain and spinal cord, and is rather like a large computer wiring network, which transmits and receives messages via a highly complex system of neurons (brain cells) and chemical transmitters.

The central nervous system

Anatomy of the brain

The brain is divided into three main parts: the forebrain, the midbrain and the hindbrain (Figure 4.1). Despite considerable advances in medical understanding of the brain, there is still a great deal that remains unknown about the brain and its structure and function.

(a)

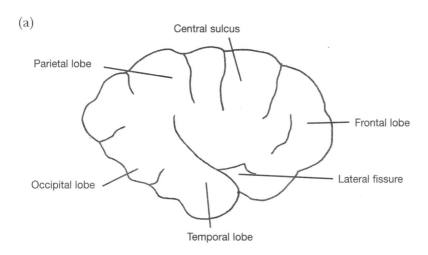

(b)

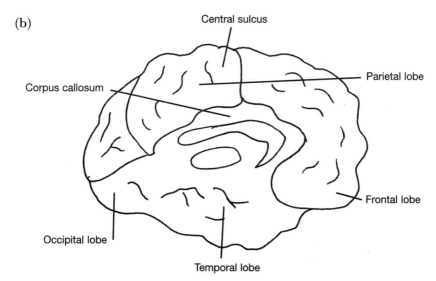

Figure 4.1 (a) Lateral view of the brain; (b) inner view of the left hemisphere.

The forebrain

This consists of the cerebrum, which is divided intro two main hemispheres connected by a large bundle of myelinated axons (nerve cells) allowing communication between the two individual hemispheres. Each hemisphere consists of an outer cortical section and the inner subcortical structure, which connects with the midbrain and hindbrain. The cortex is made up of 'grey matter' and is the main information processing area. The surfaces or lobes of the cortex are named after the bones of the skull.

The frontal, temporal, parietal and occipital lobes
The frontal lobes are responsible for the planning, execution and evaluation of the body's actions and they also control behaviour and personality. The speech centres (Broca's and Wernicke's areas) are also situated in the frontal lobes. The parietal lobes are responsible for reception and perception of the senses and make sense of sensations such as touch and pain (see Chapter 7). They are also believed to be instrumental in the creation of memory. The occipital lobes deal with most of the input from the eyes and contain the visual cortex areas. The temporal lobes also form part of the memory system and receive sensory input from the ear.

The cerebral nuclei
The white matter lies beneath the cortex. It consists of myelinated axons that convey impulses around the brain. There are also areas of grey matter that comprise thought-processing areas called the basal ganglia and the limbic system. The basal ganglia control movement and interact with the motor cortex. The limbic system consists of the hippocampus and the amygdala. This system has a role in memory, behaviour, and the control and maintenance of feeling and emotion.

The diencephalon, which consists of the thalamus and hypothalamus, lies within the forebrain. The thalamus acts as a dispatch centre for sensory input to the cortex. The hypothalamus lies at the base of the brain. This structure controls the autonomic nervous system and, via the pituitary gland, releases several of the main hormones.

The midbrain

The midbrain consists of the tectum and the tegmentum. The tegmentum helps control movement, relays sensory information and has a role in the control of sleep cycle. The tectum forms the posterior part of the midbrain. The tectum receives input from the eyes, via the thalamus, and helps control eye movement. It also receives sound input from the hearing system.

The hindbrain

The hindbrain or brain stem is composed of the cerebellum, pons varolii and the medulla oblongata. The pons varolii is part of the communication system transferring information to the cerebellum. The medulla oblongata links the brain with the spinal cord. The medulla controls respiration, cardiovascular acceleration and depression, and also transmits impulses from the body via the spinal cord. The cerebellum is a large structure at the back of the brain. This part of the brain receives input from the eyes and ears. The cerebellum controls the fine tuning of movement, and is essential to moving, walking and even standing.

The cranial nerves

The cranial nerves are part of the peripheral nervous system and connect directly to the brain rather than via the spinal pathway. Injury to the cranial nerves may disrupt certain functions, which can alert the nurse to the patient's worsening condition. There are 12 pairs of cranial nerves. Ten pairs connect with the brain stem; two pairs, the olfactory and optic nerves, connect with the area known as the forebrain. The brain has three coverings:

1. the dura, the outer covering of dense fibrous tissue that closely follows the inner wall of the skull
2. the arachnoid, a very delicate membrane sited beneath the dura mater
3. the pia mater, a layer of delicate connective tissue that adheres closely to the brain and the spinal cord.

The brain and the spinal cord are bathed in cerebrospinal fluid (CSF) in the subarachnoid space. This fluid, which is colourless and has a specific gravity of 1.007, is made in the brain from the blood in the choroid plexus.

Blood supply

Four arteries supply the brain with blood, two of which originate from the common carotid arteries. Each carotid artery divides into an internal and external branch – the internal carotid arteries supply the brain and the external carotid arteries supply the pharynx, larynx and the face. The other two arteries supplying the brain are called the vertebral arteries (Figure 4.2a).

To maintain normal activity, the adult brain requires approximately 750 ml of oxygenated blood per minute (Muxlow 2000). Of the total amount of circulating oxygen, the brain consumes an astonishing 20%. Under normal circumstances the cessation of blood flow to the brain for as short a period as 5–10 s is sufficient to cause temporary changes in neural activity, and fainting can occur. Disruption of blood flow to the brain for 5–10 minutes will result in irreversible brain damage and, ultimately, death. The major blood vessel configuration associated with the flow of blood to the brain tissue is the circle of Willis.

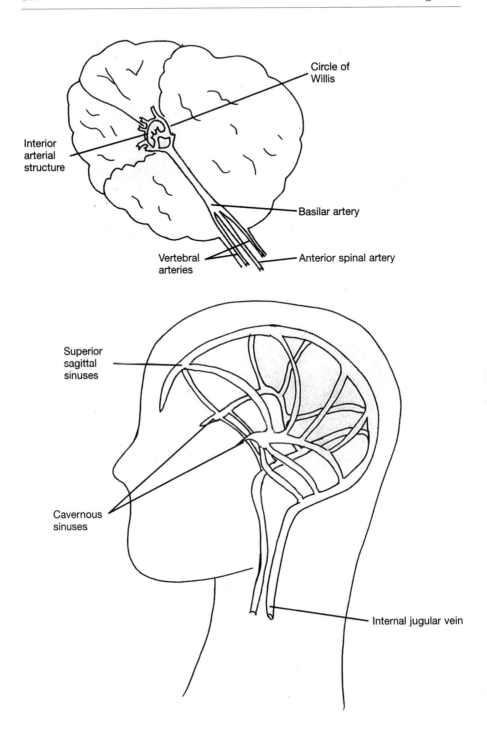

Figure 4.2 (a) Arterial supply to the brain; (b) venous return from the brain.

Assessment of the nervous system

This is an essential nursing duty; a systematic and rigorous assessment of the patient's neurological condition is the first step to good nursing care. The neurological history and assessment begin the moment the nurse first meets the patient. When admitting a patient, the nurse should note the patient's appearance and assess speech and motor function. If the patient appears to have cognitive deficits or has trouble speaking or hearing, the nurse also asks a family member or friend to stay with the patient during the history taking take to ensure that accurate information is obtained.

While collecting information on admission, the nurse can observe and assess the patient's mental status, behaviour and speech:

- Are the patient's answers appropriate?
- Are the answers complete?
- Is the speech pattern of normal tone, rhythm, rate and volume?
- Is the patient's appearance neat or untidy?
- Is the patient's behaviour appropriate?
- Is the patient co-operative, hostile or anxious?

Questions about the patient's level of activities of daily living (ADL) may highlight subtle changes in neurological function. They establish a baseline against which changes caused by improving or worsening neurological function and the effects of treatment can be measured. It is also important to identify whether the patient is left- or right-handed. This information is important for several reasons:

- The patient may be stronger on the dominant side, and this would be expected.
- The patient has a greater degree of independence if the dominant hand and arm can be free of tubing and tape.
- The effect of cerebral injury or disease can be more pronounced if the dominant hemisphere is involved.

Neurological assessment provides both the basic tool for diagnosis of neurological deficit and the means for measuring whether a patient is deteriorating or improving. It is therefore essential that it is completed accurately and any changes in a patient's neurological function is detected and reported promptly to ensure timely and appropriate patient care. A complete neurological assessment should include assessment of:

- level of consciousness
- cranial nerves
- motor function
- sensory function
- cerebellar function
- vital signs.

Current history should also be noted.

- Current symptoms
  - headaches
  - nausea or vomiting
  - blurred vision
  - numbness, tingling
  - weakness, clumsiness
  - personality changes
  - speech or swallowing difficulties
  - bladder or bowel difficulties.

This assessment should be completed on admission and then at regular intervals to monitor the patient's condition. Clinicians with neurological experience would usually perform this type of full assessment. Commonly, a reduced assessment is performed by nursing staff. This includes:

- level of consciousness
- motor function
- pupillary signs
- vital signs.

In practice, this requires an assessment of the Glasgow Coma Scale (motor and level of consciousness; Figure 4.3), a limb assessment (motor) and pupil assessment.

Assessment of consciousness level using the Glasgow Coma Scale

Assessment of the level of consciousness is critical in monitoring all patients, not just those with cerebral pathology. Historically, systems of observations

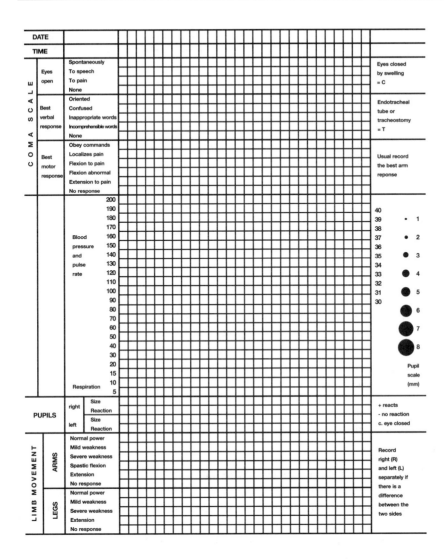

Figure 4.3 Observation chart for the Glasgow Coma Scale.

allowed inconsistency and variability in defining levels of consciousness, with no general agreement about terminology and interpretation.

Consciousness

Consciousness has been defined as a general awareness of oneself and the surrounding environment; it is a dynamic state that is subject to change. It has two components:

1. Arousal – which depends on the integrity of the reticular activating system extending from the brainstem to the thalamic nuclei in the cerebral hemispheres.
2. Cognition – which is largely a function of the cerebral cortex.

If arousal is significantly altered or absent, cognition cannot take place. Consciousness cannot be measured directly and is assessed only by observing a person's behaviour in response to different stimuli.

The Glasgow Coma Scale

Not only is it difficult to define consciousness, it is also impossible to draw a clear line between it and coma. For this reason, the Glasgow Coma Scale (GCS) was first introduced by Teasdale and Jennett in 1974. It aimed to replace the use of subjective classifications such as coma, stupor and semi-conscious, and is used throughout the world to measure levels of consciousness objectively. A GCS score below 8 has been accepted as equivalent to coma.

The GCS was never intended to stand alone, but to be used as an adjunct to an initial detailed neurological examination that would aim to 'establish the cause of the patient's condition in anatomical and pathological terms'.

The three main reasons for assessing a patient's conscious level are to determine whether it is:

1. improving
2. remaining static
3. deteriorating.

The GCS consists of three aspects of the patient's behaviour, each evaluated independently and graded according to a rank order that indicates the degree of dysfunction. The highest score that can be achieved is 15, the lowest 3. Although a single score is usually given for a patient, of greater significance is how this score is composed, for example GCS 9 (E2, V2, M5). The three areas assessed are:

1. **Eye opening**
2. **Verbal response**
3. **Best Motor response.**

Points to remember when performing the GCS evaluation are as follows:

• The arms give the widest range of responses and for this reason are always observed when performing the GCS. Spinal reflexes may cause the arms/legs to flex briskly in response to pain and must not be interpreted as a response.

- Always record the best response.
- As the GCS is an assessment of conscious level, it cannot be determined with accuracy in the patient who is receiving anaesthetic agents or drugs that may alter neurological status. Some drugs may affect pupillary reaction and the effects of any prescribed medication must be considered when assessing the pupils.
- To avoid misinterpretation and facilitate continuity, when giving verbal handover at the beginning of a new shift, an initial GCS must be performed together by both nurses.
- The GCS is recorded as a total score of between 3 and 15. A deterioration of 1 point in the GCS is of clinical significance and must be reported immediately.
- If in any doubt about the patient's level of consciousness, seek verification from an experienced member of nursing or medical staff.
- Follow local guidelines for performing the GCS if used.

Eye opening

If the patient's eyes are closed as a result of swelling or facial fractures, this is recorded as 'C' on the chart. Eye opening is meaningless under these circumstances.

Spontaneous eye opening
It is important to exclude the fact that the patient is asleep before proceeding to assess eye opening. This is recorded when the patient is observed to be awake with eyes open. This observation is made without any speech or touch.

Eye opening to speech
This is recorded when the patient's eyes open to normal clear voice. If there is no response, it may be necessary to speak in a louder voice. This observation is made without touch.

Eye opening to pain
If there is no eye opening to speech or loud clear commands, begin with touch, gradually progressing to painful stimuli. This is recorded when the patient's eyes open to a painful stimulus applied to the lateral aspect of the third finger. Nailbed pressure should not be used, as it will cause bruising and prolong residual discomfort. Sternal rubbing should also be avoided as this is unnecessary and may leave bruising.

In the patient with suspected spinal injury, it will be necessary to use supraorbital ridge pressure to elicit a response. This method involves resting the hand on the patient's head, with the flat of the thumb or finger placed on the supraorbital ridge or eyebrow, gradually increasing the pressure. Do not use this method if there is any suspicion of facial damage or fractures.

No response
This is recorded when no response to painful stimuli is observed.

Best verbal response

If the patient has an endotracheal tube or tracheostomy tube *in situ*, this is recorded as 'Y' on the chart.

If the patient is dysphasic, best verbal response cannot be determined with accuracy. This is recorded as a 'D' on the chart under 'No response'.

Orientated
To be classified as orientated, the patient must be able to identify:

• who they are
• where they are
• the month and year (day and date are not required).

All three must be identified correctly for the patient to be classified as orientated. At the end of the assessment all incorrect answers should be corrected and the patient orientated.

Confused
If one or more of the above is answered wrongly the patient is classified as confused.

Inappropriate words
The use of swear words is common. Differentiation between confusion and inappropriate words can be difficult. There are three main differences:

1. conversation is absent
2. there is a tendency to use single words more than sentences
3. replies are often elicited in response to physical rather verbal stimulation.

Incomprehensible sounds
Words cannot be identified. The patient may be mumbling, groaning or screaming.

None
The patient does not respond verbally to verbal or physical stimuli.

Best motor response

Obeys commands
Nurses should be aware of their own non-verbal behaviour as patients may only mimic what they see. This response is recorded when the patient carries out the following command: ask the patient to grip and then *let go* of your fingers. The patient must grip then ungrip to discount a reflex action. If in

any doubt, ask the patient to raise his eyebrows or stick out his tongue. If you are unsure whether there is a weakness on one side, ask the patient to lift up both arms then close his eyes. If there is any weakness, the weak side tends to fall. (Note that it is the best motor response that is recorded. Any weakness is recorded in the limb movement section of the chart.) The patient should repeat the command twice to rule out a coincidental response.

Localizes to pain

The patient is unresponsive to verbal commands. It is important to differentiate between localizing to pain and flexion to pain, as localizing is a powerful response and an indication of better brain function. Flexion is not a purposeful response and may be a reflex action. Supraorbital ridge pressure is considered to be the most reliable and effective technique to distinguish localizing from flexion or abnormal flexion, as the observed response to this method of pain stimuli is less likely to be misinterpreted.

The procedure is as follows. A painful stimulus is applied to the supraorbital ridge (to stimulate the supraorbital nerve). In the presence of facial fractures or gross eye swelling, pinching the earlobe is preferable to supraorbital ridge pressure. To be classified as localizing pain, the patient must move the hand to the point of stimulation, bringing the hand up beyond the chin and across the midline of the body.

Flexion

No localizing seen. This is recorded when the patient bends the arms at the elbow in response to painful stimuli. It is rapid withdrawal (likened to withdrawing from touching something hot) and is associated with abduction of the shoulder.

Abnormal flexion

This is classified when the patient's elbow flexes. It is characterized by internal rotation and adduction of the shoulder, and flexion of the elbow. It is a much slower response than flexion and may be accompanied by spastic wrist flexion.

Extending to pain

This is recorded when the patient presents with straightening of the elbow joint, adduction and internal rotation of the shoulder, and inward rotation and spastic flexion of the wrist.

No motor response

This is recorded when there is no response to painful stimuli.

Pupillary responses

Pupil size and reaction to light are important neurological observations.

Normal pupils

- Are round and equal in size, average 2–5 mm in diameter.
- The millimetre scale (as indicated on the neurological observation chart) is used to estimate the size of each pupil.
- The shape of each pupil should be noted in the nursing documentation. Abnormal pupil shapes may be described as ovoid, keyhole or irregular.

Reaction to light

When light is shone into the eye, the pupil should constrict immediately. Withdrawal of the light should produce an immediate and brisk dilatation of the pupil. This is called the direct light reflex. Introducing the light into one pupil should cause similar constriction to occur simultaneously in the other pupil. When the light is withdrawn from one eye, the opposite pupil should dilate simultaneously. This response is called the consensual light reaction.

Assessment

For the purposes of neurological assessment the size and reaction of the pupils to bright light are recorded.

- If the pupil reacts briskly to light, record as +.
- If the pupil does not react briskly to light, record as –.
- If the pupil is sluggish in response when compared with the other pupil, record as S.

A sluggish pupil may be difficult to distinguish from a fixed pupil and may be an early focal sign of an expanding intracranial lesion and increased intracranial pressure. A sluggish response to light in a previously reacting pupil must be reported immediately.

Procedure for the purpose of neurological assessment

- The pupils should be first observed simultaneously to determine size and equality.
- A bright light is shone into each eye and the result recorded; any external light source should be eliminated if possible.
- Pupillary responses must always be monitored and recorded in the sedated patient with neurological injury.
- The shape of the pupil should also be assessed; an ovoid pupil may be an indication of intacranial hypertension.

Points to note

- Pinpoint non-reactive pupils are seen with opiate overdose and pontine haemorrhage.

- The parasympathethic nerve fibres of the third cranial nerve (oculomotor nerve) control pupillary constriction; compression of this nerve will result in fixed dilated pupils.
- Atropine will cause dilated pupils.
- Non-reactive pupils may also be caused by local damage.
- One dilated or fixed pupil may be an indication of an expanding/developing intracranial lesion, compressing the oculomotor nerve on the same side of the brain as the affected pupil.

Limb assessment

A limb assessment is useful to assess for focal damage. Spontaneous movements are observed for equality. If there is little or no spontaneous movement then painful stimuli must be applied to each limb in turn, comparing the results. It is most appropriate to complete this while assessing the motor component of the GCS.

Signs and symptoms of increased intracranial pressure

Nursing assessment of neurological signs is directed at **early** signs and symptoms of increased intracranial pressure (ICP), when nursing and medical interventions are still effective. Therefore, the baseline neurological assessment and ongoing assessments, most importantly GCS by knowledgeable practitioners, are the most sensitive indicators of neurological change. When **late** signs appear (brain stem signs, including changes in vital signs and alterations in respiratory pattern), it may be too late to reverse cerebral deterioration or even death. This response is called Cushing's response. It is essential to observe for a deterioration in conscious level and report it urgently.

Signs and symptoms of Cushing's response

- Hypertension – this is a compensatory mechanism that tries to maintain cerebral blood flow in the brain when ICP is high.
- Bradycardia – as pressure in the brain continues to rise, the pulse drops to 60 beats per minute or less as it attempts to compensate. The pulse is described as full and bounding. The decreased rate and bounding quality are the result of an attempt by the heart to pump blood upwards into vessels on which pressure is being exerted in the brain.
- Respiratory patterns can also be affected.

As discussed, Cushing's response and its effect on vital signs is a late and potentially fatal sign of neurological deterioration. Therefore neurological assessment is directed towards identification of altered consciousness so that treatment can be commenced when the chances of control and reversal are good.

Diagnostic assessment

With the exception of the neurological examination and lumbar puncture, most neurological diagnostic procedures are performed in the radiology department or special procedure areas, rather than in the ward setting.

If at all possible, the nurse caring for the patient should accompany the patient to diagnostic procedures. Sometimes this is an absolute necessity, for example if the patient needs frequent suctioning or respiratory support. It is often necessary for the patient to co-operate, lie quietly or follow instructions. For the patient with impaired cognitive function and understanding or a high anxiety level, the nurse may make the difference between success and failure of the diagnostic procedure.

Patients undergoing a diagnostic procedure need a general explanation of the procedure with special emphasis on their participation in it. For example, patients who are about to undergo computer tomography (CT) or magnetic resonance imaging (MRI) should be told that they must remain very still while the scan is being taken to ensure accuracy and quality of the images. If the patient is restless or unco-operative, sedation may have to be given. In such cases an anaesthetist is usually required as the patient may need respiratory support whilst sedated. In such cases the patient will need to be accompanied to the procedure by a qualified nurse. The nurse may need to repeat information about the procedure several times, because neurologically impaired patients with cognitive dysfunction may have difficulty understanding and remembering what is said.

Written consent is required for many of the neurological diagnostic procedures. If patients have altered consciousness, cognitive deficit or other impairment, it will affect their ability to give informed consent. It is the doctor's responsibility to obtain written consent after explaining the procedure to the patient and a family member.

Lumbar puncture

A lumbar puncture involves the introduction of a hollow needle with a stylet into the lumbar subarachnoid space of the spinal canal using strict aseptic technique. In an adult, the needle is placed between L3 and L4 to avoid injury to the spinal cord, which ends at about L1–L2. The patient lies on his side in the fetal position, with the knees drawn up to the chest and the neck flexed forwards, so that the spine is flexed and the spinal processes are separated. If there is any suspicion of raised ICP or a space-occupying lesion, then caution is advised as either of these situations may result in brain stem compression, herniation or 'coning' through the foramen magnum. A sample of CSF can be tested for many factors to assist in the diagnosis of many neurological diseases. The standard test is bacteriology and biochemical tests, usually protein and glucose, but many other tests can also be performed:

- virology
- cytology
- fungal and parasitic tests
- HIV test
- VDRL (Venereal Disease Reference Laboratory) test.

A sample can be observed immediately for:

- blood (normal CSF is clear) – three consecutive samples are required to avoid contamination from the puncture site
- cloudiness, which can indicate infection
- pressure, by connecting a manometer (normal pressure is 100–150 mm CSF).

Follow-up care

After lumbar puncture, the patient is restricted to bed rest in a flat position for 4-8 hours or as determined by hospital policy, to prevent CSF leakage from the puncture site. A decrease in the amount of CSF may cause a severe, throbbing headache, so prescribed analgesia may be required. The patient should be encouraged to increase fluid intake for 24–48 hours to facilitate CSF production. Neurological and initial signs should be monitored and the puncture site observed for signs of leakage of CSF or bleeding.

The nurse's role in the care and management of patients with an altered level of consciousness

There are a number of patient problems associated with altered levels of consciousness:

- airway clearance impaired
- risk of aspiration
- risk of injury
- elimination pattern altered (bladder and bowel)
- mobility impaired
- nutrition altered
- sleep pattern disturbance
- communication impaired
- thought processes altered

- sensory perception altered
- individual coping impaired.

Nursing a patient with an altered level of consciousness can be very challenging; the demand on a nurse's skill is surely greater when caring for patients who cannot respond, talk or comprehend as they normally would. Someone with severe mental and physical disturbance needs to be in the care of an experienced, sensitive, multidisciplinary team, who have the skill and knowledge to ensure that these patients receive the appropriate care.

It can be difficult as a student nurse to feel confident when caring for such patients. But the following discussion of nursing interventions should help you to meet the challenge and increase your knowledge base in caring for them.

The following are some basic interventions for a patient with altered consciousness:

- Maintaining a patent airway is a major priority and patients should not be left lying on their back because of the possibility of aspiration. The position selected should allow oral secretions to be drained.
- A change in the level of consciousness is the most sensitive indicator of neurological change. When there is an alteration in neurological status it is the first neurological sign to change, so the nurse should assess level of consciousness regularly (as often as every 5–10 minutes in the acute, unstable patient and less frequently in the apparently stable patient). Despite all the technological advances in medicine, the most sensitive 'sensor' of neurological change is the nurse who is well acquainted with the patient and who can best evaluate whether behaviour changes are caused by psychological stress, pain, fatigue or neurological deterioration. The nurse has the responsibility of advising the medical staff of any changes in the patient's level of consciousness.
- When managing a patient whose level of consciousness has deteriorated, the nurse should talk to the patient in a calm, normal voice, explaining in simple terms what is being done and orientating the patient to the environment. If the patient normally uses glasses or a hearing aid, it should be worn.
- When talking to the patient, the nurse should try to screen out external environmental stimuli that could be confusing for the patient. For example, a group of people entering the room and talking to the patient can be both overwhelming and confusing, as it can result in a sensory overload for the fragile, recovering neurological circuits, causing confusion and misinterpretation of stimuli.
- Once patients regain consciousness and begin to verbalize, they can be frightened by the void of time while they were unconscious for which they cannot account. The nurse should fill in the gaps of time by briefly

recounting what has happened, and, when the patient begins to verbalize, the nurse should correct any misconceptions.

- As the level of consciousness deteriorates, the nurse must assume total responsibility for the patient's safety. The methods employed depend on the availability of staff (usually fewer staff on evening and night shifts), the patient's degree of agitation and impulsive behaviour, the location of the patient's room in relationship to the nurse station and the use of support equipment for the patient. Regardless of the circumstances, caring for this type of patient requires much more nursing time and intervention than for an alert, orientated patient. The nurse should observe the patient frequently; talk in a calm manner and ensure that the bed is kept low, unless contraindicated. Cot sides are sometimes a useful deterrent to stop the patient getting out of bed, but they may increase the height from which the patient can fall. Restraint is often resented and sometimes unnecessary, and the patient may fight continuously to escape, so you may need to try many different tactics to pacify and settle the patient. Note that if cot sides or any form of restraint is used, hospital policy should be followed.
- Night-time and darkness often lead the patient to misinterpret the environment and other stimuli. A night light and periodic visits by the nurse can help to control fear, confusion and hallucinations.
- The very disturbed patient who is constantly climbing out of bed or undressing and is abusive and noisy is upsetting to other patients and visitors, but their co-operation and tolerance can usually be gained by explanation that this is a transitory stage of recovery.
- Nurses need to be on their guard for unpredictable behaviour and avoid personal injuries. It is unwise to argue with a patient who is hallucinating, aggressive or deluded.
- The family and other visitors need help to learn how to visit a patient whose level of consciousness has deteriorated and who has cognitive deficits. The guidelines suggested will depend on the particular patient. The nurse should be available to intervene if problems occur during the visit, as well as to alleviate the effects of the visit on the patient and visitors afterwards. If the patient is upset, the possible reasons for reaction should be pursued. Family members may also need support after the visit to express their concerns and fears.

Care of the unconscious patient

In addition to the above considerations, there are several others to be aware of when caring for a patient who is unconscious. The most important thing to remember is that these patients are totally dependent on the nurse to maintain their activities of living. The specific nursing care of the unconscious patient is shown in Table 4.1.

Table 4.1 Nursing management of the unconscious patient

Problem	Nursing intervention
Inadequate airway/ poor gag reflex	Nurse patient on side with neck in neutral position to ensure clear airway. Elevate head of the bed to 30°; if appropriate an oral or nasal airway may be used. If a tracheostomy tube is *in situ*, give care as required
Poor respiration pattern and potential for deterioration in gaseous exchange	Observe and document rate, depth and pattern of respirations and observe frequently for signs and symptoms of respiratory distress. Position the patient appropriately to facilitate respiration and turn at least 2-hourly. Listen to chest sounds and provide chest physiotherapy to maintain gaseous exchange and reduce secretions. Administer oxygen as required
Airway clearance ineffective/poor cough reflex	Assess patient's requirements for suctioning and observe throughout suctioning procedure for signs of cardiovascular deterioration
Potential for deterioration in cardiovascular status	Monitor pulse rate and rhythm, and blood pressure. Observe patient's skin colour, including peripheries, for signs of cyanosis, and report any deterioration immediately
Immobility	Reposition patient regularly, avoiding positions that may cause a rise in ICP, such as hip flexion, and ensure neck is maintained in neutral alignment. Observe pressure areas for signs of deterioration and assess Waterlow score daily, using appropriate equipment to prevent pressure or skin damage. Apply thigh-high pressure stockings and monitor patient for signs of deep vein thrombosis formation. Administer passive range of motion exercises at least 6-hourly and collaborate with physiotherapist
Maintenance of hydration and nutrition	Monitor patient's weight at least weekly. Maintain an accurate input and output record. Administer fluids and nutrition as prescribed by a dietician, enterally (via nasogastric tube or if long-term feeding is required via a percutaneous endoscopically placed gastrostomy tube) where possible, to maintain gut integrity. Assess skin turgor and mucous membranes for dryness. Monitor urine and serum (blood) osmolarity. Fluid infusions should be isotonic and any electrolyte imbalance corrected (hypernatraemia promotes cerebral oedema)

Table 4.1 Nursing management of the unconscious patient (contd)

Problem	Nursing intervention
Elimination pattern altered	Monitor fluid balance. If an indwelling catheter is in place, maintain a closed system and follow protocol for catheter care. Monitor urinalysis, urine culture and sensitivity. Monitor the patient and his urine output for signs and symptoms of infection. Monitor and record the frequency of bowel movements. Monitor characteristics of the stool. Initiate a bowel programme
Potential for seizure activity	Observe for origin, sequence of events and start/finish time. The patient should be placed in the left lateral position when the seizure is over, and observation should continue. The GCS is affected by the post-ictal state, and should be completed regularly, until the pre-seizure status is regained. Anticonvulsants should be administered in an attempt to stop the seizure, and then regularly to inhibit further seizure activity. Seizures will increase the ICP, and if continuous, i.e. status epilepticus, can cause severe cerebral oedema, occasionally causing brain stem death
Maintenance of hygiene requirements	Provide regular care of skin, ensuring particular care for mouth, eyes (blink reflex may be absent) and around invasive catheters
Sensory perceptual alterations due to unconsciousness Rehabilitation	In conjunction with the multidisciplinary team, provide sensory stimuli while caring for the patient by the use of non-instrumental touch, talking to the patient and addressing the patient by name. Tell the patient about the surroundings, treatments and procedures, and orientate to time and place. Encourage family members to touch and talk to the patient. Structure sensory stimuli so periods of rest are included to prevent sensory overload. Support and prepare long-term carers and prepare discharge plans

Common disorders of the nervous system

We will now consider some of the other more common disorders of the nervous system.

Action point 2

Multiple sclerosis is a common condition that you will almost certainly come across. Write down all you know about it and how you need to care for a patient with this illness.

Multiple sclerosis

- Multiple sclerosis (MS) is a chronic and usually progressive condition affecting the CNS.
- It affects approximately 85 000 people in the UK, with a ratio of three women to every two men.
- It is the second leading cause of neurological disability in young adults after head injury.
- The peak age for diagnosis is 30, remaining high in the 40s but then starting to decline.
- The annual cost of MS care in the UK is estimated at £1.2bn pounds and is a significant healthcare problem.
- Although people can lead a normal life span when suffering from MS, it is the psychosocial impact of living with the disease that has an impact on the lives of the individual and the family.
- Although there have been many advances in the treatment of MS, especially with disease-modifying drugs, the mainstay of treatment is symptomatic treatment by a multidisciplinary team of healthcare professionals.

Pathophysiology

MS is characterized by episodes of inflammation leading to demyelination of the brain or spinal cord. Myelin is the fatty sheath that protects nerve fibres (axons) and forms the white matter in the brain. Demyelination is the destruction or removal of the myelin sheath, which affects the conduction of electrical impulses along or between nerves. Any damage to the myelin will delay or interrupt the transmission of impulses as they travel from the brain to the spinal cord and out to various parts of the body. Inflammatory lesions can be seen as white plaques on an MR image. During an acute exacerbation of MS, the nerve becomes inflamed and oedematous, the blood–brain barrier is disrupted, and demyelination and gliosis (overgrowth of cells of the nervous tissue in an area of damage in the brain or spinal cord) occur. In the early stages of MS there is a capacity for the myelin to regenerate, and it is probably this process of remyelination that plays a part in disease remission. However, as the disease progresses, there are repeated attacks on the myelin, which is then unable to regenerate, leading to myelin loss (demyelination). The myelin is replaced by fibrous scar tissue (sclerosis). Recent findings indicate that, at this stage, axonal loss can also occur. Axonal loss is irreversible and it is this process that accounts for permanent disability.

What causes MS?

MS has been described for over 170 years and, despite many theorists' attempts to explain its cause, none has been substantiated. However, immunological and epidemiological studies have provided clues to the causes of MS, which include the following:

- *Immune*: there is increasing evidence that MS is an immune-mediated condition, and people with MS have been found to have specific immune system abnormalities compared with healthy individuals.
- *Genetic*: although MS is not a hereditary disease, there is believed to be an inherited genetic predisposition, with siblings and parents of people with MS showing an increased susceptibility to developing the disease. Up to 20% of people with MS have at least one relative with the condition. Children with a parent who has MS have a low risk of developing the disease, at around 2–5%. However, this is a much higher risk than that of the general population, which is approximately 0.01%.
- *Environmental*: different studies have identified that rates of MS vary in different countries. The prevalence in the UK is significantly higher in the north east of Scotland than in the south of England. The reasons behind the geographical distribution of MS remain unclear, but studies have shown that the incidence of MS is at its highest in countries furthest from the equator.

Diagnosis

There is no single test to confirm a diagnosis of MS. The patient's past medical history, clinical (neurological) examination, MRI, visual evoked responses and lumbar puncture are all used in the diagnosis. The advent of MRI and increased knowledge and development of its use have reduced the need for invasive procedures such as lumbar puncture.

Common symptoms

One or more symptoms might be evident at the initial presentation of MS. These include:

- limb weakness
- paraesthesia (numbness)
- diplopia (double vision)
- vertigo.

Patients with MS can experience a range of symptoms, but not everyone who is diagnosed with the condition will experience all the symptoms outlined in Table 4.2.

Table 4.2 Symptoms of multiple sclerosis

- Weakness
- Fatigue
- Visual disturbance
- Vertigo
- Pain
- Trigeminal neuralgia
- Bowel problems
- Tremor
- Cognitive dysfunction (e.g. memory loss, impaired judgement)
- Sensory disturbances
- Spasticity
- Ataxia (unsteady gait)
- Dysarthria (impairments of articulation, resonance or voice)
- Headache
- Bladder problems
- Sexual problems

What are relapses?
A relapse is an acute episode of disease activity where the individual experiences a worsening of existing symptoms and/or emergence of new ones. They can occur spontaneously or be triggered by a viral illness.

The pattern of MS

MS follows a variable pattern over time, but there are four main types:

1. Benign – 20% of people with MS have this type and demonstrate no active disease or clinical deterioration for several years. They have few episodes of mild attacks and there is minimal or no disability.
2. Relapsing–remitting – occurs in 25% of MS sufferers and is characterized by clearly defined disease relapses with full recovery or with residual deficit on recovery. An individual will still be classed as having relapsing–remitting disease even if there is incomplete recovery from a relapse if, between attacks, neurological condition is stable.
3. Secondary progressive – occurs most frequently and is similar to the relapsing–remitting MS. It is characterized by the absence of periods of remission and the patient's condition does not return to baseline. Progressive, cumulative symptoms and deterioration occur over several years.
4. Primary progressive – approximately 10% of people will follow this pattern and are usually over the age of 40 when they first experience symptoms. The disease progresses without distinct relapses, although some people do have occasional plateaus and temporary minor improvements.

Treatment

Current treatment options are aimed at:

- disease modification
- treating relapses
- symptom management.

Disease-modifying treatments

All of these treatments are aimed at regulating the immune system to suppress the faulty immune response that triggers the attack on myelin. Drugs such as interferon-beta and more recently glatiramer acetate are being used for this purpose but their use in the UK is restricted. The National Institute for Clinical Excellence reviewed their cost and efficacy, and concluded that there was insufficient evidence to support the widespread use of interferon-beta in the treatment of MS.

Experience with other disease-modifying agents such as azathioprine, mitozantrone, methotrexate, immunoglobulins and plasma exchange is developing.

Treating relapses

Glucocorticoids (steroids) given either intravenously or orally are used to treat relapses by reducing inflammation around the MS plaque and also suppressing the immune system. Although they do not have any long-term effect on the disease itself, they do shorten the relapse.

Symptom management

As demyelination can occur in any part of the CNS, the symptoms vary, but can usually be attributed to the specific area of the CNS that has been damaged. Therefore, people with MS can have a variety of unpredictable symptoms that can alter from day to day, making MS a very frustrating condition.

Motor symptoms

Motor symptoms can be very disabling for people with MS. They can suffer from movement difficulties due to increased muscle tone, tremor, lack of co-ordination and muscle weakness (usually in lower limbs); the last is especially evident after exertion.

Spasticity is a common symptom of MS and is an involuntary increase in muscle tone identified clinically as an increased resistance to passive stretching of a muscle. As spasticity occurs in patients with muscle weakness, it may be beneficial in keeping them mobile, as the stiffness can keep the joints straight, helping them to stand and walk. However, it can have a severe impact on everyday life and can be both painful and disabling, hampering personal care and preventing sexual activity. Spasms can occur when someone is sitting down, and a violent spasm could cause a person to fall or be ejected from a chair. Many factors, including infections, pressure sores and constipation, can aggravate the problem. Therefore, assessment to exclude such 'noxious stimuli' and to assess seating is crucial. Muscle spasms can also occur as a hyper-reactive response to a stimulus, such as touch. Lesions in the cerebellum can impair balance and co-ordination, and ataxia of the trunk or lower limbs results in a 'wide-based', unsteady gait. These symptoms may be improved by physiotherapy and walking aids.

Treatments for spasticity include the following:

- Botulinum toxin given intramuscularly to disrupt activity at the neuro-muscular junction, and phenol given intramuscularly or intrathecally as a peripheral nerve blocker.
- Oral drug treatments such as baclofen, tizanidine, dantrolene and benzo-diazepines can be effective. However, 25–30% of people with MS develop intolerable side effects or an unsatisfactory response.
- Intrathecal baclofen (delivered directly into the spinal subarachnoid space via an implanted pump) can be used to treat intractable spasticity, but financial implications limit its widespread use.
- Irreversible surgical procedures such as rhizotomy or tenotomy may be used as a last resort for severe spasticity when intrathecal baclofen is not effective.
- Trials are currently being undertaken to establish whether oral cannabis has a significant effect on reducing spasticity in MS.

Tremors

Tremors caused by MS can be mild, but in some patients they are severe and incapacitating. Intention tremors, where the tremor amplitude increases as the 'target' is approached, are most common, and are usually caused by a lesion in the cerebellum or cerebellar outflow pathway. Unfortunately, treat-ments for tremors are not very successful. Drug treatments (beta blockers, isoniazid, clonazepam) can cause side effects and have a limited effect. Lycra skin splinting has the potential to reduce the tremor in some patients.

Sensory symptoms

Sensory symptoms arise from damage to the sensory cortex or from the spinal pathways, such as the spinothalamic tract and dorsal columns. The symptoms (common early in the disease) include pins and needles, numb-ness, tingling and Lhermitte's sign (brief electrical sensations shooting down the spine, occurring on neck flexion).

Pain affects about 30–65% of people with MS at some point. It is usually described as a 'shooting' or 'burning' pain and traditional analgesia is not effective. However, tricyclic antidepressants (such as amitriptyline) and/or anticonvulsants (e.g. gabapentin or carbamazepine) can offer some relief, along with TENS (transcutaneous electrical nerve stimulation) machines.

Bowel problems

Bowel problems are also common, with 68% of people with MS experiencing incontinence or constipation. It is unclear what is responsible for these problems. Spinal cord lesions are not the cause of all bowel symptoms, because constipation does not always correspond with bladder problems, and constipation occurs in people with little disability. Constipation may be due to pelvic floor spasticity or poor colonic motility, and may be made worse by reduced mobility, side effects of medication and poor fluid or fibre intake.

Faecal incontinence is usually linked to a lack of rectal or perineal sensation and poor pelvic floor contraction, and often occurs in conjunction with constipation and overflow. Effective bowel management depends on the assessment of all relevant factors. Advice on fluids, diet, positioning, abdominal massage and establishing a bowel regimen can help, but serious constipation requires medication.

Bladder symptoms

Bladder dysfunction is common in MS, with up to 90% of people affected at some stage. It is caused by loss of the complex control of the bladder, which involves long spinal cord pathways and the pontine micturition centre. As bladder dysfunction is usually a result of spinal cord disease, there is a strong link between bladder problems and spasticity in the lower limbs.

The type of bladder problem depends on which part of the pathway is damaged, and may present as:

- detrusor areflexia: failure to empty bladder resulting in symptoms of urgency and frequency, with a residual volume
- detrusor–sphincter dyssynergia: lack of co-ordination between detrusor muscle and sphincter, resulting in the bladder contracting against a closed sphincter. Symptoms are urgency and hesitancy and there may be post-void residual volume
- detrusor hyper-reflexion: failure to store urine, resulting in frequency, urgency and urge incontinence.

Treatment of bladder problems

Treatment depends on the type of dysfunction, which can be determined by thorough investigation, e.g. bladder ultrasound. Patients should be referred to a specialist continence service, but fortunately bladder symptoms are some of the most treatable for MS patients.

Visual disturbances

Diplopia (double vision) can be relieved by wearing an eye patch, and swapping it from one eye to the other every few hours. If the patient has peripheral visual deficits, scanning techniques (moving the head from side to side) can help. In a hospital environment, nursing staff need to orientate the patient to the surroundings, which must be kept free from clutter.

Dysphagia and dysarthria

Dysphagia (difficulty swallowing) due to brain stem (lower cranial nerve) plaques can occur at any stage of MS, such as during an acute relapse, but is more common in advanced MS. If it is not effectively managed it can be life threatening, because of the risk of aspiration pneumonia and nutritional compromise. Swallowing difficulties need to be assessed as a priority by a speech and language therapist, who, in conjunction with a dietician, can give advice on the correct posture for eating, altered-texture diets and the timing of meals to avoid fatigue.

If the dysphagia is severe, then other methods of feeding need to be used. The preferred method for longer-term enteral feeding is via a percutaneous endoscopic gastronomy (PEG) tube. Ensuring nutritional needs are met will not only reduce the risk of aspiration but also improve nutritional status, bladder and bowel function and general health.

Dysarthria (loss of control of the muscles of the lips, tongue and face) is present in about 40% of people with MS, owing to cerebellar involvement. Speech and language therapists can assess and advise on methods to improve intelligibility and can provide appropriate communication aids and amplifiers.

Intracranial haemorrhage

Action point 1

From your knowledge of the brain's anatomy and how it is protected, try to think of potential problems for a patient who suffers from a bleed into the brain.

The term intracranial haemorrhage describes the concept of bleeding within the head. More specifically, however, it may be one or a combination of the following:

- intracerebral – bleeding into brain tissue
- intraventricular – bleeding into the cerebral ventricles

- subarachnoid – bleeding into the subarachnoid space
- subdural – bleeding from vessels beneath the dura
- extradural – bleeding from vessels outside the dura.

The common causes of intracranial haemorrhage are:

- hypertension
- vascular abnormality, e.g. aneurysm, arteriovenous malformation (AVM) and vasculitis
- trauma, tumour
- pathogenic problems with coagulation
- drug abuse, e.g. cocaine.

In most cases, the diagnostic pathway will begin in the Accident and Emergency (A&E) department. The diagnosis of intracranial haemorrhage will consist of the following:

- patient history
- signs and symptoms
- full neurological assessment
- CT
- angiogram for suspected vascular abnormality.

Psychological, social and family support play a major part in care, but are not discussed in detail in this chapter.

Intracerebral haemorrhage

Intracerebral haemorrhage most commonly occurs as result of trauma, or in the older adult with a history of poorly controlled hypertension or anti-coagulant therapy. A smaller percentage of cases, affecting younger people particularly, may be due to rupture of an AVM. The bleeding is into the brain tissue itself and can occur anywhere in the brain. Patients will experience common symptoms of intracranial haemorrhage (Table 4.3), plus other symptoms specific to the location of the bleed. For example, hemiparesis and third-nerve palsy indicate bleeding above the tentorium, severe ataxia, nystagmus and hydrocephalus indicate bleeding in the cerebellar region, and quadraplegia and abnormal respiratory patterns can indicate brain stem involvement. Treatment depends largely on the size of the bleed and its effects on the patient. The conscious, stable patient with a small haematoma and minimal midline shift may be managed conservatively, allowing the haematoma to resolve itself over a period of weeks. But the unconscious, unstable patient with a large haematoma and significant brain shift requires emergency craniotomy for evacuation of the haematoma.

The size and location of the bleed, its effect on the patient, and the speed of diagnosis and management all affect outcome.

Table 4.3 Common signs and symptoms of intracranial bleed

- Headache
- Reduction in score on Glasgow Coma Scale
- Neck rigidity
- Limb weakness, usually down one side
- Speech deficits
- Unequal pupils
- Papilloedema
- Seizures
- Vomiting
- Agitation
- Changes in respiratory pattern

Subarachnoid haemorrhage

Subarachnoid haemorrhage (SAH) occurs in approximately 10–15 per 100 000 people a year, most commonly women aged between 40 and 60. This prevalence is not fully understood, although there may be familial, probably genetic, factors involved. There is also a link with smoking, hypertension and alcohol.

Classic symptoms are acute onset of severe headache (often described as 'the worst ever') and vomiting, associated with some degree of impaired consciousness. Further symptoms of epilepsy, neck stiffness, reactive hypertension, pyrexia and coma may follow.

The severity of the symptoms is related to the severity of the bleed, which in turn is related to patient outcome. The World Federation of Neurosurgeons has formulated a grading system for SAH, which acts as a good prognostic indicator, estimating likely patient outcome, where grade 1 patients fare best and grade 5 fare worst (see Figure 4.4).

Table 4.4 World Federation of Neurosurgeons grading system for SAH

WFNS grade	Glasgow Coma Score	Motor deficit
1	15	Absent
2	14–13	Absent
3	14–13	Present
4	12–7	Present or absent
5	6–3	Present or absent

Over 70% of SAHs are due to the rupture of a berry aneurysm within the arterial blood supply to the brain around the circle of Willis. Other causes include bleeding from an AVM, haemorrhage from a tumour, vasculitis or as a result of anticoagulant therapy. About 15% of cases have no identified cause.

To put all this in context, 10–15% of patients die before reaching hospital. A further 20% will die during the next 48 h from hydrocephalus, secondary haematoma causing brain damage and brain shift, or a brain stem event. Those who survive for 48 h run a high risk of rebleeding or developing complications from cerebral vasospasm, which can lead to delayed cerebral infarct. Quick accurate diagnosis proceeding to prompt treatment is essential.

Diagnosis

The diagnosis of SAH is confirmed by performing a CT scan, where the presence of blood in the ventricles, basal cisterns and/or sylvian fissures will be apparent. Angiography will locate the exact cause of the haemorrhage. Angiography is performed as soon as possible, but may be delayed if the patient is particularly unstable. It involves the injection of contrast medium into the cerebral circulation via a catheter fed up the femoral artery from the groin. X-rays of the circulatory network of the head can then be examined. At this point, the presence and precise location of an aneurysm or AVM can be determined.

Management

The patient is nursed flat with one pillow (although there is no scientific evidence to suggest that this reduces the incidence of rebleeding) and closely monitored neurologically for signs of deterioration.

Historically, the analgesia of choice was codeine phosphate, and more recently DF118, as these do not depress neurological signs. However, there is now increasing support for controlled use of morphine for pain management. Patients will require assistance with all activities of daily living, and strategies designed to reduce the incidence of rebleeding and vasospasm must be implemented. Cerebral vasospasm is thought to be caused by substances released following red blood cell breakdown after the initial bleed. This results in decreased blood flow to the brain. These treatments involve administrating the calcium antagonist nimodipine, which has been shown to reduce the incidence of delayed cerebral infarction and improve outcome, and triple 'H' therapy (hypertensive, hypervolaemic, haemodilution). A daily fluid intake of 3 litres produces a degree of hypervolaemia and haemodilution, which aids capillary passage and helps maintain cerebral perfusion in the face of cerebral vasospasm. If the patient deteriorates neurologically despite these measures, then the use of inotropes may be necessary to restore cerebral perfusion by increasing blood pressure.

For patients with a ruptured aneurysm, treatment may be surgical, endovascular or conservative. The traditional option of clipping the aneurysm via a craniotomy allows the fragile structure to be excluded from the circulation, thus avoiding further bleeding. Relatively new, less invasive procedures using an endovascular approach insert platinum coils into the aneurysm via its neck, initiating thrombosis and obliteration. In some cases where the aneurysm is deeply embedded in vital centres or the patient's condition is too unstable, conservative management may be most appropriate. Whichever form of treatment is used initially, the patient will require continued close neurological monitoring, nimodipine, triple 'H' therapy and gentle rehabilitation.

Various methods are used to treat AVM. Excision via a craniotomy is the most effective, but success depends on age, the location of the AVM, its size and precise anatomy. The endovascular approach allows acrylic glues to thrombose feeding vessels, while stereotactic radiotherapy offers a localized high dose of radiation that, over time, shrinks small AVMs.

For those patients presenting with SAH and a negative angiogram, treatment is conservative: symptom relief, rest and then a gentle mobilization programme. A repeat angiogram is usually offered 3 months later to check that no abnormality has been overlooked.

Long term, approximately half of all patients admitted to a neurosurgical unit after a SAH make a good recovery and return to work, but changes in personality and cognitive ability are not uncommon.

Intraventricular haemorrhage

Intraventricular haemorrhage occurs secondary to a SAH or following an intracerebral bleed, where the location of the primary bleeds results in blood flushing into the ventricles or rupture of the ventricle wall. It also occurs in pre-term infants of less than 32 weeks' gestation where there is an increase in cerebral blood flow from hypoxia, respiratory distress or a rise in central venous pressure. Treatment may be conservative. However, in the event of obstructive hydrocephalus, where the flow of CSF is inhibited due to excessive blood, the temporary insertion of an extraventricular drain or more long-term ventricular peritoneal shunting may be necessary.

Subdural haematoma and extradural haematoma

These different types of haematoma are usually associated with a traumatic incident. Subdural haematomas can be either acute or chronic. Chronic haematomas are linked more commonly with infants or elderly people, where there are several predisposing factors; acute ones can affect all age groups.

A subdural haematoma usually results from the rupture of small bridging veins within the subdural space. This results in the slow build-up of a subdural haematoma, which can become chronic. Acute subdural haematomas are nearly always the result of a traumatic cortical laceration.

Extradural haematoma occurs in association with skull fracture, as blood from the fracture itself or from a torn meningeal vessel accumulates in the extradural space.

Both subdural and extradural haematomas carry significant risk to the patient, due to the presence of the space-occupying clot, brain shift and subsequent rise in ICP. In acute cases where there is a clear diagnosis and neurological deterioration, treatment will involve emergency surgical evacuation of the clot via craniotomy or a burr hole, relieving the pressure on the brain.

Nursing implications

Caring for this particular client group requires not only an understanding of the conditions themselves, but also insight into the concept of raised ICP and the significance of neurological observations.

Preoperatively, most of these patients will be experiencing some degree of raised ICP or have the potential to deteriorate as a result of further bleeding or vasospasm. Preoperatively, postoperatively and postembolization, patients require close monitoring, reporting and accurate handover of details of their level of consciousness, pupil reaction, motor function and vital signs to detect deterioration.

These patients require significant nursing input to manage a severe headache, often with photophobia and vomiting. Most will be nursed in bed with one pillow, to reduce strenuous activity or an acute rise in ICP. They will, therefore, need assistance with all aspects of hygiene, bladder and bowel management, eating and drinking, and pressure area care. Constipation is a problem, compounded by the use of analgesics including codeine. Patients' bowel function should be assessed regularly and preventive action taken according to patient need. Psychological, social and family support are also essential.

Future developments

Future developments within this field lie predominantly in the care of people with SAH. Much research is currently under way into understanding and improving medical management of cerebral vasospasm and refining endovascular techniques for obliterating aneurysms.

This will potentially reduce the need for the more invasive surgical treatments and limit the morbidity from complications. The development of more sophisticated neurosurgical techniques may also facilitate minimally invasive approaches for the management of other forms of haemorrhage. In addition, advances in therapies that assist with neuroprotection in the event of brain injury and ischaemia would have a significant impact on patient prognosis and outcome. A current untapped area is genetic predisposition to brain disease, and the way that individual brains react to injury. It may be that, in future, developments in gene therapy will enable prevention of brain disease itself or help to control the effects of brain injury.

Epilepsy

Epilepsy is a common condition with up to 100 people diagnosed with epilepsy every day. An epileptic seizure is defined as a brief, usually unprovoked, disturbance of behaviour, emotion, motor function or sensation, which is caused by an abnormal, sudden, excessive discharge of electrical activity in the brain. At some time in their life, one person in every 100 suffers a seizure. Periods between seizures can vary widely, but they must recur to constitute epilepsy.

Classification of seizures

How the nervous system is affected depends on whether the seizures are generalized or partial. The area of the brain where the seizure originates will also determine the types of seizures the individual experiences.

- Parietal lobe – transient sensory symptoms, tingling and numbness.
- Motor cortex – motor focal jerking.
- Occipital lobe – transient visual symptoms, such as flashing lights.
- Frontal lobe – complex behavioural disturbances.
- Temporal lobe – olfactory (smell) or gustatory (taste) symptoms, visual disturbances and déjà-vu experiences.

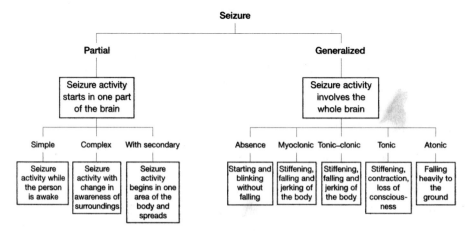

Figure 4.5 Classification of seizures.

Aetiology

Idiopathic (no known cause) epilepsy accounts for up to 75% of cases of epilepsy. When a cause can be found, it is referred to as symptomatic epilepsy caused by:

- drugs and alcohol (2%)
- anoxia (lack of oxygen) (2%)
- neoplasms (tumours) (2%)
- congenital disorders (4%)
- head trauma (5%)
- vascular disease (stroke, aneurysm, AVM) (5%)
- CNS infection (5%).

Precipitating factors

For those diagnosed with epilepsy, it is worth noting that the following factors can induce seizure activity:

- fever
- menstruation
- emotional stress
- metabolic disturbances
- poor drug compliance
- constipation
- sleep deprivation
- excessive alcohol or withdrawal
- toxins and drugs.

Diagnosis and investigations

Blood tests
Routine haematology and biochemistry investigations and toxicology screening may provide useful information in isolating the cause of epilepsy. Prolactin levels can be used as a marker, as they rise after a seizure.

CT scan
This is used to identify if there is a structural cause for the seizures (such as a tumour or abscess).

MRI
Similar to a CT scan and used for the same reason, but can give better anatomical detail and identify very small abnormalities.

Electroencephalogram (EEG)
This records the minuscule electrical discharges generated by the nerve cells. It also helps to classify the seizure type. It can be carried out in the clinic or

may be ambulatory, with the encephalograph worn by the patient over a period of time.

Telemetry
The individual is admitted to a specialist unit where he will be simultaneously recorded on video and EEG, possibly until a seizure has occurred. Comparisons can then be made between the video footage and the EEG recording.

Current medical treatment

The main form of treatment for epilepsy is with anticonvulsants, which often have to be taken for life. The aim is to prevent seizures, while ensuring that the individual suffers minimal side effects. If the correct medication is selected, a good remission rate of seizures can be obtained. Therefore finding the right treatment or right combination for an individual is paramount and may require close observation or a stay in hospital. Generally, one drug is introduced at a time and, if the chosen drug is not effective, the dosage may be increased or another drug introduced. The dosage of medications is adjusted to achieve therapeutic blood levels without causing major side effects. The nurse administers the medications at the correct time to maintain therapeutic blood levels and maximum effectiveness, and observes for side effects or adverse reactions. The patient should be instructed to avoid drugs and food that might interfere with the absorption or metabolism of the medication, e.g. warfarin should not be given with phenytoin. If medication is withdrawn or not taken, it can increase seizure activity and may cause status epilepticus, a medical emergency. For those free of seizures for a number of years, discontinuation of medication may be an option, but it should be carried out very gradually, one type of medication at a time, and under strict supervision.

For more information on drugs most commonly used and their side effects, refer to the *British National Formulary* (BNF).

Surgical options

The patient with seizures that do not respond to medication may benefit from surgical excision of the seizure area in the brain. However, this intervention is a last resort when all other options have failed. A very new surgical procedure involves a scanning technique that identifies the area in the brain with higher water content, which is normal for brain-damaged tissue. Surgery is then performed on that isolated area, using electrodes to identify electrical activity. Once abnormal electrical activity has been identified, the damaged brain tissue is removed surgically.

Prognosis

The risk of further seizures decreases with the length of the interval from the initial event. Most recurrences happen within 6 months of the first seizure. With long-term drug treatment, up to two-thirds of people with epilepsy may stop having seizures within 2–3 years of onset. Complete remission is achieved in less than 20% of cases, with prolonged control more likely if the epilepsy is of recent onset and if the seizures tend to be the generalized absence type. A less favourable prognosis is generally given if:

- there is a brain lesion
- seizures start in childhood and are associated with brain damage
- seizure control is difficult and a combination of drug therapy is required.
- there are other neurological factors, e.g. cerebral palsy or learning difficulties.

Mortality figures for someone with epilepsy are not particularly high, but a diagnosis of epilepsy will have an impact on the individual and their family. There are certain activities in which the individual will not be able to participate, such as driving a vehicle or doing a job that involves operating heavy machinery.

Caring for a patient with epilepsy in hospital

The nurse's aim is to monitor the patient and protect them from injury. This will involve the following:

- The individual should be nursed in an area where they can be observed easily (and cot sides should be used as necessary).
- The bed area should have an oxygen and suction supply.
- The nurse should be aware of the individual's usual pattern of medication time and any warning signs of impending seizures (e.g. auras/feelings).
- Nursing staff must be aware of the individual's whereabouts at all times.
- Nurses must ensure compliance with medication (taken on time and witnessed).
- Any triggers (e.g. flickering lights, TV) should be removed.
- The patient should be educated about the condition and any necessary lifestyle changes.

Care of the patient during a tonic–clonic seizure

- Ensure safety; only move the patient if they are in danger.
- Provide privacy.
- If in a chair, assist the person to the floor.

- Cushion and protect the head.
- Loosen restrictive clothing.
- Turn the patient on to their side.
- Do not restrain; guide the patient's movements if necessary.
- Maintain the patient's airway.
- Do not force anything into the patient's mouth.
- If the seizure lasts a long time (more than 5 minutes) ask for some assistance and call for medical help.
- At the completion of the seizure:
    - stay with the person until they recover (place in recovery position when appropriate)
    - check the mouth for injury as a result of tongue biting
    - take the patient's vital signs and GCS
    - allow the patient to rest
    - document the seizure (see below).

Accurate documentation

Accurate documentation following a seizure is vital, as this will allow clinicians to plan and implement treatment. Nurses should note:

- the circumstances leading up to the seizure
- the sequence of seizure progression (where the seizure began and body part first involved)
- any movements/twitching made during seizure (which limbs/parts of the body were involved)
- eye movements (eyes shut or open, pupil size, eye deviation)
- whether the patient was conscious
- whether the patient was incontinent
- length of seizure
- oxygen saturation: if saturation levels are low the patient may require oxygen therapy.

Status epilepticus

Status epilepticus is seizure activity that lasts longer than 30 minutes or a series of seizures that occur in rapid succession. It is a potential complication of all types of seizures. The usual causes of status epilepticus include:

- sudden withdrawal from anticonvulsant medication
- infections
- acute alcohol withdrawal
- head injury

- cerebral oedema
- metabolic disturbances.

It is classed as a medical emergency, and these episodes have a mortality rate of between 3 and 20%. It also carries the risk of irreversible brain damage. Therefore it is vital that the individual receives adequate oxygenation and treatment.

Care for the patient in status epilepticus

- Support the ABCs (Airway, Breathing, Circulation).
- Prepare for possible endotracheal intubation.
- Protect the patient from injury.
- Do not force an airway into the patient's mouth: provide oxygen via a facemask.
- Establish intravenous access if not already available and begin an infusion of 0.9% saline.
- Administer drugs as prescribed (usually diazepam or lorazepam to stop motor movement, and an anticonvulsant) and observe the patient for side effects or signs of toxicity from the medications.
- Monitor vital signs, cardiac rhythm and oxygen saturation.

Raised intracranial pressure

Many acute neurological conditions can cause a rise in ICP; therefore it is important for the nurse to have an understanding of the pathophysiology of raised ICP and how it affects the patient, to ensure appropriate and effective patient care.

The physiology of raised intracranial pressure

The brain is composed of brain tissue (80%), blood (10%) and CSF (10%). It is encased in the relatively rigid skull. Within this space, there is little room for any of the components to expand or increase in volume. Through the processes of accommodation and compliance, the ICP is maintained at its normal level of 0–15 mmHg (average 10 mmHg) despite transient increases in pressure that occur with straining during defecation, sneezing or coughing. According to the Monro–Kellie hypothesis, any increase in the volume of one component must be compensated for by a decrease in the volume of one of the other components.

As a first response to an increase in volume of any of these components:

- the CSF is shunted or displaced from the cranial compartment to the spinal subarachnoid space

- the rate of CSF absorption is increased
- the rate of CSF production is decreased.

An additional response, if needed, is:

- a decrease in cerebral blood volume by the displacement of cerebral venous blood into the sinuses.

As long as the brain is able to compensate for the increase in volume and to remain compliant, there are minimal increases in ICP. However, once the compensatory mechanisms have been exhausted, a small additional change in volume results in a large pressure rise. As the ICP increases, cerebral blood flow decreases, leading to tissue hypoxia, a decrease in serum pH level and an increase in CO_2 levels. This process causes cerebral vasodilatation and oedema, resulting in further increases in the ICP, and the cycle continues.

If the condition is not treated, the brain, as it swells within the rigid box of the skull, herniates downwards towards the brain stem, causing irreversible brain damage and eventually brain-stem death.

Early detection of raised ICP may be life saving and may also reduce the risk of further brain damage by preventing secondary damage to the brain. Secondary damage is potentially irreversible and can occur as a result of:

- cerebral oedema
- haematoma
- ischaemia
- infection.

Contributory factors also include:

- hypoxia
- hypercapnia (high levels of CO_2 in the blood)
- hypotension.

Damage to the brain tissue occurs primarily because the delivery of oxygen and glucose to the brain is interrupted.

Symptoms of raised ICP

These include:

- reduction in GCS
- headache
- nausea and/or vomiting
- limb weakness, usually down one side

- alteration in pupil reactions
- papilloedema
- seizures
- speech deficits
- agitation.

Late signs include:

- bradycardia
- rise in blood pressure
- changes in respiratory pattern.

Nursing care of a patient with raised ICP

The aim of care for these patients is to avoid further increases in ICP and to prevent or limit any secondary damage. Thorough assessment is essential to gather as much early information as possible, followed by continuous assessment of the patient's neurological state.

ICP can rise during nursing care, especially when there is no break between procedures. Therefore the patient's care should be planned to ensure a break of at least 15 minutes between activities. Clustering of procedures, such as mouth care, eye care, bed bath and linen changes, should be avoided, and you will need to work closely with other members of the multidisciplinary team to ensure this can be achieved.

The patient's head should be slightly elevated (no more than 30° of tilt) to promote venous drainage via the neck veins. Flexing and extending the neck can inhibit drainage, so the patient should be nursed in natural alignment at all times. This involves log-rolling the patient when changing position and using pillows and rolls to keep the head in alignment when the patient is lying on one side. Hip flexion must also be avoided as it can increase intrathoracic pressure, which in turn adversely affects cerebral venous drainage. Oropharyngeal suction also increases ICP and should be avoided if possible. Straining on defecation can raise ICP, so great care must me taken to ensure that the patient does not become constipated.

Other aspects of nursing care are aimed at minimizing the factors that can cause secondary brain damage. As these factors include hypoxia and hypercapnia, the nurse must ensure that the patient's respiratory function does not deteriorate. If oxygenation is compromised, then appropriate treatment, such as physiotherapy, oxygen therapy or antibiotics for chest infections, must be instigated promptly. Any pyrexia should be treated immediately, as a rise of 1°C above normal body temperature (37°C) increases the brain's metabolic demands by 10%, which could further compromise the brain's oxygen supply. This could result in increased cerebral ischaemia.

Communication has been shown to reduce the ICP of patients with head injury, as has therapeutic touch, although overstimulation should be avoided. The nurse will need to educate the patient's family about the benefits and dangers of overstimulation and encourage them to talk to the patient in a quiet and calm manner. Many patients with raised ICP are unconscious or have an altered level of consciousness, so the earlier sections describing the care of these patients also need to be considered.

Meningitis

Action point 4

Meningitis is quite a common condition. What do you know about it? How can you tell that someone may be suffering from meningitis?

Meningitis is an inflammation of the meninges that covers the brain and spinal cord. Bacterial and viral organisms are most often responsible for meningitis, although fungal and protozoal meningitis also occurs.

- Bacterial meningitis occurs most frequently and early detection and treatment are associated with a more favourable outcome.
- Viral meningitis is usually self-limiting, and the patient makes a complete recovery.

The organisms responsible for meningitis enter the CNS via the blood-stream at the blood–brain barrier. Direct routes of entry occur as a result of penetrating trauma, surgical procedures or a ruptured cerebral abscess. Otorrhoea (ear discharge) or rhinorrhoea (nasal discharge), which may be caused by a fracture of the base of the skull, can lead to meningitis, owing to the direct communication of the CSF with the environment.

Common types of meningitis

- Meningococcal: caused by the meningitis bacterium. This infection is transmitted through respiratory droplets.
- Haemophilus: caused by the *Haemophilus influenzae* organism. This bacterium is transmitted via direct contact with respiratory secretions.
- Pneumococcal: caused by the *Steptococcus pneumoniae* bacterium. This is also transmitted through secretions of the respiratory tract, and may be by either direct or indirect contact.
- Viral: this is not transmitted from person to person and can be caused by most viral infections.

Meningococcal meningitis is the most virulent form of meningitis and is most prevalent among children and teenagers. One of the most important signs in diagnosis is the now well-publicized rash that does not blanch when compressed by a drinking glass. This form of meningitis is accompanied by blood coagulation problems and may result in circulatory collapse.

Diagnosis

Diagnosis is confirmed through a lumbar puncture, where CSF is obtained for culture. Blood cultures, nose and throat swabs are also taken. If the cause of meningitis is not clear, occasionally CT or MRI may show the original site of the infection. Complications include the development of seizures caused by cerebral irritability, and blocking of the arachnoid villi with debris of white cells, which will result in the prevention of CSF flow and lead to the development of hydrocephalus. This will be indicated by the patient becoming increasingly drowsy, the blood pressure rising, and the pulse and respiration rates decreasing (raised ICP).

Patient symptoms

- General discomfort, including severe, unrelenting headache.
- Photophobia.
- Limb pain, backache and fever.
- Meningeal irritability causing:
    - nuchal rigidity – a stiff neck, particularly when neck is flexed
    - positive Kernig's sign – to elicit this sign the nurse flexes the patient's leg at the hip, brings the knee to a 90° angle, then attempts to extend the knee. If meningitis is present, the patient will experience pain and spasm of the hamstring muscle when the leg is straightened
    - positive Brudzinski's sign – to test, the nurse gently flexes the patient's head and neck on to the chest. A positive response is indicated by flexion of the hips and knees.
- Nausea due to cerebral/meningeal irritation.
- Deterioration in conscious level, disorientation, drowsiness.
- Meningeal irritability may lead to seizures.
- Fever and chills, tachycardia
- Red, macular, non-blanching, widespread rash (in meningococcal meningitis).

Nursing care of the patient with meningitis

The most important nursing intervention for patients with meningitis is the accurate monitoring and recording of their neurological status, vital signs and vascular assessment. In addition, it is vital that the patient receives the appropriate antibiotics as soon as possible. Other areas of nursing care are summarized below:

- Take vital signs and perform neurological observations (GCS) every 2–4 h or as instructed.
- Give prescribed analgesia and antiemetics as soon as possible to reduce the patient's discomfort.
- Give medications as ordered, and document the patient's response.
- The patient will be sensitive to noise and light, and therefore should be nursed in a quiet environment without bright lights.
- Treat pyrexia.
- Fluid balance should be recorded, and the patient who is nauseated may require intravenous fluids.
- Safety precautions to prevent patient injury should be taken if the patient is drowsy or if seizures occur.
- Barrier nursing is indicated until the diagnosis is confirmed, including the type of infection.
- Perform vascular assessment to prevent and detect early vascular compromise from septic emboli by assessing extremities for temperature, colour, pulses and capillary refill. If vascular compromise is left unrecognized and untreated, gangrene can develop quickly, leading to the possible loss of the involved extremity.

Brain tumours

Brain tumours are relatively rare, with approximately 4000 new cases a year in the UK, so the average GP will see a new case once every 9 years. It is essential that patients are treated at specialist centres where experienced and knowledgeable healthcare professionals can provide effective care for the patient and their family. The impact of such a diagnosis is immense and begins a journey of uncertainty, fear and hope for patients and families. The effects of a brain tumour on an individual can be devastating, as the tumour can affect control of the body's vital systems, movement, sensation, intellect, memory and personality. Therefore such patients and their families need to be cared for in a compassionate, sensitive and humanistic manner.

Pathophysiology

Primary brain tumours occur as a rapid proliferation or abnormal growth of cells normally found within the CNS. Neurons stop dividing and multiplying at birth and do not give rise to tumours. However, the support cells (glial cells) carry on reproducing, so they are susceptible to tumour formation.

The most common tumour of this 'intrinsic' type is the astrocytoma. Tumours can also arise from the cells of the dura mater, which lines the skull, or from the cells sheathing the cranial nerves. These are called meningiomas and neuromas respectively. Secondary brain tumours occur when malignant cells from other tumours outside the CNS metastasize to the brain.

Classification of tumours

Brain tumours are generally classified as malignant or benign.

Benign

- Slow rate of growth.
- Do not infiltrate healthy tissue.
- Easy to differentiate from normal tissue.

Malignant

- Rapid growth.
- Infiltrate healthy tissue.
- Difficult to separate from normal tissue.
- May spread through the CSF pathways.

Although benign tumours are generally associated with a favourable outcome, this is often not the case with malignant tumours. However, benign tumours may be malignant by virtue of their location, if they are situated near a vital structure within the brain. If the tumour cannot be completely removed or treated, it continues to grow. As it invades other brain tissue, cerebral oedema, focal neurological deficits and an increased ICP occur. Herniation of the brain tissue eventually leads to death. In addition, benign tumours may undergo histological changes and become malignant.

Signs and symptoms

The particular clinical presentation of a brain tumour in a patient depends on:

- the compression or infiltration of specific cerebral tissue
- the related cerebral oedema
- the development of increased ICP.

The patient with a brain tumour can complain of a wide variety of symptoms, many of which can be mistaken for signs of other, more common diseases. Onset may be slow and insidious (e.g. with personality change) or it may be rapid and dramatic, as with epilepsy. Headache is one of the most common presenting signs. Headaches may be localized or more general and are frequently worse in the early morning.

Focal symptoms

The tumour infiltrating or pressing on nearby structures causes focal symptoms. This effect is compounded by oedema in the compressed tissue. Even very small tumours can cause major problems in a crowded area. For example, a tumour may press on the seventh (facial) cranial nerve, leading to a one-sided facial weakness. Focal symptoms include:

- dysphasia (speech areas)
- unilateral weakness or altered sensation (motor and sensory strips)
- memory impairment (temporal lobes)
- personality change (frontal lobe)
- disordered co-ordination (cerebellum and brain stem)
- tunnel vision (optic nerve pathways)
- deafness and vertigo (eighth cranial nerve)
- cortical blindness (occipital lobe)
- hormonal derangement (hypothalamus and pituitary gland).

Epilepsy

Epilepsy is a common presenting symptom in tumours above the tentorium and affects 30% of patients (Lindsay et al. 1997). It is caused either when the tumour presses on healthy tissue or when the tumour takes away the blood supply from healthy tissue, damaging it. The seizures are usually partial, affecting only one part of the body, but they can become generalized.

Hydrocephalus

Hydrocephalus is usually the result of a tumour blocking the CSF flow through the narrow aqueducts (infratentorial tumours such as medulloblastomas are most likely to do this). Patients with hydrocephalus complain of headache (common first thing in the morning), nausea and vomiting. Children under 2 years may have an enlarged head circumference and 'sunset eyes', where only the upper half of the iris is visible above the lower eyelid. Untreated hydrocephalus causes a dangerous rise in ICP.

Increased ICP

As a tumour enlarges, it occupies space that should be occupied by brain tissue, a situation made worse by the swollen tissue around the tumour. Since the skull cannot expand, ICP rises. Blood supply is reduced, as the blood vessels are squeezed and healthy tissue becomes ischaemic. The damaged tissue then becomes swollen resulting in the ICP rising further. If a tumour and surrounding oedematous tissue grow large enough, they will have what is called a mass effect, pushing the brain's structures out of alignment. The affected side pushes across the midline, compressing the non-affected side (midline shift). This can occur without warning – even in people with no previous symptoms – if one of the fragile blood vessels in or around the tumour ruptures. The patient will have signs of a dangerously high ICP and will be close to death.

Investigations

Initial investigation centres on the history and presentation. CT and MRI will show the location of the tumour and its position, and the way it responds to radio-opaque contrast dye will reveal much about its type. However, the only accurate way to identify the type and malignancy of a tumour is by taking a biopsy. These are usually obtained by stereotactic biopsy, a technique that uses a special external frame and CT to map three-dimensional co-ordinates of the lesion. This allows a biopsy to be taken through a small burr hole, resulting in minimal disruption to normal tissue.

Prognosis

The prognosis depends on the type, grade and location of the brain tumour. The most malignant tumours, e.g. the glioblastoma multiforme, carry a very poor prognosis, and the patient's life expectancy may be only a matter of months. This has implications for the treatment options offered to the patient and the care and support required.

Treatment

The treatment needed depends on the type of tumour and its location. If a cure is not possible, the aim of treatment is to improve the patient's quality of life by reducing the size of the tumour, which will relieve symptoms. Unfortunately, the improvement may be only temporary.

Steroid therapy, in particular dexamethasone, is used to reduce the oedema in the tissue around the tumour. This can result in a dramatic improvement in symptoms, which can lead to false optimism for the patient and family.

The treatment for the majority of brain tumours is still surgery. If the tumour is benign, complete removal may be possible. Malignant tumours are hard to distinguish from brain tissue and may be impossible to remove entirely. In such cases, the tumour is partially removed or debulked.

Location is also important: the surgeon will be more cautious when operating around critical zones, such as the speech areas or the brain stem. One option is the 'awake craniotomy' in which the patient's anaesthetic is reversed during surgery so that the function of particular areas can be assessed during the operation. This technique aims to remove as much of the tumour as possible, while minimizing damage to important parts of the brain.

If surgery is not possible, radiotherapy is used, but is more commonly combined with surgery when total removal is not an option. Malignant tumours, which grow rapidly, are more susceptible to radiation than the slower-growing benign tumours, although the tendency of malignant growths to infiltrate makes it difficult to target tumour cells without disrupting normal tissue. As the blood–brain barrier buffers the brain's environment from the rest of the body, chemotherapy is not a very effective treatment because of the toxic levels of drugs that have to be given to have any real impact on the tumour cells.

Nursing care of a patient with a brain tumour

One of the main priorities in the care of patients with brain tumours is patient safety. All brain tumours pose the risk of a sudden and life-threatening rise in ICP, as well as such symptoms as epilepsy or hemiparesis. Regular observation of the GCS and vital signs is essential.

Some dangers can be less obvious and therefore require careful assessment based on knowledge of the individual patient's disease. Pain is often a problem, so needs to be managed quickly and effectively. Although strong analgesia may be required, it is important not to make the patient drowsy (which can make accurate assessment of their GCS very difficult) or suppress respiration. Codeine phosphate and dihydrocodeine are commonly used, although morphine is now often used in the immediate postoperative period. Nausea and vomiting are also common and should be treated with antiemetic medication and intravenous fluids.

After the patient's safety and immediate comfort are assured, a full nursing assessment should be made and the nursing care planned to meet the individual needs. This needs to be re-evaluated frequently. For example, a patient with a tumour around Broca's speech area in the temporal lobe may be expressively dysphasic. The patient knows what he wants to say but cannot find the words, using the wrong ones or even makes them up. This can cause difficulties over a wide range of activities, e.g. the patient may not eat properly if he cannot ask for the food he likes, he may have continence problems if he cannot ask for a bottle when he needs one, and so on.

Psychological care

Perhaps no role is more important than that of providing sensitive, supportive care for the patient and family throughout the course of the illness. As much of the anxiety of any illness is associated with loss of control, it is not surprising that a diagnosis of a brain tumour is particularly frightening. In addition, there is a social stigma associated with cognitive and neurological illness, which can leave the patient and family feeling isolated.

When a brain tumour, especially one such as glioblastoma multiforme, is diagnosed, the patient and family may experience denial, as well as anger and acceptance.

The patient, who may have been the breadwinner and head of the family, becomes dependent and, as a result of the illness, family dynamics and relationships may change. These changes to established family roles can be made worse if the location of the tumour produces cognitive or memory problems in the patient. For example, it can be very stressful to have to remind someone every few minutes where they are and it is distressing when a loved one's personality has changed.

Although patients with brain tumours share many treatments and experiences with patients who have other forms of cancer, many brain tumours are very aggressive, and this often leads to a rapid decline in cognitive function not seen in other cancers.

Conclusion

The care of the patient with a cerebral condition can be very demanding for the nurse, but with clear guidelines and focused treatment and nursing care, the patient and family can be helped through the often disturbing and frightening effects of these types of illness.

References and further reading

Ackerman KD (2000) Stress and its relationship to disease activity in multiple sclerosis. International Multiple Sclerosis Journal 7(1): 20–29.

Addison C (2001) Systems and diseases: the nervous system 10. Nursing Times 97(22): 43–46.

Addison C, Shah S (1998) Neurosurgery. In Guerrero W (ed) Neuro-oncology for Nurses. London: Whurr.

Barker EC (1994) Neuroscience Nursing, St Louis, MO: Mosby.

Barker R (1999) Neuroscience at a Glance. Oxford: Blackwell Science.

Bassett C, Makin L (2000) Caring for the Seriously Ill Patient. London: Arnold.

Bickerstaff E (1995) Neurology. London: Hodder & Stoughton.

Boskwick J, Sneade M (2001) Nursing a patient after subarachnoid haemorrhage. Nursing Times 97(34): 36–37.

British Society of Rehabilitation Medicine (1993) Working Party Report Multiple Sclerosis. London: BSRM

Brunker C , Shah S (2001) Systems and diseases: the nervous system 11. Nursing Times 97(26): 43–46.

Campbell P, Edwards S (1997) Hyperdynamic therapy: the nurse's role in the treatments of cerebral vasospasm. Journal of Neuroscience Nursing 29(5): 318–324.

Caplan I (1992) Intracerebral haemorrhage. The Lancet 339: 656–658.

Davis S (1999) Rehabilitation Nursing: foundations for practice. Edinburgh: Baillière Tindall.

Donnan GA, Davies SM, Chambers BR et al. (1996) Streptokinase for acute ischemic stroke with relationship to time of administration. Journal of the American Medical Association 276(12): 961–966.

Drake C (1988) Report of the World Federation of Neurological Surgeons Committee on a Universal Subarachnoid Haemorrhage Grading Scale. Journal of Neurosurgery 68(6): 985–986.

Fairley D, Cosgrove J (1998) Leeds General Infirmary Neuroscience Unit: Clinical guidelines for Performing Glasgow Coma Scale and Pupillary Responses. Leeds: ULTH Trust.

Fairley D, Cosgrove J (1999) Glasgow Coma Scale: improving nursing practice through clinical effectiveness. Nursing In Critical Care 4(6): 276–279.

Fisher JS (2000) Neuropsychological effects of beta interferon 1a in relasping multiple sclerosis. Annals of Neurology 48(6): 885–892.

Fox S, Lantz C (1998) The brain tumour experience and quality of life; a qualitative study. Journal of Neuroscience Nursing 30(4): 245–252.

Hickey JV (1997) The Clinical Practice of Neurological and Neurosurgical Nursing. Philadelphia, PA: Lippincott.

Hinds J (1990) Prevalence of bowel dysfunction in multiple sclerosis: a population survey. Gastroenterology 98(6): 1538–1542.

Hutchinson P (1998), Factors implicated in details from subarachnoid haemorrhage: are they available? British Journal of Neurosurgery 1(1): 37–40.

Iacono RP (1995) The results, indications, and physiology of postventral pallidotomy for patients with Parkinson's disease. Neurosurgery 36(6): 118–125.

Ignatavicious DD, Warkman ML, Misher MA (1996) Medical-Surgical Nursing across the Health Care Continuum, 3rd edn. Philadelphia, PA: WB Saunders.

Kyriazis M (1994) Devlopments in the treatment of stroke patients. Nursing Times 90(29): 30–32.

Lampl Y (1995) Neurological and functional outcome in patients with supratentorial haemorrhages. A prospective study. Stroke 26(12): 2249–2253.

LaRocca NG (1995) Employment and Multiple Sclerosis Health Service Research Reports. New York: National Multiple Sclerosis Society Information for Nurses and Health Professionals, Herts: MSRT.

Lindsay KW, Bone I, Callender R (1997) Neurology and Neurosurgery Illustrated, 3rd edn. Edinburgh; Churchill Livingstone.

Lubin FD, Reingold SC (1996) Defining the clinical cause of multiple sclerosis: results of an international survey. Neurology 46(4): 907–911.

Multiple Sclerosis Research Trust (1999) Multiple Sclerosis Information for Nurses and Health Professionals. Herts. MSRT.

Muxlow J (2000) Caring for the neurological system. In Bassett C, Makin L (eds) Caring for the Seriously Ill Patient. London: Arnold.

Phadke JG, Downe AW (1987) Epidemiology of multiple sclerosis in the north east. (Grampian region) of Scotland – an update. Journal of Epidemiology and Community Health 41(1): 5–13.

Quiney N et al. (1996) Pain after craniotomy. A time for reappraisal. British Journal of Neurosurgery 10(3): 295–299.

Russell A (1995) Epilepsy. Nursing Standard 10(3): 33–38.

Sadovinick AD (1992) Life expectancy in patients attending multiple sclerosis clinics. Neurology 42(5): 991–994.

Shorvon S (2000) Handbook of Epilepsy Treatment. Oxford: Blackwell Science.

Smith M (1999) Rehabilitation in Adult Nursing Practice. Edinburgh: Churchill Livingstone.

Stoneham M, Walters F (1995) Post-operative analgesia for craniotomy patients: current attitudes among neuroanaesthetists. European Journal of Anaesthesiology 12(6): 571–575.

Teasdale G, Jennett B (1974) Assessment of coma and impaired consciousness. The Lancet ii: 81–83.

Viney C (1996) Nursing the Critically Ill Patient. London: Baillière Tindall.

Watkiss K , Ward N (2001) Systems and diseases: nervous system 8, 9. Nursing Times 97(14): 43–46.

Widdows K (2001) Systems and diseases: nervous system 12. Nursing Times 97(30): 45–48.

Youdium BH, Riederer P (1997) Understanding Parkinson's disease. Scientific American Medicine 39(1): 52–59.

CHAPTER FIVE

The renal system

ROBERT DONALD

Introduction

This chapter explores the assessment of the renal system. It considers the physiology of the kidney and bladder and discusses issues concerned with medical and surgical interventions. Fluid balance and replacement therapy are discussed in relation to other chapters, and nursing care and medical treatment are described.

The renal system is often regarded simply as the means by which the body removes the end products of protein metabolism and excess water, in the form of urine. However, it is a highly sophisticated collection of physiological functions, which has an impact on all the systems of the body. The effects of renal dysfunction reflect that complexity and the student nurse may well be faced with such a diverse range of symptoms that it may sometimes be difficult to distinguish cause and effect, with subsequent life-threatening clinical situations developing rapidly. The linking of seemingly disparate signs and symptoms to the patient's diminishing renal function can serve to speed diagnosis and prevent further renal damage, which could prolong recovery of adequate renal function in acute renal failure or preserve what residual renal function remains in chronic renal failure.

After an initial brief overview of the anatomy and physiology of the renal system, there is a more detailed consideration of the physiology as each aspect of dysfunction is explored. This should enable the student nurse to recognize the genesis of renal dysfunction as well as to distinguish the potential causes from the symptomatic effects of dysfunction.

Anatomy and physiology: an overview

Action point 1

Write down all you can remember about the anatomy and functions of the renal system.

The renal system (Figure 5.1) consists of two bean-shaped structures – the kidneys – which lie either side of the spine in the retroperitoneal space at the level of the twelfth thoracic and third lumbar vertebrae. Each kidney is approximately 10–12 cm in length and 5–7 cm in width, or about 'the size of the owner's fist'. The left kidney sits behind the spleen and the right behind the liver, slightly lower than the left kidney. Each weighs approximately 150 g. Both kidneys are heavily protected. The upper poles are covered by the lower ribs, and they are further protected by three outer layers. The renal fascia, a fibrous layer of connective tissue, anchors the kidneys to the inferior abdominal wall, and each kidney is enclosed in a tough fibrous capsule of connective tissue.

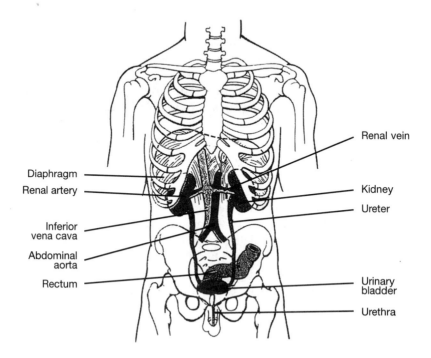

Figure 5.1 The renal system in the male.

Exiting each kidney via its inner concave surface is the ureter, and at a fissure in the central portion – the hilus – the renal blood vessels enter and leave. These blood vessels comprise the renal arteries and the renal veins. The kidneys require a tremendous volume of blood to function – approximately a quarter to a third of the cardiac output.

The ureters are tubes about 25–30 cm in length, which extend from the renal pelvis to the posterior wall of the bladder. They are made up of three layers: an inner mucous membrane; a middle section of smooth muscle, which contracts and propels urine in peristaltic spurts; and an outer, fibrous coat.

The bladder lies in the lower abdomen and can be described as a collapsible bag, with walls made up of two sets of smooth muscle. The detrusor muscle is tremendously flexible, with the ability to stretch to the thickness of one cell, and is under the control of the autonomic nervous system. The trigone, a triangular-shaped muscle which also responds to autonomic nerve stimuli, lies between the entry points of the two ureters. It differs from the detrusor muscle in that it does not expand during bladder filling.

Contraction of the detrusor and relaxation of the trigone lead to the bladder emptying into the urethra. This is controlled by the smooth muscle of the internal urinary sphincter and the external urinary sphincter.

The structure of the kidney

The kidney comprises the cortex, medulla, major and minor calyces, and the renal pelvis (Figure 5.2).

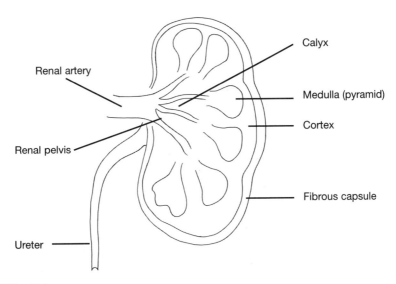

Figure 5.2 The kidney.

The cortex is made up of nephrons, which number approximately 1 million per kidney. These nephrons are 'blind-ended' tubes extending from the collecting ducts, which themselves make up the medulla and which drain into the major and minor calyces, emptying into the renal pelvis.

The renal vasculature is formed from the renal artery entering the kidney at the hilus and then segmenting into branches between the calyces. Venous drainage, which runs alongside the arteries, leaves the kidney at the point of the hilus, in the form of the renal vein, which joins the inferior vena cava.

At the microscopic level, the combination of nephrons (Figure 5.3) and associated arterioles forms the functioning parts of the kidney. It is the arrangement of the cellular structure and permeability of the nephron, arteriole and peritubular capillaries that enables the kidney to produce urine and regulate several homeostatic functions.

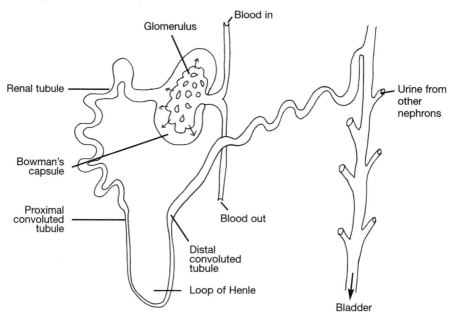

Figure 5.3 The renal system (nephron).

The blind end of the tubule distends to form the Bowman's capsule, which can be likened to a half-inflated balloon into which a tuft of small blood vessels from the intralobular arteries has been pushed. The Bowman's capsule and these small blood vessels form the glomerulus, where the first stage of urine production occurs, that of filtration.

Running from the Bowman's capsule is the proximal convoluted tubule, which is composed of highly permeable epithelial cells. These cells also have microvilli on their inner surface, which present the maximum possible surface area to the filtrate. The tubule then dips down from the cortex into the medulla and back up again into the cortex, forming the loop of Henle. The descending limb of the loop is thin and permeable, while the ascending limb becomes thicker and less permeable. Finally, before the nephron joins the collecting ducts, it forms a distal convoluted tubule.

Urine formation

Urine formation is a product of the application of three forces within the tubule. The first is hydrostatic pressure in the glomerular capillaries. Approximately 1 litre of blood per minute flows through the collective surface area of the glomerulus. The glomerular capillaries against which this pressure is applied are highly permeable; therefore there is a shift of fluid and substances from the blood into the Bowman's capsule, in the form of filtrate. The composition of this filtrate is determined by the molecular size of the substances being driven across the glomerulus. Substances of the same molecular weight as serum albumin or larger are too large to pass through the glomerular capillaries. Substances smaller than serum albumin will pass through and so form the filtrate.

The second force being applied is plasma oncotic pressure, which is the osmotic force created by the relative strength of the fluid in the glomerulus according to the concentration of plasma proteins it contains. In this case, as the blood passing through the glomerulus loses fluid by filtration, the concentration of the remaining blood increases and the plasma oncotic pressure rises, drawing fluid back from the filtrate. However, as long as hydrostatic pressure exceeds plasma oncotic pressure within the glomerulus, there will be a flow of filtrate from the blood into the nephron. The importance of plasma oncotic pressure becomes more critical in the proximal convoluted tubule, where the next stage of urine production occurs – reabsorption.

Approximately 120 ml of filtrate are produced per minute, which equates to approximately 180 litres per day. Yet, under normal circumstances, urine volume is only about 1 litre per day. Thus over 99% of the filtrate is reabsorbed.

In the proximal convoluted tubule, the relative difference in 'strength' of the filtrate and the blood in the peritubular capillaries means that the oncotic gradient is from the relatively weak filtrate to the relatively 'strong' blood. The highly permeable tubule wall and the increased inner surface area of the tubular cells facilitate reabsorption, and there is passive reabsorption of water and substances vital for normal metabolism. About two-thirds of the water and electrolytes and all the filtered glucose and amino acids are reabsorbed here.

The loop of Henle takes the forces generated by osmotic and oncotic pressure differences and creates a countercurrent mechanism, by which filtrate is concentrated and sodium (Na^+) and water are conserved. This is achieved by the movement of water from the filtrate in the descending limb of the loop to the interstitial space between the descending and ascending limbs. In the ascending limb, the permeability of the wall is reduced, and water is unable to move back into the filtrate. However, Na⁺ and chloride (Cl⁻) ions move from the filtrate to the interstitial space by the process of diffusion. The blood vessels surrounding the tubule then reabsorb this water and the electrolytes. In this way, the volume of filtrate is reduced by approximately 15%, while the relative strength of the filtrate and blood becomes more even.

The distal convoluted tubule is where the homeostatic balances of the body are achieved and where the third force – active transport – plays a significant role, resulting in selective reabsorption. This area of the nephron reabsorbs small and variable volumes of filtrate, mainly under the influence of hormone control systems.

The volumes reabsorbed depend on the needs of the body as a whole either to conserve water and electrolytes or to excrete them. The feedback mechanisms that determine these needs are changes in systemic blood pressure (BP), the autoregulation of blood flow to the kidney and changes in blood osmolarity. These changes result in the release of antidiuretic hormone (ADH) and aldosterone.

When blood osmolarity increases, ADH is released from the posterior pituitary gland at the base of the brain. In the presence of ADH, the permeability of the distal convoluted tubules increases and water passes from the filtrate to the blood by osmosis, whereas in the absence of ADH water remains in the tubule and so more urine is passed. Therefore, blood osmolarity regulates the selective reabsorption of water.

Aldosterone is produced by the adrenal glands, which are located one on top of each kidney: Two factors stimulate its production: an increase in plasma concentration of potassium (K⁺) and a decrease in BP. As with ADH, in the presence of aldosterone, the distal convoluted tubule becomes more permeable to water. At the same time, active transport mechanisms within the tubule cells secrete K⁺ and hydrogen (H⁺) ions back into the filtrate. In this way, excess ions are excreted while the circulatory volume, and therefore BP, increases.

Several other functions take place within the tubule, as well as those of the excretion of urea nitrogen waste, conservation of vital substances, regulation of blood osmolarity and regulation of BP. These are:

- the production of the hormone erythropoietin, which stimulates the production of red cells in the bone marrow
- the regulation of calcium and phosphate homeostasis via the conversion of vitamin D to its active form in order to absorb calcium from the diet and effect the mobilization of calcium and phosphate in bone.

By the time the filtrate arrives at the collecting duct it is finally urine, i.e. water, salts, acids and nitrogenous wastes, all at concentrations determined by the body's needs to maintain its homeostatic state.

Action point 2

What types of renal problems have you heard of or come across in your patients?

Causes and classifications of renal dysfunction

Renal dysfunction is classically divided into acute renal failure and chronic renal failure, with considerable differences in their presentation and potential clinical outcomes. Acute renal failure forms the main focus of this chapter, with chronic renal failure discussed in less detail.

Acute renal failure is characterized by the abrupt cessation of renal function, resulting in retention of nitrogenous waste products in the body. In addition, there is a failure to regulate fluid and electrolyte homeostasis adequately. The condition is potentially reversible provided the patient is treated successfully for the cause or causes and receives prompt treatment for the potentially lethal effects of the renal dysfunction. The mortality associated with acute renal failure is most commonly due to the effects of fluid overload, hyperkalaemia (raised serum K^+ level) and acidosis (Donald 2000).

Chronic renal failure, on the other hand, is characterized by usually slow and insidious onset, as the causative disease process destroys the renal structure. The development of the symptoms of renal dysfunction will depend on the extent and progression of the renal destruction, until eventually the residual renal function is insufficient to maintain life without mechanical renal replacement therapy. This is known as end-stage renal failure (ESRF), and the patient will be faced with the prospect of haemodialysis or continuous ambulatory peritoneal dialysis for the rest of his life unless he receives a kidney transplant.

The causes of acute renal failure are usually divided into three groups:

1. those that decrease the blood flow to the kidney (prerenal)
2. those that attack the structure of the kidney itself (intrarenal)
3. those that obstruct the flow of urine along the renal tract (postrenal or obstructive).

These are listed in Table 5.1.

Table 5.1 Causes of acute renal failure

Causative conditions	Potential conditions
Prerenal causes	
Hypovolaemia	• Haemorrhage – trauma, surgery • Gastrointestinal loss – vomiting, diarrhoea, gastric infections, bowel obstruction • Polyurea – diuresis, nephritic syndrome, excess diuretic use • Fluid redistribution – hypoalbuminaemia, hypoproteinaemia, malnutrition, pancreatitis, peritonitis • Vasodilatation – excess antihypertensive use, septic shock, anaphylaxis • Burns • Dehydration
Decreased cardiac output	• Left ventricular failure • Right-sided heart failure • Valvular disease • Pericarditis and pericardial tamponade • Myocardial infarction • Pulmonary embolism • Arrhythmias • Cardiomyopathy • Cardiogenic shock
Renal vascular disease	• Renal artery stenosis • Dissecting aortic aneurysm • Vasoconstriction – effect of non-steroidal anti-inflammatory drugs on the afferent arterioles
Intrarenal causes	
Glomerular damage	• Acute glomerulonephritis – post-streptococcal, rapidly progressive glomerulonephritis • Secondary to systemic disease – systemic lupus erythematosus, papillary necrosis, Goodpasture's syndrome, Wegener's granulomatosis, endocarditis
Tubular damage	• Ischaemic – acute tubular necrosis (mean systemic blood pressure <60–70 mmHg in the afferent arteriole) caused by shock, heart failure, effects of 'prerenal' causes • Nephrotoxic – acute tubular necrosis caused by antibiotics (sulphonomides, methicillin, cephalosporins, aminoglycosides, gentamicin, vancomycin), radiological contrast medium

Table 5.1 Causes of acute renal failure (contd)

Causative conditions	Potential conditions
Tubular damage (contd)	• Intratubular obstruction caused by casts and debris from myoglobulinuria and haemoglobinuria resulting from crush injury, hyperthermia, sepsis, alcohol and drug abuse, or mismatched blood transfusion; immune complex; uric acid; calcium • Infective nephritis caused by acute pyelonephritis, necrotizing papillitis, bacterial infections of the kidney and renal pelvis
Vascular damage	• Severe (malignant) hypertension • Disseminated intravascular coagulation • Scleroderma
Postrenal causes Urinary tract obstruction	• Structural obstruction – ureteric strictures, calculi, blood clots, retroperitoneal fibrosis and tumours compressing ureters, prostatic hypertrophy, urethral strictures, obstructed urinary catheters • Functional obstruction – drugs interfering with autonomic nerve activity to the bladder or ureters, e.g. antihistamines • Spinal cord damage • Diabetic neurological damage

The causes of chronic renal failure can be divided into two groups.

1. Primary renal disease: those disorders of the renal system itself in which the microscopic structure of the nephron is progressively destroyed, or where the gross structure of the kidney is damaged.
2. Secondary renal disease: those systemic disease processes that have a destructive impact on the kidney structure.

Systemic effects of renal dysfunction

Whatever the disease processes that cause the renal dysfunction, which have their own signs and symptoms, the effects of renal failure will have an impact on all the systems of the body (Table 5.2). These effects can be subtle or obvious, depending on the severity of the renal failure, and the patient may present with few outward symptoms or be severely ill, requiring high dependency or intensive care.

Table 5.2 Systemic effects of renal dysfunction

Renal function	Problems of renal dysfunction	Systems affected
Excretion Nitrogenous waste (urea, creatinine) Drugs and toxins	'Uraemia' and azotaemia (raised blood urea nitrogen) Raised internal toxic environment Increased metabolic rate Suppressed immunological response Retention of drugs or metabolites Nephrotoxic destruction of residual renal function	All systems
Fluid homeostasis	Fluid overload Oedema Pulmonary oedema Congestive cardiac failure Increased metabolic rate	Skin Tissues Cardiovascular Respiratory
Electrolyte homeostasis (Na^+, K^+)	*Hypernatraemia* Exacerbation of fluid retention and oedema Thirst Hypertension *Hyperkalaemia* Increased excitability of nerve tissue Coarse muscle twitching Grand mal convulsions Cardiac arrhythmias Ventricular tachycardia Ventricular fibrillation Exacerbation of acidosis	Haematological Tissues Skin Cardiovascular Central nervous system Respiratory
Control of blood pressure Control of circulating blood volume Control of renin/angiotensin cycle	Fluid-dependent hypertension Renin/angiotensin-dependent hypertension *Both:* CVA, hypertensive encephalopathy, retinopathy, bleeding, left ventricular hypertrophy, cardiac failure, increased reabsorption of sodium and water, increased metabolic rate	Cardiovascular Respiratory Tissues Skin Central nervous system

Table 5.2 Systemic effects of renal dysfunction (contd)

Renal function	Problems of renal dysfunction	Systems affected
Erythropoiesis (hormonal control of red cell production in bone marrow)	Renal anaemia: hypoxia, tiredness and lethargy, increased cardiac effort and angina, left ventricular hypertrophy, cardiac failure, increased metabolic rate, pallor, exacerbation of acidosis	Haematological Cardiovascular Tissues Respiratory Skin Central nervous system
Acid–base balance	Metabolic acidosis: tiredness and lethargy, confusion, grand mal convulsions, coma, 'air hunger' (Kussmaul's respiration), acetone on the breath, dry and coated tongue, increased metabolic rate, exacerbation of hyperkalaemia Increased ammonia in the blood Gastric irritation, ulceration Pleural irritation, rubs, effusions Pericardial irritation, rubs, effusions, tamponade	Haematological Central nervous system Respiratory Tissues Gastrointestinal Cardiovascular
Calcium and phosphate homeostasis in conjunction with vitamin D conversion	Renal bone disease associated with hyperphosphataemia: osteopenia, osteoporosis, osteomalacia, fractures, bone pain Calcification of soft tissues associated with hypercalcaemia (calcification of large vessel vascular tree), loss of control of BP, calcification of small vessels, ischaemia and occlusion, calcium nodule formation in tissues, skin, sclera, nerve tissue, clotting problems, puritus (itching), cardiac arrhythmias, confusion and disorientation	Skeletal Skin Tissues Haematological Central nervous system Cardiovascular

Action point 3

In what ways do you think we need to plan our care for the patient with renal problems?

Care planning for patients with renal disease

Care planning for the patient with renal dysfunction should centre around three key areas.

1. Treat the cause or causes of the renal dysfunction. This is particularly true in acute renal failure. However, in chronic renal failure the disease could have resolved a long time ago and no longer present an active problem. This would not be the case in renal failure secondary to such disease processes as diabetes, for example. Here, the ongoing management of the primary disease will have great benefit for the preservation of any residual renal function.
2. Protect the patient from the effects of renal dysfunction:
    – In acute renal failure, the symptoms of the dysfunction usually worsen rapidly, leading to death, and require vigorous intervention.
    – In chronic renal failure, the usually slow and progressive nature of the destruction of renal tissue may well produce symptoms that will cause increasing problems for all the body systems as they seek to adapt, leading to multiple pathology.
3. Preserve and enhance any residual renal function. This is particularly true in chronic renal failure, where any improvement in residual renal function will diminish the systemic effects of the failure. The longer the body can be helped to maintain its own homeostatic balances and residual renal function, the longer the patient can avoid the advent of ESRF, in which there is insufficient function to maintain life. At this point, mechanical means of replacing renal function are required, such as haemodialysis or continuous ambulatory peritoneal dialysis. The only way the patient can be free of such interventions is through a successful kidney transplantation.

Care planning for acute renal failure

Acute renal failure has a sudden onset, over hours or days, and results in a rapid and severe decline in glomerular filtration, which causes:

- oliguria or anuria
- retention of blood urea nitrogen (BUN)

- electrolyte and fluid imbalance
- acid–base imbalance
- haemodynamic instability.

Acute renal failure is both treatable and reversible. It has been reported as occurring in 5% of hospitalized patients, with a mortality rate ranging from 7% to as high as 80% in patients compromised by infection or cardiopulmonary complications (Thadhani et al. 1996). Control of the patient's hydration status, reversal of acidosis and correction of hyperkalaemia will significantly improve the patient's prognosis through the course of the failure to eventual renal recovery.

The course of acute renal failure has been described as having four phases: onset, oliguric, diuretic and recovery, each with distinct care planning requirements.

The onset phase is the period from the initial 'insult' to the beginning of the loss of control over urine production. This may take from 1 h to 2 days and is characterized by a decrease of renal perfusion to 25% of normal, a fall of urine output to 20% of normal, and clearance of BUN and solutes to 10% of normal.

The oliguric phase, which may also present as anuria, may last for 8–14 days and is characterized by the life-threatening effects of renal failure, fluid overload, acidosis and hyperkalaemia. The longer the patient remains in this phase, the lower the chances of survival.

Following the oliguric phase the nephrons begin to recover and the patient starts to pass increasing amounts of dilute urine, as the kidney slowly begins to take control of the concentration of urine. This then is the diuretic phase, with early diuresis producing an output volume 150–200% greater than normal, while clearance of BUN and solutes remains at 10% of normal. As diuresis continues, BUN and solute clearance normalize and urine volume gradually reduces.

The final phase is that of recovery, in which all the functions of the kidney return to normal or acceptable limits and the patient is asymptomatic. This phase may last for up to 6 months and the extent of the original 'insult' and the renal effects of dysfunction will determine the extent of any permanent damage.

Hydration status

First we must consider the three components of the maintenance of normal hydration status.

Intake mechanisms

Thirst is the driving force controlling fluid intake. It is produced by an increase in the tonicity of the blood due to loss of water from the circulating volume. As fluid is lost, serum Na^+ concentration increases, stimulating osmoreceptors in the hypothalamus of the brain. This 'thirst centre' then stimulates the release of ADH from the pituitary gland. ADH travels to the distal convoluted tubule, where it increases the permeability of the tubule walls, thus increasing the uptake of water from the filtrate back into the circulation.

Output mechanisms

An increase or decrease in the volume of urine produced and its relative 'strength' (high or low solute concentration) is dependent on the presence or absence of ADH and aldosterone. When these hormones are not secreted, the kidneys produce more dilute urine and fluid output increases. If the patient is dehydrated, ADH is released as described above. And in response to the fall in BP that accompanies dehydration, baroreceptors in the aortic arch and the macula densa of the renal tubules stimulate the adrenal cortex to secrete aldosterone. The action of the macula densa in the tubules is to stimulate the juxtaglomerular apparatus cells of the afferent arteriole to release renin, which converts to angiotensin I and II in the presence of oxygen and an enzyme from the liver. This leads to systemic vasoconstriction and an increase in Na^+ reabsorption by the distal convoluted tubule. As water follows the Na^+, there is a corresponding increase in water uptake from the filtrate to the blood. In addition, K^+ is secreted into the filtrate for excretion.

Location of fluid within the body compartments

The location of fluid within the body determines its availability for removal or retention by the action of the kidney under the influence of ADH or aldosterone. For its removal, the fluid must be in the circulation.

The forces that determine the location of fluid are:

- capillary hydrostatic pressure (blood pressure at the capillary level) forcing fluid from the circulation into the tissues
- capillary osmotic/oncotic pressure (the osmotic forces created by the concentration of plasma proteins within the circulation) drawing fluid from the tissues back into the blood
- interstitial fluid hydrostatic pressure (the force exerted by the volume of fluid in the tissues), which is determined by such factors as the rate and efficiency of lymphatic drainage versus the volume forced out of the capillaries.

Therefore, the BP, relative tonicity of the fluid and the plasma oncotic pressure of the blood will constantly be changing according to the body's hydration status as homeostasis is maintained.

Care and management of hydration in the onset phase

In the onset phase of acute renal failure, the patient's hydration status will depend on the cause of the renal dysfunction. In hypovolaemia and dehydration, it is essential to replace the circulatory volume. In cardiogenic failure (see Chapter 1), the removal of excess fluid and the possible use of inotropic agents play a role in stabilizing the cardiac output and BP. The aim is not only to address the physiological demands of the causative disorder, but also to protect the glomerular hydrostatic pressure and therefore the glomerular filtration rate. The shorter the period of renal hypotension, the swifter the recovery of renal function.

Care and management of hydration status in the oliguric/anuric phase

Oedema is one of the main features in the oliguric and anuric phases of acute renal failure. It can lead to peripheral oedema, 'overspill' of fluid from the circulation into the alveoli of the lungs causing pulmonary oedema, and an increase in cardiac effort causing left ventricular failure. Loss of control of the ability to regulate Na^+ will contribute greatly to the accumulation of fluid, as salt attracts fluid.

The aim in this phase is to regulate the patient's intake of fluid and restrict the intake of Na^+. Respiratory function should be supported to ensure adequate oxygenation of the tissues and to reduce the cardiac embarrassment caused by circulatory overload. Fluid restriction is based on the careful measurement of fluid balance on a day-by-day basis. Fluid intake and urine output are notoriously difficult to measure accurately, and so such information should be triangulated with changes in the patient's weight (if it is possible to weigh the patient). One litre of fluid is equivalent to 1 kilogram, so changes in weight can give a far more accurate indication of the fluid status over 24 h.

To estimate the fluid allowance for a patient, a volume of 500 ml is given to account for insensible loss (that from sweat, water vapour on the breath, etc.), and the total allowance is made up with the volume of the previous 24 h urine output. However, further considerations must be made for the overload volume of oedema, as the approach outlined would merely maintain such an overload. A target of fluid loss over the next 24 h must be made and this volume subtracted from the total allowance. This becomes the fluid restriction for the next 24 h (Donald 2000).

Other considerations in the correct estimation of fluid balance will centre on the level of Na^+ and plasma proteins in the body, as both will affect the availability of fluid for removal from the circulation. If the fluid is trapped in the tissues by hypernatraemia (raised serum Na$^+$ level) or is unable to re-enter the circulation because of low plasma oncotic pressure, then it cannot get to the kidney for removal by any residual renal function that may still be available. Restriction of Na$^+$ intake from any source – salt in food, condiments, Na$^+$ content of drugs, etc. – must be made. In addition, the patient's nutritional status must be addressed to prevent or reverse the catabolic effect of the acute renal failure and the associated increased utilization of protein in conjunction with its reduced intake due to anorexia.

In the oliguric patient with a residual renal function, that function may be enhanced with the use of diuretics. The use of furosemide or bumetanide is particularly useful, as these are loop diuretics and so enhance the removal of both salt and water.

Care and management of hydration status in the diuretic phase

Once renal function starts to recover, the patient enters the diuretic phase and fluid output increases. This cannot be regarded as a return to normal function, however, as the regulation of solutes and the efficient removal of BUN have not yet been achieved, despite the diuresis. The danger to the patient is as acute during this period as in the anuric phase, but for exactly the opposite reasons. There is a distinct possibility of dehydration if adequate replacement of fluid is not achieved. In addition, in the initial diuretic phase where solute removal remains inefficient, there is a possibility of an increase in the levels of both Na$^+$ and K$^+$ as a result of dehydration. A further potential complication can occur in patients who are poorly nourished and have low serum protein levels. In such cases, the circulatory volume may be reduced while plasma oncotic pressure is insufficient to draw fluid from the tissues to replace the volume loss. This will result in a circulatory hypovolaemic state with intractable tissue oedema.

Whatever the cause of the hypovolaemia in the diuretic phase, the effect will be the same – the nephron will be driven back into acute tubular necrosis. To ensure this does not happen, it is vital to maintain fluid balance, using the method described for the anuric phase. Where the volume loss exceeds 2–3 litres per day, the patient may require intravenous fluid support in addition to as much oral fluid as can be tolerated. In the case of the malnourished patient with low serum proteins, it may be necessary to provide additional supplement protein drinks, or even total parental nutrition (TPN).

As the diuretic phase continues, careful monitoring of serum Na$^+$ and K$^+$ levels is necessary, as these solutes will start to return to normal levels and so can be reintroduced to the patient's diet to avoid hyponatraemia or hypokalaemia.

Potassium status

There are three main causes of mortality in acute renal failure: the cardiac effect of fluid overload, acidosis and hyperkalaemia. Therefore it is essential to know the normal homeostasis of K^+.

Intake mechanisms

Potassium is the major cation of intracellular fluid and is acquired from the average diet at a rate of between 50 and 150 mmol/day (Sloan 2000). As K^+ is always found in association with protein, a protein-rich diet is a significant contributor to the daily K^+ intake. Other foods high in K^+ include:

- potatoes
- fruit and fruit juices
- vegetables and pulses
- chocolate
- coffee.

Output mechanisms

The renal control of K^+ excretion is based on glomerular filtration and passive reabsorption in the proximal tubule and selective reabsorption from, or secretion into, the distal convoluted tubule. This secretion occurs under the influence of the hormone aldosterone, which itself is part of the interlinked process of Na^+ regulation involving the renin–angiotensin cycle. This cycle is stimulated when there is a decrease in BP and a corresponding decrease in renal perfusion. Cells in the afferent arteriole release renin, which converts to angiotensin under the influence of an enzyme from the liver. Angiotensin brings about systemic vasoconstriction, while also stimulating the release of aldosterone from the adrenal gland. The action of aldosterone is to increase Na^+ reabsorption and, as a consequence, increase K^+ excretion by the distal tubule (Edwards 2001).

Location of K^+ within the body compartments

Concentration of K^+ within the cells is 28 times that of extracellular fluids. In conjunction with Na^+, it is responsible for the correct functioning of excitable cells such as muscles, neurons, sensory receptors, etc., through the action of the 'Na^+ pump mechanism'. It is also involved in the regulation of fluid levels within the cells and in maintaining the correct pH balance within the body.

K$^+$ enters the cells more readily than Na$^+$ and instigates a Na$^+$-K$^+$ exchange across the cell membrane. In nerve cells, this Na$^+$ pump mechanism generates the electrical potential that aids the conduction of nerve impulses. It is also important in cellular biochemical reactions and energy metabolism, in particular the synthesis of protein from amino acids. And it plays a role in carbohydrate metabolism in the conversion of glucose to glycogen, which is stored in the liver for future use (Merck 2001).

Care and management of the potassium status

Three factors need to be considered in the management of K$^+$ status:

- controlling the intake of K$^+$ from all sources
- enhancing the output of K$^+$ via the residual renal function
- regulating the patient's metabolic rate to reduce the K$^+$ loss from the intracellular compartment.

The range of K$^+$ levels that the body will tolerate is very narrow – 3.5–5.5 mmol/l – and a level exceeding 5.5 mmol/l is a potential cause of cardiac arrhythmia and death through ventricular fibrillation. Therefore, swift and decisive action is required in the face of hyperkalaemia.

The dietary intake of K$^+$ can be regulated by the avoidance of foods containing high levels of the electrolyte. However, patients in acute renal failure may be nutritionally challenged owing to anorexia and require TPN or nasogastric feeding, which makes this more difficult. Careful monitoring of serum K$^+$ levels is required throughout such nutritional support.

The patient's own residual renal function is the best way of reducing K$^+$ concentrations if such function can be enhanced with the use of diuretics. Again, care must be taken to avoid K$^+$-sparing diuretics, and the use of furosemide as a loop diuretic is favoured. If the residual renal function is insufficient to excrete the level of intracellular K$^+$ released, then a rapid, life-threatening hyperkalaemia occurs. This calls for two actions. First, the patient must be protected from the effects of the hyperkalaemia and, second, metabolic functioning must be brought under control. An intravenous infusion of dextrose 50% in conjunction with soluble insulin can effect a shift of K$^+$ back into the cells within 15 minutes, with the effect lasting 4–6 h while the infusion continues. Alternatively, an intravenous administration of 10–20 ml 10% calcium gluconate will have a similar effect, with the effect lasting approximately 1 h. With this 'breathing space', the cause of the hyperkalaemia can be addressed.

In the case of fluid-induced cardiac embarrassment, the removal of fluid and the reduction of the cardiac load will reduce the catabolic status. In the case of acidosis, sodium bicarbonate given intravenously will not only reduce the H⁺ concentration and return the blood pH to acceptable limits, but also reduce the stimulus to the cell walls by H⁺ inducing the release of potassium.

Continuous cardiac monitoring and ECG parameters may be required over this period and any ventricular tachycardia or extrasystole must be reported immediately to the senior staff.

In situations where K^+ is between 5.5 and 6 mmol/l, it can be controlled with the use of an ion-exchange resin. These work by binding K^+ in the gastrointestinal tract. As exchange resins have a tendency to cause constipation, the initial dose is often combined with a laxative agent such as sorbitol.

Acid–base balance

The lungs and the kidneys play vital roles in the physiological control of the body's pH, maintaining the homeostasis of the acids and bases. The respiratory control of pH is determined by changes in respiratory activity in response to the concentration of H⁺ in the blood. This is covered in Chapter 2.

The renal control of pH is concerned with metabolic acids as well as carbonic acid, and involves the removal of H⁺ by secretion and the creation and maintenance of substances that form buffers when combined with acids. In this way, the neutral pH of the body is maintained, despite the continual production of H⁺ by metabolic processes.

Respiratory compensation of acid–base imbalance with Kussmaul's breathing (deep rhythmic, sighing breaths) leaves the patient's mouth dry and coated, further complicating the ability to correct nutritional deficit. Extensive mouth care, especially in the face of fluid restriction, is required on a continuing basis.

Muscular weakness and cardiac depression due to the acidosis will respond to the administration of sodium bicarbonate. However, the liberation of K^+ from the intracellular compartment in response to acidosis can cause a rapid and fatal hyperkalaemia, and close observation and treatment must be instigated at the first symptoms.

Ultimately, the success of the conservative correction of the effects of acute renal failure depends on the degree of severity of the failure.

Care planning for patients with chronic renal failure

Chronic renal failure has been defined as the progressive, irreversible loss of the nephrons and nephron function. This can occur over a number of years, with dysfunction ranging from mild to severe kidney failure and ultimately progressing to ESRF. There are many systemic disease processes that can lead to chronic renal failure; however, the signs and symptoms will depend on the extent of the nephron damage, which is classified according to the amount of glomerular filtration that has been lost. ESRF is said to have occurred when virtually all renal function is lost and residual renal function is so inadequate that the patient's life cannot be sustained without mechanical renal replacement therapy.

The nurse could be faced with a patient in chronic renal failure who is not yet at end stage, and the care planning will have a great influence on the speed of the progression and the preservation of residual renal function. Once again the aim is to:

• treat the cause or causes of the renal dysfunction if it is still active
• protect the patient from the effects of renal failure
• preserve and enhance any residual renal function.

Three aspects of CRF are particularly threatening to the patient's survival: loss of control of BP, anaemia and calcium–phosphate imbalance.

Action point 4

Why do some patients have alterations in their blood pressure?

Blood pressure status

Blood pressure is created from three components:

1. the cardiac output (consisting of the stroke volume and the heart rate)
2. the peripheral resistance (the pressure exerted on the systemic blood vessel walls and their corresponding state of vasodilatation or vasoconstriction)
3. the viscosity of the blood itself (the ratio between the fluid volume and the cells).

There are several complex mechanisms used to maintain BP: the heart and circulation play a major role (Macintosh 2000); fluid and electrolyte concentrations stimulate factors that affect circulatory volume; and the kidney produces the stimulus for the hormonal control via the renin–angiotensin cycle.

In chronic renal failure, the predominant problem with BP is hypertension (raised arterial BP). However, this is something of a 'chicken and egg' situation in that essential hypertension can be a cause of renal failure, while chronic renal failure can ultimately lead to hypertension as a result of renal damage. In this section we will consider the two causes of BP disruption in chronic renal failure – that induced by fluid overload and that induced by overproduction of the hormone renin.

Care and management of blood pressure status

The major consideration in the management of the patient's BP status in chronic renal failure is the pharmacological control of hypertension. The patient's cardiac status will also need attention, in terms of either reducing the strain on the heart through the control of the hydration and Na^+ status, or the improvement of cardiac efficiency in the case of hypovolaemia induced by cardiac failure.

A consensus has been reached on the acceptable range of BP in patients with chronic renal failure (Table 5.3), but with targets individualized for patients' differing circumstances (Turner 1995).

Table 5.3 Acceptable range of blood pressure in patients with chronic renal failure

	Age	18–24	25–34	35–44	45–54	55–64	65–74
Male	Systolic	124	133	137	143	152	173
	Diastolic	79	83	87	89	89	87
Female	Systolic	119	122	130	141	160	179
	Diastolic	75	79	83	87	92	91

The patient's own independence and continuing self-care is vital in the attempt to maintain BP at an acceptable level. Compliance with dietary restrictions to modify fluid and sodium intake, and also with medication, can prove problematic, especially in the face of side effects of antihypertensive medication. Hypertension has often been described as the 'silent killer' (Goldsmith 2000), and if the patient associates the symptoms with the drug regimen and does not see the benefit of maintenance of such strict treatments then the motivation to comply with treatment will be severely reduced.

Patient education is the key factor in nursing this aspect of care. The accent should be on enabling the patient to read and understand his own BP and be aware of the benefits of maintaining its control. The assessment of the patient's perceptions of health status will give insight into the level of educational input required and the likelihood of the patient taking responsibility for lifestyle changes essential for BP control. These will include the modification of fluid and Na^+ intake, as highlighted in the section on the management of hydration status. Controlling hypertension will preserve residual renal function and avoid the potentially fatal secondary effects of uncontrolled high BP such as cardiac failure, strokes, etc.

Anaemia status

The patient in chronic renal failure will inevitably have the single overarching symptom of anaemia, varying in degree depending on the severity of the renal damage. Anaemia is not a disease in itself; rather it is a manifestation of underlying disease processes resulting in a reduced number of normal red blood cells, a reduced quantity of haemoglobin and a reduced haematocrit (volume of packed red cells per 100 ml of blood).

Chronic renal failure and anaemia

In chronic renal failure, the primary cause of the anaemia is the failure of the damaged kidneys to produce erythropoietin (EPO). The amount of erythropoietin produced in the liver is inadequate to meet the body's demands. In addition, the toxic internal environment, caused by uraemia and azotaemia, destroys whatever erythropoietin is produced and reduces red cell survival.

The patient's haemoglobin can fall to below 8–10 g/dl and, although the slow progress of chronic renal failure allows for compensatory mechanisms to reduce the effect, eventually primary signs and symptoms will arise. These include chronic fatigue, pallor, reduced exercise tolerance, breathlessness and muscular weakness.

Care and management of anaemia

Management of the renal patient's anaemia is based on reducing the demand for oxygen, maximizing the availability of oxygen carriage and improving the production of red blood cells. The first thing to note is any potential bleeding problems that would exacerbate the anaemia. Eventually, blood transfusions may become the only option and, in those patients who are potential candidates for a kidney transplant, this can prove detrimental to the success of such an operation. With repeated blood transfusions the patient's immune system is sensitized to the presence of foreign proteins and the risk of rejection of a transplant is increased manifold. Therefore, the conservative control of renal anaemia becomes even more important.

Medication to treat renal anaemia is based on an artificial source of EPO, recombinant human EPO, which provides a ready supply of iron for the production of haemoglobin and ensures there is sufficient folic acid and vitamin B_{12} to stimulate stem cell proliferation within the bone marrow.

Ferrous sulphate is the iron supplement most widely used. Oral iron can cause gastric upset and so should be taken with food.

Vitamin B_{12} and folic acid are common micronutrients with few, if any, side effects reported.

Calcium–phosphate status

One of the most disturbing features of long-term chronic renal failure for the patient is the loss of control of calcium and phosphate homeostasis, which leads to renal bone disease and the calcification of soft tissue.

Renal control of calcium and phosphate has two aspects: enabling dietary calcium to be absorbed in the gut; and, subsequently, the regulation of calcium and bone to maintain sufficient levels of serum calcium. The body needs calcium to enable nerve conduction and muscle contraction, especially the heart muscle. It also plays a role in blood clotting, stimulates hormone secretion and affects plasma membrane permeability. Therefore, the conservation of calcium in bones and teeth, and by implication the regulation of bone metabolism, is of vital importance to ensure a constant supply in the face of a varied dietary intake of calcium. In this way, the kidney has a major function in the maintenance and building of bone.

The challenge in the control of calcium and phosphate is one of prevention of imbalance. The early recognition of patients at risk is essential and so serum levels of calcium and phosphate should be monitored.

In addition, restricting protein in the diet will reduce nutritional intake of phosphates and thus reduce the serum phosphate and, coupled with the use of diuretics, will enable the phosphate levels to be reduced. Serum phosphate can be further controlled with phosphate-binding agents, such as aluminium hydroxide. However, the toxic effect of aluminium on bone needs to be taken into consideration and its use restricted to overwhelming need. Newer forms of binding agents that do not contain aluminium are now available and should be considered as an alternative.

Mechanical renal replacement therapy

Patients whose renal function falls below 10% of normal are said to be in ESRF. At this point, the only two ways in which life can be sustained are mechanical replacement of the renal function or transplantation. There are two main forms of mechanical renal replacement therapy available within specialist care centres – haemodialysis and peritoneal dialysis (the permanent form being continuous ambulatory peritoneal dialysis, CAPD). Both forms can be used in the acute situation, but haemodialysis is far more common, with a similar system, haemofiltration, being used extensively in intensive care areas as a supplement to or replacement for haemodialysis.

In chronic renal failure, haemodialysis and peritoneal dialysis offer the only means of survival until transplantation can occur or, for those patients who are not transplant candidates, for the rest of the patient's life.

Peritoneal dialysis was the first system used to treat renal failure mechanically, with the permanent form (CAPD) introduced in the 1970s. It works using the principles of osmosis and diffusion across a semipermeable membrane to remove excess fluids, electrolytes and nitrogenous waste. The semipermeable membrane is the patient's own peritoneum. This is a thin, highly vascular structure covering approximately 1–2 m², which lies below the abdominal wall and forms an 'envelope' around the abdominal organs. It offers support to the organs and, with a small quantity of serous fluid between its folds providing lubrication, it acts as a 'frictionless' surface.

A catheter is introduced through the abdominal wall (a permanent one in the case of CAPD) and a hypertonic fluid is infused into the peritoneal cavity. Osmosis of water and diffusion of solutes from the blood to the solution then takes place. The hypertonic solution is removed and replaced regularly to achieve dialysis. Peritoneal dialysis is not as aggressive as haemodialysis and is not as efficient in the acute situation. However, as a permanent treatment, it offers a considerable advantage over haemodialysis because it provides continuous dialysis as long as the hypertonic solution is in place.

Haemodialysis also utilizes a semipermeable membrane to remove fluids, electrolytes and waste products, but in this case the membrane is contained within an artificial kidney and the blood is pumped from the patient to the kidney and back to the patient in a circuit. The semipermeable membrane is formed from millions of hair-fine 'hollow fibres' through which the blood flows. On the opposite side of the membrane to the blood, the dialysis fluid (dialysate) is pumped from the dialysis machine to the dialyser, and as it flows through the artificial kidney it carries the waste products, water, etc. back to the machine and to a drain.

Unlike peritoneal dialysis, which relies on osmosis and diffusion as the forces to produce dialysis, haemodialysis utilizes hydraulic forces. Blood is pumped from the patient into the confined space of the artificial kidney; therefore within the blood compartment there is a positive pressure. The dialysate, on the other hand, is being 'drawn' through the kidney and so there is a negative pressure on the dialysate side of the membrane. These two forces drive fluids, solutes and waste from the blood to the dialysate and so increase the efficiency of the treatment greatly. Although the dialysate is still hypertonic, it utilizes the differences in fluid content between the blood and the fluid to regulate the volume of loss of vital substances between them.

Patients on haemodialysis usually receive three treatments per week, each lasting 4–6 hours. To achieve sufficient blood flow through the artificial kidney, a permanent vascular fistula is created in the patient's wrist, joining an artery to a vein. The high-pressure arterial blood inflates the low-pressure veins on the patient's forearm, allowing large-bore needles to be inserted for each treatment.

Mechanical renal replacement therapy is a complex and highly sophisticated treatment, yet it still cannot replace all the functions of a healthy kidney efficiently. It is only through a combination of the care principles explored here and the patient's continuing independent participation in their own care that some semblance of health can be achieved.

Conclusion

The renal system is extremely complex and can be a difficult system to understand. However, it is important for the nurse to make sure she is familiar with it, as she has a key role to play in the care and successful management of the renal patient. This will involve monitoring the patient's vital signs, including fluid balance. The nurse acts not only as a provider of care, but also as a facilitator and educator of the patient's own health practices through the principles of assessment, planning, implementation and evaluation.

References and further reading

Agrawal M, Swartz R (2000) Acute renal failure (online). American Family Physician. Available at www.aafap.org/afp/20000401/2077.html (accessed 24 March 2001).

Anaizi N (2000) Renal pharmacology (online). The Drug Monitor. Available from www.home.eznet.net/~webtent/RIT97.html (accessed 8 June 2001).

Brady HR, Singer GG (1995) Acute renal failure. The Lancet 346: 1533–1540.

Challinor P and Sedgewick J (1998) Principles and Practice of Renal Nursing. London: Stanley Thornes.

Donald B (2000) Caring for the renal system. In Bassett C, Malkin L (eds) Caring for the Seriously Ill Patient. London: Arnold.

Edwards S (2001) Regulation of water, sodium and potassium. Implications for practice. Nursing Standard 15(22): 20–24.

Gilbert BR, Leslie BR, Dorracott Vaughan E (1992) Normal renal physiology. In Walsh PC (ed) Cambell's Urology, 6th edn. pp 70–90. Philadelphia: Lippincott.

Goldsmith C (2000) Hypertension: still the silent killer (online) Nurseweek 6 March. Available from nurse.cyberchalk.com/nurse/courses/nurseweek/nw1860new/courses/articles/ce35a.htm (accessed 19 August 2001).

Graber MA, Martinez-Bianchi V (1999) Genitourinary and renal disease. Renal failure (online). Virtual Hospital: University of Iowa Family Practice Handbook. Available from www.vh.org/providers/clinref/fphandbook/chapter11/ 10–11.html (accessed 8 April 2001).

Groszek B (2001) Hyperkalaemia (online). Department of Clinical Toxicology, Jagiellonian University, Krakow, Poland. Available from www.intox.org/pagesource/treatment/english/hyperkalaemia.htm (accessed 8 July 2001).

Harden RM, Jackson AC, Hall M (1999) Care Information for Clinical Management of Patients with Renal Anaemia. Centre for Medical Education, University of Dundee.

Harnett JD (1995) Cardiac function and haematocrit level. American Journal of Kidney Disease 25(4): 53–57.

Harper A (1990) Drug treatment in patients with renal impairment. Pharmaceutical Journal 20(4): 12–15.

Kapit W, Macey RI, Meisami E (1987) Physiology Colouring Book. London: Harper Collins, pp 54–66..

Krause RS (2000) Renal failure, chronic and dialysis complications (online). Emergency Medicine. Genitourinary. Available from www.emedicine.com/ emerg/topic501.htm (accessed June 2001).

Kutchai H (1998) Renal physiology (online). Medical Education. University of Virginia Health System. Available from hsc.virginia.edu/med-ed/phys/handouts2.htm (accessed 17 April 2001).

Macintosh M (2000) Caring for the cardiovascular system. In Bassett C, Makin L (eds) Caring for the Seriously Ill Patient. London: Arnold.

Marieb EN (1999) Human anatomy and physiology. In The Urinary System. Menlo Park: Benjamin Cummings.

Merck (2000) Potassium metabolism (online). The Merck Manual. Available from (www.merck.com/pubs/mmanual/section2/chapter12/12c.htm (accessed 17 July 2001).

Moses S (2000) Acute renal failure management (online). Family Practice Notebook. Available from fpnotebook.com/RENCh8.htm (accessed 8 August 2001).

Sloan E (2000) Constituents of food important in renal disease (online). EdRen handbook. University of Edinburgh Renal Unit. Available from renux.dmed.ed.ac.uk/ EdREN/Handbookbits/HDBKdiet.html (accessed 8 July 2001).

Smith T (1997) Renal Nursing. London: Baillière Tindall.

Swanson P (1990) Drug treatment of chronic renal failure. Pharmaceutical Journal 20(5): 41–49.

Thadhani R, Pascual M, Bonentre JV (1996) Acute renal failure. New England Journal of Medicine 334: 1448–1460.

Totora GJ, Grabowski SR (1996) The urinary system. In Introduction to the Human Body. New York: John Wiley & Son.

Turner N (1995) Blood pressure in renal disease (online). American Journal of Kidney Disease 25: 103–106. Available from renux.dmed.ed.ac.uk/EdREN/Handbookbits/ HDBKBP.html (accessed 8 July 2001).

Wharton S (1997) Applied anatomy and physiology. In Smith T (ed) Renal Nursing. London: Baillière Tindall.

Wolfson AB and Singer I (1998) Haemodialysis related emergencies. Part II. Journal of Emergency Medicine 6(1): 60–70.

Wright JR, Foley RN (2000) Cardiac dysfunction in renal failure (online). National Library of Medicine. PubMed. Available from www.medicinaintensiva-online.org/opexpertos/openefro/foley/heartdisfunctarf.html (accessed 18 December 2000).

CHAPTER SIX

The metabolic and hepatic system

HELEN HAND AND SARAH STARR

Introduction

This chapter explores the assessment and care of the patient's metabolic system. The normal anatomy and physiology of the thyroid gland, gallbladder, liver and pancreas are discussed briefly. You may wish to supplement this with reference to an anatomy and physiology textbook. Specific aspects of the medical and surgical treatment of some of the common thyroid, gallbladder, liver and pancreatic diseases are described, together with the nursing care.

> **Action point 1**
>
> Write down what you know about the metabolic system; consider the organs and their functions.

What is metabolism?

In a powerstation, a fuel such as coal is burned to produce heat. The heat is then used to drive the generator, which in turn produces electricity. The electricity is then utilized for a variety of different functions. Heat has been converted into usable energy.

Like a machine, the body needs energy to carry out its vital functions. The body obtains this energy by consuming and burning fuels in the form of carbohydrates and fats. The oxidation of these foodstuffs produces heat. However, in contrast to the powerstation, the body is not able to convert the heat directly into work. Instead, the body's cells couple the oxidation of food-

221

stuffs with the generation of the energy-rich chemical intermediate adenosine triphosphate (ATP). ATP is then used in a variety of chemical (e.g. synthesis), mechanical (e.g. muscle contraction) and electrical (e.g. nerve activity) body functions that the cells need to carry out in order to thrive. Like all machines, the body is not totally efficient. Some of the energy liberated during the oxidation of foodstuffs is released as heat, which maintains the body temperature.

Every cell in the body obtains its energy from reactions that break down chemical bonds and thus release energy. At the same time, cells also take up chemicals from the blood and use them to synthesize other molecules. The process of using chemicals to obtain energy is called catabolism. The process of synthesizing new compounds is called anabolism. All the reactions that take place produce heat, and the total heat produced per unit of time is known as the metabolic rate.

Many factors affect the metabolic rate, including age, body temperature, ingestion of food and exercise, but it is the endocrine system that has the greatest effect. Various hormones, including adrenaline, testosterone and human growth hormone, can speed up the metabolic rate. However, the most significant ones are those produced by the thyroid gland.

The thyroid gland

The thyroid gland is a butterfly-shaped gland situated in the neck. The gland is composed of two types of hormone-producing cells. The bulk of the cells, known as follicle cells, produce two thyroid hormones – thyroxine (T_4) and triiodothyronine (T_3). Interspersed between these cells are the parafollicular cells that produce the hormone calcitonin, which is responsible for the normal metabolism of calcium.

Thyroid hormones are transported via the bloodstream and affect almost all tissues, as shown in Table 6.1. T_4 is normally secreted in greater quantities than T_3, although T_3 is the more potent. More than 99% of the T_3 and T_4 that circulate in the blood is bound to specific proteins. In this protein-bound form, the hormones are inactive but serve as a reservoir or store of thyroid hormones. Just 0.05% of total T_3 and T_4 in blood is present in a free (unbound to protein) and therefore physiologically active form (Higgins 2000). Both hormones increase the speed of cellular metabolic reactions and are therefore vital regulators of homeostasis. It is essential that levels of the thyroid hormones are maintained within appropriate limits (Table 6.2).

The production of thyroid hormones is controlled by a negative feedback mechanism (Figure 6.1). Figure 6.1 shows that normal concentrations of thyroid hormones are dependent on:

- a normally functioning thyroid gland
- adequate amounts of iodine in the diet for the manufacture of thyroid hormones
- normal production of thyroid-stimulating hormone (TSH) by the pituitary gland
- normal production of TSH-releasing hormone (TRH) by the hypothalamus.

Table 6.1 Effect of thyroid hormones

Tissue	Effect
Fetal development	Before 11 weeks the fetus is dependent on small amounts of maternal T_3
Heat production	T_3 increases oxygen consumption and therefore heat production
Skeletal effects	T_3 increases bone reabsorption and, to some extent, bone formation
Gastrointestinal effects	Gut motility is stimulated by thyroid hormones
Neuromuscular effect	Thyroid hormones are essential for normal growth and for development and functioning of the nervous system
Cardiovascular system	Thyroid hormones increase the number of beta-adrenergic receptors on the heart, thereby increasing contractility
Pulmonary effect	Thyroid hormones maintain a normal response from the respiratory centre

Table 6.2 Normal range for serum thyroid hormone

Hormone	Normal range
Total thyroxine (T_4)	50–141 nmol/l
Triiodothyronine (T_3)	0.8–2.4 nmol/l
Free T_4 (FT_4)	9.0–24 pmol/l
TSH	0.4–4.7 mU/l

Hypothyroidism

Hypothyroidism is a condition in which the thyroid gland is underactive and therefore causes a reduction in the metabolic rate. In its most severe form,

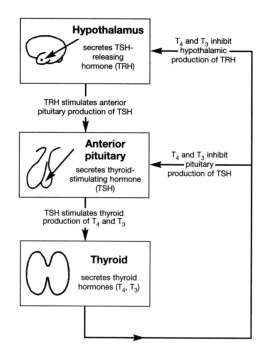

Figure 6.1 Negative feedback control of thyroid hormone secretion.

it is known as myxoedema. The symptoms of hypothyroidism are listed in Table 6.3. Onset is slow and insidious, and it may therefore be some time before the patient seeks a doctor's opinion.

Table 6.3 Symptoms of thyroid disorders

Hyperthyroidism	Hypothyroidism
Weight loss	Weight gain
Increased appetite	Decreased appetite
Intolerance to heat	Intolerance to cold
Increased heart rate (tachycardia)	Decreased heart rate (bradycardia)
Palpitations	Puffy face, particularly below the eyes
Diarrhoea	Constipation
Nervousness and anxiety	Lethargy and depression
Inability to concentrate	Slowing of mental agility
Fine hand tremor	Hoarse, gruff voice
Staring prominent eyes	Dry, coarse skin
Menstrual disturbances, impaired fertility	Impaired fertility
Decreased libido	Decreased libido,
Breathlessness on exertion	Dry, thick, coarse hair

Table 6.4 Investigations for thyroid dysfunction

Blood tests	Radioactive tests	Other investigations
T_4 T_3 Thyroid stimulating hormone (TSH) TSH-releasing hormone (TRH) Free T_4 concentrations	Radioactive iodine uptake test Radionuclide thyroid imaging	Ultrasound test Computed tomography (CT) Magnetic resonance imaging (MRI)

The most common cause of hypothyroidism in the UK, according to Higgins (2000), is autoimmune destruction of thyroid tissue, and Hashimoto's disease is the most common autoimmune disorder to give rise to this. The second most common cause is the effect of treatment for hyperthyroidism. Both radioactive iodine treatment and surgical intervention for hyperthyroidism can result in hypothyroidism. Other rare causes can include a lack of iodine in the diet, inherited disorders and disorders of the hypothalamus or the pituitary gland, which interfere with the production of factors necessary to stimulate the thyroid gland.

Diagnosis is usually based on blood tests, although other investigations may be needed (Table 6.4). Treatment of hypothyroidism is relatively straightforward, and consists of oral replacement of the thyroid hormone. Treatment starts with a low dose, gradually increasing until the desired effect is achieved.

Myxodematous coma

Myxodematous coma is the most severe form of hypothyroidism and is a severe medical emergency. In the absence of sufficient thyroid hormones, the body slows down to the extent that the patient becomes comatose. Intubation and ventilatory support may be required. It is characterized by coma, hypothermia and cardiovascular collapse. Treatment involves aggressive management of factors and supportive therapy. Aspects of nursing care may include:

- care of an unconscious patient
- observations of blood pressure (BP), pulse and respirations
- care of pressure areas
- care and maintenance of an intravenous infusion.

Prognosis is good, provided the disease is recognized early and appropriate treatment commenced (Bassett and Makin 2000).

Hyperthyroidism

Primary hyperthyroidism

By far the most common form of primary hyperthyroidism is Graves' disease, which is more common among women than men, and affects around 1–2% of the adult population. The thyroid gland becomes enlarged and hyperactive, resulting in increased thyroid hormone production. The disease is caused by the production of an abnormal antibody by the immune system, which acts like TSH to stimulate the thyroid. The action of this antibody continues despite rising thyroid hormone levels. Less common causes of primary hyperthyroidism include toxic nodular goitre, Plummer's disease and thyroiditis. Whatever the cause, primary hyperthyroidism is characterized by increased production of thyroid hormones, which results in the symptoms listed in Table 6.3. Because increased levels of thyroid hormones lead to suppression of TSH, a low concentration of TSH is diagnostic of primary hyperthyroidism.

Secondary hyperthyroidism

Secondary hyperthyroidism may be caused by overproduction of TSH by the pituitary gland, usually as a result of disease or a tumour. The thyroid gland is therefore responding appropriately to the increased amount of TSH, resulting in increased levels of circulating thyroid hormones.

Diagnosis and treatment of hyperthyroidism

Diagnosis is based on the tests listed in Table 6.4. There are three forms of therapy available for the treatment of hyperthyroidism:

1. antithyroid drug therapy
2. radioactive therapy
3. surgery.

Antithyroid drug therapy

Antithyroid medication, typically carbimazole, is commonly used to treat hyperthyroidism. It works by suppressing the synthesis of thyroid hormones. The patient should continue to take the medication until a euthyroid state (one of normal thyroid function) is achieved. After this, the levels of T_4 and the dose of the drug are carefully monitored to maintain the euthyroid state. A patient who is tachycardic may need to take beta blockers until the thyroid hormone levels are normal.

Radioactive therapy

Radioactive iodine therapy is an effective alternative to prolonged drug therapy or surgical intervention. This usually takes the form of a single oral dose of radioactive iodine, administered in an outpatient setting. It is considered appropriate for older patients and those with compliance problems. It is not suitable for women of childbearing age or children.

During treatment, the thyroid gland picks up the radioactive elements as it would normal iodine. The radioactivity then destroys some of the cells that normally concentrate iodine and produce T_4, thus decreasing T_4 production. In most patients, symptoms usually disappear within 6–8 weeks of treatment; some, however, require a second dose. Patients are advised not to eat for 3 hours after administration to ensure adequate absorption of the iodine. They are also advised to drink at least 2 litres of fluid over the next 24 h to rid the body of excess iodine not taken up by the thyroid gland. It may take up to 3 months to achieve the euthyroid state (Torrance and Serginson 1999). Patients may be instructed to avoid contact with others during the 2–3 days after treatment, as they present a radiation risk.

Surgery
Partial thyroidectomy is performed only after a euthyroid state has been achieved. Before surgery the patient may be given a course of medication to inhibit thyroid hormone release and reduce the size and vascularity of the gland, thereby reducing the risk of postoperative haemorrhage. Surgery is the usual option for the following patients:

- those with large or unsightly goitres
- those for whom medication or radioactive treatment is not appropriate or has not been successful
- those at risk from haemorrhage or the effects of pressure from the enlarged gland.

Specific preoperative nursing considerations
- It is important that the patient is euthyroid, so it is vital to observe BP pulse and respirations. Sleeping pulse may be requested. If this is repeatedly over 80 beats per minute, suitability for surgery should be reassessed.
- Administer antithyroid medication as prescribed.
- Observe for anxiety.
- Promote rest and quiet. Limit visitors if necessary.
- Consider whether night sedation is required.
- Assess the patient's nutritional status and record weight.
- The patient should eat a diet high in protein, with adequate fluid intake.
- Assess the patient's voice to determine whether there is damage to the vocal cords or recurrent laryngeal nerve that supplies the vocal cords.
- Teach the patient how to support the neck to reduce stress on the surgical wound postoperatively.
- Assess the patient's response to the effect of impending neck surgery on body image.

- Make sure the patient is aware of what to expect after the surgery, including the presence of an intravenous infusion, the types of sutures to be used and any drains that may be inserted. The patient will also be required to sit upright postoperatively and oxygen should be prescribed.
- Discuss discharge arrangements with the patient. The length of stay in hospital is usually around 4 days, and support may need to be arranged from family or social services.

Postoperative care

Postoperative treatment involves the usual range of nursing observations and interventions. If complications arise following a partial thyroidectomy, more specific aspects of care are required (Table 6.5).

Table 6.5 Care required for complications following partial thyroidectomy

Potential complication	Nursing care
Airway obstruction following surgery to the neck	Encourage the patient to sit upright with support for the neck, to increase comfort and reduce anxiety. Give prescribed oxygen, observe respiratory effort and monitor respiration.
Postoperative haemorrhage	Record the BP, pulse and respirations at half-hourly intervals. Observe for tachycardia and difficulty breathing and ensure that equipment for removing the staples/sutures is available
The risk of tetany due to accidental removal of the parathyroid gland	Observe for signs of tetany, such as tingling in the fingers and feet, as a consequence of the disruption in calcium regulation. If not treated this will lead to airway obstruction, fitting and possible death
Damage to the laryngeal nerve	Observe the patient's breathing and swallowing, and listen for signs of hoarseness. Nerve damage may result in vocal cord spasm and paralysis of the larynx, causing respiratory obstruction, which may require a tracheostomy

Thyrotoxic crisis

A fifth complication known as a thyrotoxic crisis or storm can occur, either in patients with pre-existing, though unrecognized, thyrotoxicosis, or during surgery for partial thyroidectomy. It is thought to be a result of the massive release of thyroid hormones into the blood. It can occur during surgery or up to 6–24 h afterwards, although, with the emphasis on establishing the euthyroid state prior to surgery, its occurrence is now rare.

Initially the patient may have marked tachycardia, vomiting and stupor. If left untreated, vascular collapse, hypotension, coma and death will follow.

Other findings include a combination of irritability and restlessness, visual disturbances, tremor and weakness, angina, shortness of breath, cough and swollen extremities. There may also be palpitations and pyrexia that begin insidiously and rise to dangerous levels.

As well as frequent assessment of the patient's BP, pulse temperature and respiration rate, Springings and Chambers (2001) suggest that specific treatment for thyrotoxic crisis should include the following:

- Cardiac monitoring, oxygen therapy and pulse oximetry.
- If heart failure is not present, beta blockade may be commenced to reduce the heart rate.
- Steroids may be administered to inhibit the conversion of T_3 to T_4 and to replace depleted cortisol.
- Antithyroid medication in the form of carbimazole or propylthiouracil, and oral iodine to inhibit the secretion of thyroxine, given as prescribed.
- Antipyretics may be required if the patient has a fever.
- Supportive measures such as the administration of fluids, nutrients and vitamins may also be required.

Action point 2 – case scenario

Mrs Jones is 39 years old and has two children aged 5 and 7. She visits her doctor complaining of difficulty sleeping, increasing anxiety and palpitations. When questioned, she also states that she has lost weight recently. On the basis of the following blood results, the doctor makes a diagnosis of primary hyperthyroidism:

> TSH 0.01 mU/l
> FT_4 40 pmol/l
> T_3 5 nmol/l.

- From what you have read, can you explain why the level of TSH is so low? Try to explain the reason for the development of Mrs Jones' symptoms and describe the treatment options available for her.

The gallbladder

The gallbladder plays an important role in metabolism through its ability to store and secrete bile. Bile is produced by the liver and passed to the gallbladder via the hepatic duct. Within about 30 minutes of eating a meal, particularly one containing fats, the gallbladder is stimulated to contract and expel bile. The bile flows through the common bile duct, through the sphincter of Oddi and into the duodenum. The signal to contract comes from both the parasympathetic nervous system and the hormone cholecystokinin (CCK), which is released by the duodenum in response to the arrival of amino acids and fatty food.

Bile function

Bile contains 97% water, organic salts such as sodium chloride and sodium bicarbonate, and inorganic constituents in the form of bile salts formed from cholesterol and bile pigments. To form the bile pigments, bilirubin, which is a product of the destruction of old red blood cells, is taken up from the blood and converted into a more water-soluble substance known as bilirubin glucuronide, which gives bile its yellow/green colour. The bile salts are the most important constituent, and their role is to increase the solubility of fat. In the presence of bile salts, large fat droplets disperse and form smaller fat particles, a process known as emulsification. In this emulsified state, the fats can be digested more easily by the pancreatic enzyme lipase into smaller molecules – glycerides and fatty acids – which are small enough to be absorbed through the walls of the small intestine. In the absence of bile, fat digestion decreases markedly, even though the pancreatic enzyme is still present.

Cholecystitis

Cholecystitis (inflammation of the gallbladder) is usually caused by the presence of stones in the gallbladder (cholelithiasis), although as illustrated in Table 6.6 there are several other causes.

Table 6.6 Causes of cholecystitis

- Tissue damage due to trauma, massive burns or surgery
- Gram-negative septicaemia
- Multiple blood transfusions
- Hypertension
- Overuse of opiate analgesia
- Prolonged fasting

There are three different types of gallstone formed from the constituents of bile:

1. Cholesterol stones – the most common type, accounting for up to 80% of all stones in the UK, thought to form in bile that is supersaturated with cholesterol. Pure cholesterol stones are usually white in colour.

2. Pigment stones – black pigment stones are more common in patients with haemolytic disease, such as sickle cell anaemia.
3. Mixed stones – with characteristics of cholesterol and pigment stones.

Gallstones are the most common abdominal reason for admission to hospital in developed countries and account for an important part of healthcare expenditure. As many as 5.5 million people in the UK have gallstones, and over 50 000 cholecystectomies are performed each year (Beckingham 2001). Gallstones are twice as common in women as in men, and are often associated with advancing age and obesity, although according to Alexander et al. (2000) gallstones are now affecting people at a younger age than previously, for unknown reasons.

Once formed, the stones may:

- remain in the gallbladder without causing any problems
- block the cystic duct, leading to inflammation of the gallbladder (cholecystitis) and a compensatory increase in gallbladder contraction and peristalsis within the duct. The inflamed, obstructed gallbladder may now become distended and ischaemic and, if it perforates, may lead to peritonitis
- leave the gallbladder and block the hepatic duct leading from the liver to the gallbladder. This causes retention of bile within the liver and increased release of bilirubin into the bloodstream for eventual excretion by the kidneys
- leave the gallbladder and obstruct the common bile duct (choledocholithiasis), or obstruct the opening of the pancreatic duct into the common bile duct. This leads to retention of pancreatic enzymes in the pancreas, which may contribute to pancreatitis. Bacterial infection can also occur, producing cholangitis (inflammation of the bile duct).

Although gallstones can be asymptomatic, more often than not they cause an attack of acute or chronic cholecystitis. In both types, inflammation causes the gallbladder wall to become thickened and oedematous, and the lumen of the cystic duct to increase in diameter. Table 6.7 lists the signs and symptoms of cholecystitis and the nursing care required.

Figure 6.2 shows the common locations of gallstones.

Investigations for acute cholecystitis

- Diagnosis is usually made on the basis of ultrasound investigation. Beckingham (2001) reports that this has 95% sensitivity and specificity for stones over 4 mm in size. It can identify stones in the gallbladder, thickening of the gallbladder wall and dilatation of the hepatic duct. It can also be used on patients with jaundice.

Table 6.7 Signs and symptoms of cholecystitis

Patient issues	Nursing care
Pain in the upper right quadrant, commonly after a high-fat meal. The pain may radiate through to the back or right shoulder	Carry out regular pain assessment using a recognized pain assessment tool. Administer prescribed analgesia and monitor the effect
Nausea and vomiting	Administer prescribed antiemetic and monitor the effect. Record the amount and frequency of vomit on an intake and output chart. Attend to patient comfort; supply tissues, vomit bowl and mouthwash. If vomiting is persistent, a nasogastric tube may be inserted. This should be aspirated as directed and all aspirate recorded on the intake and output chart
Patient nil by mouth and requires an intravenous infusion	Assess the patient's hydration status regularly. Ensure that the infusion is administered as prescribed and recorded on the fluid balance chart. Regular observation of the cannula site is required
Patient observations	Observations of pulse, BP and respiration rate must be made. This acts as a baseline and evidence of improvement or deterioration. If the patient is pyrexial, temperature should be recorded hourly
Urine and stool changes	Lack of bile pigment results in pale faeces, and urine will be dark due to the excretion of bile pigment by the kidneys. Observe for changes in the colour and record appropriately
Presence of infection	Intravenous antibiotics may be prescribed. Record the patient's temperature to assess the effect of medication
Obstructive jaundice may develop if the inflamed gallbladder presses on the common bile duct	Hygiene needs should be attended to to promote comfort and allow skin assessment. Changes in the level of jaundice should be noted (if present), and the patient encouraged to refrain from scratching. Antihistamines may be prescribed
Diet	When the patient resumes eating, a nutritional needs assessment should be undertaken. A diet high in carbohydrate and low in fat should be encouraged. The dietician may need to speak with the patient and family

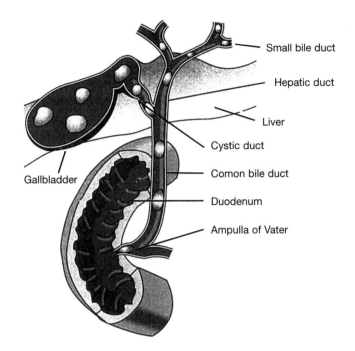

Figure 6.2 Common locations of gallstones.

- Blood tests for white cell count, liver function test (LFT) and serum amylase.
- Endoscopic retrograde cholangiopancreatography (ERCP).

Cholecystectomy

Acute cholecystitis is usually treated by removal of the gallbladder. Some surgeons choose to operate immediately, while others may choose to wait until the symptoms have settled. Cholecystectomy can be performed as either a laparoscopic or an open procedure.

Specific nursing care following open cholecystectomy

Nursing care following an open cholecystectomy encompasses all aspects of care associated with major abdominal surgery, which should have been discussed with the patient prior to surgery. Specific aspects include the following:

- The patient may experience abdominal discomfort when breathing or coughing, depending on the location of the wound. The patient should be taught how to support the wound and encouraged to breathe deeply to prevent pulmonary complications. Mobilization should also be encouraged to avoid venous stasis.

- If there were stones in the common bile duct, they will have been removed and a T-tube inserted in the common bile duct attached to a drainage bag, to ensure that bile is now flowing. This tube should drain up to 500 ml of bile in the first 24 h (Torrance and Serginson 1999), the amount reducing as the duct heals. A T-tube cholangiogram may be performed 7–10 days after the operation to ensure patency of the duct. If it is stone free, the tube will be removed. Analgesia will be required 30 minutes before the removal of the tube.
- A wound drain may also be inserted during the operation. This will usually be removed within 24–48 h. All drainage should be observed and amounts recorded on the intake and output chart. Excessive amounts of bright red blood should be reported immediately.
- Analgesia should be given as prescribed following the operation and a pain scoring system utilized. The patient may be able to manage the pain using patient-controlled analgesia (PCA).
- An intravenous infusion will be commenced. This will be discontinued when free fluids are tolerated.
- Sutures are generally removed after 7–10 days and, depending on the patient's age and condition, discharge usually takes place between 6 and 10 days postoperatively.
- The patient should be instructed to avoid heavy lifting for up to 6 weeks. If the recovery is uncomplicated, the patient may be fit to return to work after 4 weeks.

Laparoscopic cholecystectomy

Laparoscopic cholecystectomy is the preferred approach in 80–90% of current cholecystectomies (Beckingham 2001). The benefits are:

- lower mortality than the standard procedure
- lower incidence of cardiac or respiratory postoperative complications
- smaller incisions cause less pain, reducing the requirement for opiate analgesia
- patients are often treated as day-case surgery or overnight stay
- most patients are usually able to return to work between 7 and 11 days postoperatively
- there is less risk of paralytic ileus.

There are some reported problems with the laparoscopic approach. These include puncture of the bile duct, abdominal wall haematoma and puncture of organs, such as the liver or intestines. The unexpected presence of stones in the common bile duct also complicates the procedure.

Nursing care following laparoscopic cholecystectomy

- Usual preoperative observation of BP, pulse and respiration.
- Observe wound sites for leakage.
- Utilizing an appropriate pain tool, ensure that the patient has adequate and effective pain relief. The patient should be told that pain from the retention of gases used in the operation might persist for up to a week.
- Commence clear fluids slowly when ready. Avoid carbonated drinks. Recommence normal diet when fluids have been tolerated.
- Ensure that the patient has specific instructions prior to discharge to observe for signs of intra-abdominal complications, e.g. loss of appetite, vomiting, distension of the abdomen and temperature elevation.
- Ensure that the patient has transport home following the procedure.
- Ensure that the patient has assistance at home during the first 48 hours.

The pancreas

The pancreas is a large gland situated underneath the stomach. It has both endocrine and exocrine functions. The endocrine pancreas consists of the pancreatic islet cells, which secrete the hormones insulin and glucagon. It will be discussed later in this chapter. This section looks at the exocrine part of the gland, which makes up more than 98% of its bulk. It produces pancreatic juice – an alkaline substance (pH 8), consisting mainly of water, enzymes and electrolytes (primarily bicarbonate ions) – which plays a role in digestion. The enzymes include:

- lipase, which acts on triglycerides already emulsified by bile, to break them into fatty acids and glycerol
- amylase, which assists in the breakdown of carbohydrates
- proteases, including trypsin, chymotrypsin and elastase, which continue the breakdown of protein into smaller peptides and amino acids.

The pancreatic acinar cells synthesize, store and secrete approximately 1200–1500 ml of clear pancreatic juice each day (Marieb 1998). It passes along the pancreatic duct to the duodenum, where it acts to neutralize the acidic contents (known as chyme) delivered from the stomach.

The stimulus for the production of pancreatic juice is the presence of fats and protein in the duodenum. This triggers the release of the duodenal hormone CCK, which, along with stimulation from the parasympathetic vagus nerve, promotes the release of pancreatic juice. Most of the enzymes are secreted in an inactive form, and are activated just before entering the digestive tract. This is important, because the pancreatic enzymes are extremely powerful and could digest the pancreas in a short time if not inhibited. Inflammation of the pancreas is known as pancreatitis. It may be either acute or chronic.

Chronic pancreatitis

Chronic pancreatitis is a progressive inflammatory condition of the pancreas. Both the endocrine and exocrine cells are progressively destroyed and replaced with fibrous tissue, causing increased pressure within the pancreas. Eventually this may result in mechanical obstruction of the pancreatic duct, common bile duct and duodenum, giving rise to repeated attacks of pancreatitis, which may last a few days.

Chronic pancreatitis typically results from repeated episodes of acute pancreatitis, and sensitivity to even small amounts of alcohol is the most common cause. Other causes include narrowing of the pancreatic duct and the presence of gallstones.

Many patients have only mild and occasional symptoms. However, chronic pancreatitis is a potentially serious condition and as such must be investigated and treated (Table 6.8).

Acute pancreatitis

Acute pancreatitis is a potentially life-threatening disorder, associated with the escape of activated pancreatic enzymes into the pancreas and surrounding tissues. It may occur as an isolated attack, or recur in distinct episodes with reversion to normal histology between attacks. By definition, acute pancreatitis is reversible. It is therefore distinguished from chronic pancreatitis by the absence of continuing inflammation, irreversible structural changes, and permanent impairment of endocrine and exocrine function.

Eighty per cent of all cases of acute pancreatitis are caused by either alcohol misuse or gallstones (Mergener and Baillie 1998). Table 6.9 lists other known causes of acute pancreatitis.

The manifestation of acute pancreatitis varies with each individual, from mild and self-limiting to rapid, severe and potentially fatal. In its most severe form it is likely that invasive monitoring will be required and the patient will need to be nursed on a high dependency unit (HDU) or ICU. It is therefore important to be able to assess the severity of an episode of acute pancreatitis as rapidly as possible so that patients can receive optimal treatment. There

Table 6.8 Investigation and treatment of chronic pancreatitis

Presenting signs and symptoms	Nursing intervention
Pain Although there is occasionally no pain, usually the patient suffers severe recurrent epigastric and left upper-quadrant pain, which may last for hours or days. Pain may subside as the acinar cells that secrete pancreatic digestive enzymes are progressively destroyed	Medication should be given to relieve pain. Morphine has been known to increase biliary and pancreatic pressure in some patients by inducing constriction or spasm of the sphincter of Oddi. This pain may therefore be mistaken for deterioration in the patient's condition
Diet and nutritional status Many patients complain of feeling generally unwell, and weight loss, anorexia, nausea, vomiting, constipation and flatulence are also common	Medication should be administered to control nausea and vomiting. The patient will also require digestive enzyme replacement, and supplemental fat-soluble vitamins (A, E, D, K) may also be prescribed Fasting and intravenous fluids may prove beneficial Antacids or H_2-receptor blocking agents may be used to reduce acid-stimulated release of secretin, which increases the flow of pancreatic juice Alcohol is forbidden
Diabetes mellitus When the disease progresses to the extent that exocrine and endocrine function are affected, signs of diabetes mellitus will develop	Oral hypoglycaemic medication rarely helps to treat diabetes mellitus caused by pancreatitis and insulin is therefore the drug of choice. Because of the coexisting deficiency of glucagon secretion by the pancreas, the hypoglycaemic effects of insulin are unopposed and prolonged. As diabetic ketoacidosis rarely occurs in chronic pancreatitis it is therefore better to maintain the patient slightly hyperglycaemic than to risk hypoglycaemia caused by overzealous insulin administration

are two commonly used scoring criteria, described by Coad (1999) – Ransom's criteria and the APACHE II scoring system. Systems such as these are useful as a basis for monitoring progress and deciding whether admission to HDU/ICU is necessary.

Investigations for acute pancreatitis

- Endoscopic retrograde cholangiopancreatography (ERCP) is indicated in patients with recurrent episodes of acute pancreatitis of unknown cause,

Table 6.9 Causes of acute pancreatitis

- Drugs (including azathioprine, furosemide, oestrogen, tetracyclines, sulphonamides, valproate, corticosteroids, paracetamol overdose)
- Trauma to the pancreas
- Endoscopic retrograde cholangiopancreatography
- Major abdominal surgery (particularly stomach, biliary tract and after coronary artery bypass grafting)
- Hypercalcaemia
- Hyperlipidaemia
- Penetrating gastric or duodenal ulcer
- Pancreatic tumours
- Familial pancreatitis
- Vascular disease (especially severe hypotension)
- Pregnancy
- Renal transplantation
- End-stage renal failure
- Viral infections (viral hepatitis, mumps, coxsackie B, etc.)
- Idiopathic (no known cause)

to look for biliary stones or problems such as unsuspected obstructive lesions. Not all patients with acute pancreatitis will require ERCP.
- Cross-sectional imaging of the pancreas, liver, gallbladder and biliary tree by ultrasound, computed tomography (CT) and magnetic resonance imaging (MRI) are all useful in identifying the specific cause of acute pancreatitis.
- Laboratory tests cannot confirm a diagnosis of acute pancreatitis, but can support the clinical picture. Plasma amylase and lipase concentrations increase on the first day of acute pancreatitis and return to normal in 3–7 days. Both plasma amylase and lipase can be increased in other disorders, such as renal failure and abdominal conditions requiring urgent surgery (perforated ulcer, intestinal obstruction associated with ischaemia).
- Further blood tests may reveal raised white cell count, indicating inflammation.
- Third space fluid losses may increase the haematocrit, indicating severe inflammation.
- Urea and electrolytes are important in determining the state of hydration.
- Hyperglycaemia may also be present.
- Arterial blood gases may reveal hypoxia.

Table 6.10 lists the clinical manifestations of acute pancreatitis and the appropriate treatment and nursing care.

Once the immediate episode is over, the patient can begin to return to normal. Education and support will be required, particularly if the episode was alcohol related. The patient is likely to be weak and lethargic and unable to resume work for at least 4–6 weeks.

Surgical intervention during the first few days is justified in severe blunt or penetrating trauma. Other indications for surgery include uncontrolled biliary sepsis and inability to distinguish acute pancreatitis from a surgical emergency. With severe acute gallstone pancreatitis that does not improve rapidly with supportive care, ERCP and sphincterotomy may be needed to extract the stones. If the condition does not improve, cholecystectomy will need to be performed.

Action point 3 – Case scenario

Mr Smith, a known heavy drinker, is admitted to your ward in acute pain with suspected acute pancreatitis. He is vomiting, pale and clammy, and his respirations are shallow and rapid. His pulse is rapid and he is hypotensive. Blood tests reveal amylase 1700 U/l, blood glucose 15.6 mmol/l.

1. How will Mr Smith describe his pain? From what you have read, what is the cause of the pain?
2. Explain why the raised amylase is diagnostic of acute pancreatitis.
3. Acute pancreatitis represents a medical emergency. Make a list of your priorities in caring for Mr Smith during the early stages of the admission.

The endocrine pancreas

The endocrine part of the pancreas, called the islets of Langerhans, consists of one to two million round clusters of cells scattered throughout the gland between the exocrine acini. A rich bed of specialized capillaries with large pores surrounds the islets. The endocrine pancreas is critical to glucose homeostasis, which in turn is essential to energy metabolism.

The two most important types of cells in the islets in terms of glucose regulation are the alpha cells and the beta cells. The alpha cells are located peripherally and secrete the hormone glucagon. The beta cells are located centrally and are more numerous. They secrete the hormone insulin.

Insulin and glucagon regulate the metabolism of carbohydrates in tissues and ensure the maintenance of optimal blood sugar levels. The primary action of insulin is to facilitate and promote the transport of glucose across the plasma membranes of cells in certain tissues, chiefly muscle (heart, skeletal and smooth) and adipose tissue (fat). In the absence of insulin, these cells are impermeable to glucose, regardless of how much glucose is present in the blood. Normal fasting glucose levels are in the range 3.5–5.0 mmol/l.

Table 6.10 Management of pancreatitis

Clinical manifestation	Treatment and nursing care
Pain Pain is almost always present. It is often excruciating and continuous, in the epigastric region, poorly localized, often worse when supine, sometimes radiating into the back. The pain is often described as 'boring' Pain usually develops suddenly in gallstone pancreatitis, whereas pain from alcoholic pancreatitis may develop over a few weeks	Nursing care involves accurate assessment of pain and monitoring the effect of medication, using a reliable pain assessment tool Conventionally, strong analgesia such as pethidine (100–150 mg given intramuscularly) is used, although continuous infusion is preferable according to Johnson (1998), as this avoids the peaks and troughs of analgesia. Johnson (1998) also suggests that morphine should be avoided if possible as it causes the sphincter of Oddi to contract and thus increases pain
Hypovolaemia Pancreatic exudate containing toxins and activated pancreatic enzymes permeate the retroperitoneal cavity and at times the peritoneal cavity. This increases the permeability of blood vessels, resulting in the extravasation of large amounts of protein-rich fluid from the systemic circulation into 'third spaces', which produces hypovolaemia and shock. On entering the systemic circulation, these toxins and activated enzymes increase capillary permeability throughout the body and may reduce vascular tone, thereby increasing hypotension	Good nursing observations are essential in detecting the progress of the disease. The patient will be tachycardic, respirations will be shallow and rapid, blood pressure may be low with significant postural hypotension In the most severe form, a central venous pressure (CVP) line will be required to allow continuous pressure monitoring and to assess to response to treatment Dehydration can also be noted by assessing the patient's skin and mucous membranes. Good oral hygiene is important. An intravenous infusion will be commenced to correct both fluid and electrolyte disturbances. Intake and output monitoring are essential A urinary catheter may also be inserted to allow accurate measurement of urine output. Johnson (1998) suggests that any fall below 0.5 ml/kg per h that does not respond to fluid replacement may require more aggressive treatment
Nausea and vomiting Nausea and vomiting are usually present and a nasogastric tube will be inserted to facilitate either continuous or intermittent aspiration. Theoretically, this also prevents the passage of acidic gastric contents into the duodenum and therefore allows the pancreas to rest	The procedure should be explained to the patient before the insertion of the tube, to relieve anxiety and gain co-operation. The tube should be securely fastened to prevent it being dislodged. All volumes of aspirate should be recorded on the fluid balance chart. Antiemetic medication should be given as prescribed

Table 6.10 Management of pancreatitis (contd)

Clinical manifestation	Treatment and nursing care
Pyrexia The patient may present with a low-grade pyrexia and a raised white cell count. Bacterial infection associated with acute pancreatitis is common and is a cause of increased mortality. However, the inflammatory response initiated by pancreatitis may also result in pyrexia. Although the use of anti-biotics for proven infection is not disputed, the use of prophylactic antibiotics appears to be controversial. Coad (1999) suggests that there is evidence that patients with severe pancreatitis and evidence of necrosis would benefit from it	Regular recording of temperature
Respiratory problems Pain may interfere with respiratory effort, and sputum retention may promote pulmonary collapse or pneumonia	Frequent respiratory assessment is crucial Deep breathing should be encouraged
Hypoxia If arterial blood gases reveal hypoxaemia, humidified oxygen should be given via a facemask or nasal prongs. If hypoxaemia does not respond, assisted ventilation may be required	Administer oxygen as prescribed, ensuring that the patient understands the reason for it in order to maximize compliance. Pulse oximetry and regular blood gas monitoring are important
Nutrition Administration of appropriate nutrition is an essential part of management of severe acute pancreatitis. The disease may last several weeks and is characterized by a massive catabolic response in the early stages. Nutrition is usually administered parenterally because it is traditional to rest the pancreas to minimize stimulation of pancreatic secretions	Total parenteral nutrition should be administered as per regimen and recorded appropriately Blood sugar levels should be recorded 4–6 hourly because of the risk of secondary diabetes

When this level is exceeded, the glucose detectors in the beta cells release insulin into the blood. This increases the permeability of the cells to glucose, resulting in increased uptake. Once inside a muscle cell, the glucose can either be used to produce energy, or stored in the form of glycogen to be used during muscle activity.

Insulin also promotes uptake of glucose into fat cells. It is not used to provide energy in these cells, but instead is converted into glycerol, which is used to form triglycerides (the storage form of fat) from fatty acids. Insulin acts directly on liver cells. However, this action does not promote increased uptake by the liver cells, because liver cells are normally permeable to glucose. Instead, it stimulates glucose storage in the form of glycogen.

The action of insulin on the muscle, liver and fat cells results in a decrease in the level of glucose in the blood. This is sensed by the beta cells, and the production of insulin ceases.

The primary stimulus for the release of glucagon is a fall in blood sugar level, such as occurs during fasting or between meals. Glucose detectors in the alpha cells now release glucagon into the blood. Glucagon binds to specific receptors in the liver, stimulating the conversion of glycogen back into glucose. This process is known as glycogenolysis. The resulting increase in blood glucose now acts on the pancreas to reduce the secretion of glucagon. This method of glucose regulation is known as a negative feedback mechanism.

Diabetes mellitus

Diabetes mellitus is a disorder of carbohydrate, protein and fat metabolism. It results from an imbalance between insulin need and insulin availability. Because diabetes is closely linked with a number of common medical conditions, reasons for encountering diabetes in hospital will vary. The admission may be directly related to the diabetes, or it may require management as part of a different presenting illness. Good glycaemic control is also required for patients with diabetes as part of their pre- and postoperative care regimen. The nurse is therefore often presented with a dual challenge: to manage the primary problem and to ensure that the patient's diabetic control does not have an adverse effect on the eventual outcome.

Two main types of diabetes have been recognized. Type 1, or insulin-dependent diabetes (IDDM), occurs when there is an absolute insulin deficiency. Type 2, or non-insulin-dependent diabetes (NIDDM), occurs when there is impaired release of insulin by the pancreatic beta cells, or where the tissues themselves are resistant to the actions of insulin, because of inadequate or defective insulin receptors. Diabetes can, however, also occur as a result of other conditions or syndromes, such as acute pancreatitis, or it may occur during pregnancy, when it is known as gestational diabetes.

Whatever the cause, the end result is hyperglycaemia (raised blood sugar levels) as a consequence of absolute or relative insulin deficiency.

Type 2 diabetes

Type 2 diabetes is a common and serious problem believed to affect 2 million people in the UK, only half of whom are currently diagnosed. In 1997, the Chief Medical Officer identified type 2 diabetes as a priority condition for treatment and management, and in April 1999 diabetes was selected as the subject for a National Service Framework to be effective from April 2001.

The most common clinical features of type 2 diabetes are shown in Table 6.11. Diagnosis is usually confirmed with the following blood tests:

- Random plasma glucose: diabetes is confirmed if the random sugar is greater than 11.1 mmol/l.
- Fasting plasma glucose: diabetes is confirmed if the fasting sugar is greater than 7.0 mmol/l.
- Two-hour post-prandial: blood sugar should be falling back to the normal fasting level.
- Glycosylated haemoglobin (HbA1c): this is a test of long-term blood glucose control. Around 5–8% of the haemoglobin circulating in the red cells of the blood has a glucose molecule attached and is said to be glycated. The degree of glycation is dependent on the amount of circulating glucose that red cells are exposed to during their 120-day life span. This test therefore provides a good overview of blood glucose control over the preceding month. The higher the glycated haemoglobin, the poorer the control. Glycated haemoglobin is composed of three fractions: HbA1a, HbA1b, and HbA1c. Good control has been defined by Higgins (2000) as an HbA1c of less than 6.5%.

Table 6.11 Clinical features of type 2 diabetes

- Presentation usually in middle or later life
- Obesity common (present in over 75% of cases)
- Symptoms are often mild or unrecognized
- There is relative rather than absolute insulin deficiency
- Insulin resistance is common
- Ketoacidosis is rare
- Even with antidiabetic therapy the disease is progressive
- Insulin is often required to maintain long-term glycaemic control
- High risk of microvascular complications, often evident on diagnosis
- Tisssue damage often present at diagnosis

Treatment of type 2 diabetes

The UK Prospective Diabetes Study (UKPDS 1998) confirmed that intensive glycaemic control is associated with a reduction in microvascular complications. The National Service Framework for diabetes also states that the key principles in reducing complications are:

- early detection, meticulous control of blood sugar
- early detection and management of cardiovascular risk factors
- early detection and management of long-term complications, particularly of the eye, foot and kidney.

As a result of the UKPDS study, the diabetes association Diabetes UK recommends that treatment should aim at achieving a fasting blood glucose level of 4–7 mmol/l and a HbA1c of 7% or below. Treatment of type 2 diabetes is based on dietary control, with or without oral hypoglycaemic medication. Diet is beyond the scope of this chapter, but you may wish to explore this issue further by visiting the diabetic clinic or a dietician. The Diabetes UK website is also very informative

Antidiabetic medication

Current treatment of type 2 diabetes involves a range of medications. Some patients may require a single oral agent, others may be stabilized using a combination of different acting oral agents. Insulin may also be prescribed, either with or without the addition of an oral agent. The most commonly prescribed antidiabetic medications include the following:

Sulphonylureas
These include glibenclamide and glicazide. The mode of action is to stimulate the secretion of insulin from functioning pancreatic beta cells. Although they are effective initially, they do not influence the inevitable decline in glycaemic control over time. The main concern is hypoglycaemia and therefore the lowest dose should be prescribed initially.

Biguanides
Biguanides act by inhibiting glucose production by the liver and increasing glucose uptake into the muscle. The most common in this class is metformin. This has a similar efficacy to sulphonylureas in lowering blood glucose, but has a high incidence of gastrointestinal symptoms that make it more difficult to tolerate. The UKPDS (1988) favours metformin as initial oral therapy, particularly in obese patients as it does not promote weight gain, thereby reducing the risk of complications. The tablet should be taken with or immediately following food. Lactic acidosis has been reported as a side effect, and although rare, has a high mortality rate.

Alpha-glucosidase inhibitors
The only medication currently available in the UK from this class is acarbose. Acarbose acts by reducing post-prandial peaks of glucose through retarding glucose absorption from the intestines. Common side effects include diarrhoea, flatulence and abdominal bloating, which make it less desirable for some patients.

Prandial glucose regulators (meglitinides)
The first of these, repaglinide, is a derivative of the sulphonylurea glibenclamide but is more rapidly absorbed. It increases the secretion of insulin by the beta cells. It should be taken before a meal and has a short duration of action reducing post-meal hyperglycaemia and HbA1. There may be a reduced risk of hypoglycaemia and weight gain compared to glibenclamide.

Thiazolidinediones (glitazones)
These work by combining with an intranuclear receptor, which has an effect on carbohydrate and lipid metabolism similar to the effects seen when insulin combines with its receptor. The main drug in this category is rosiglitazone, currently licensed in the UK for use in combination with either metformin or a sulphonylurea. There is evidence of sustained effect of this class for up to 2 years. They appear to be well tolerated, taken once a day with no significant drug interactions. They do not cause gastrointestinal problems and do not increase the risk of hypoglycaemia.

Assessing the patient with diabetes

An abundance of complications can occur as a result of poor glycaemic control (Figure 6.3). Therefore, whatever the reason for the admission, the nurse is presented with an excellent opportunity both to carry out a thorough assessment of the patient and to undertake health promotion.

Initial assessment

On admission, it is important to establish baseline observations. The following points therefore need to be considered in relation to a client with diabetes:

- The blood sugar level: this should be taken using a blood glucose meter in accordance with the manufacturer's instructions, utilizing the correct technique and ensuring that the device has been appropriately calibrated.
- The patient's usual regimen: the usual medication type and dose as well as method of administration should be identified. The time and amount of the last medication should also be ascertained.
- Diet: it is important to discover the patient's usual dietary habits and the time and content of the last food intake. The patient's knowledge of dietary principles should also be established.

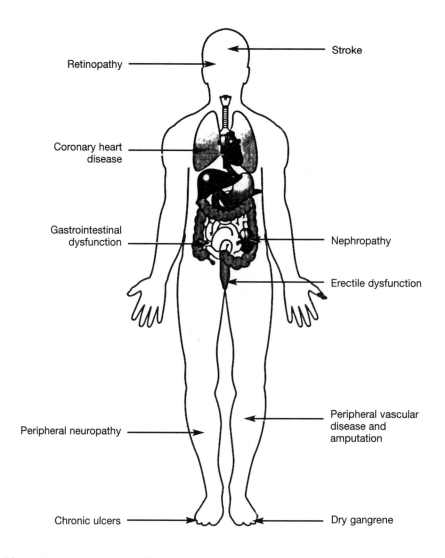

Figure 6.3 Complications of type 2 diabetes.

- Observations: other observations should be undertaken including pulse, BP, temperature, respiration rate and oxygen saturation levels. Urine should be routinely tested on admission.
- Skin: all pressure areas must be inspected and any dressings on the skin should be removed to allow observation and assessment to take place.
- Feet: the feet should be carefully examined for sensation, lesions, and signs of necrosis or infection. If possible, the patient should be asked whether they experience pain or loss of sensation, and whether they follow a foot care regimen. Foot pulses can also be assessed at this time.
- Infection: the patient should be asked about the presence of any infection.

- Eyes: the patient should be asked about any visual problems or disturbances and whether they have a regular ophthalmic assessment.
- Exercise history.
- Lifestyle factors: this should include details of any cultural, psychosocial, educational and economic factors that might affect glycaemic control.
- Risk factors for heart disease: factors such as smoking, alcohol intake, weight and family history should be assessed.
- General health: it is important to find out about the patient's general health. Factors such as general control of the diabetes and frequency of diabetes-related problems, and prior or current infections, assist in presenting an overall picture of the diabetes.

Type 1 diabetes

In type 1 diabetes there is little or no naturally occurring insulin, and in 90% of cases it is an autoimmune disorder (Krentz 2000). An autoimmune disorder is one in which the body creates antibodies that will attack its own insulin hormone and the pancreatic cells that produce insulin. Diabetes will develop when 80–90% of the beta cells have been destroyed. Type 1 diabetes is always treated with insulin.

Insulin therapy

There are a variety of insulins available. They are categorized as short acting, intermediate and long acting.

- Short-acting insulin is a clear solution with a rapid onset of action. When injected subcutaneously, its maximal effect occurs in 3–4 hours.
- Intermediate insulins are cloudy. The onset of action is delayed for 1–2 hours. Intermediate insulins achieve maximal effect in 4–6 hours and have a duration of action of 12–20 hours.
- Long-acting insulins are also cloudy, and have a greatly extended period of action which means they can be given once a day. However, control is more difficult to achieve and they may be more suited to patients with type 2 diabetes who can no longer achieve control with diet and/or oral hypoglycaemic agents.

Insulin should be stored in a fridge. However, as injecting cold insulin is more likely to be painful, if using a pen device, the device can be left at room temperature. People who have to inject insulin are encouraged to rotate between different injection sites and to inject slowly but firmly. There is no need to clean the skin with a swab before injection unless the area is excessively dirty.

Nurses will undoubtedly encounter patients in both medical and surgical environments who must fast before investigations or surgery. For further information and protocols on how to manage them, refer to Springings and Chambers (2001, Chapter 39).

Acute complications of type 1 diabetes

There are two major life-threatening complications for clients with type 1 diabetes hypoglycaemia and ketoacidosis. Although mainly a problem for patients taking insulin, hypoglycaemia can also occur as a result of type 2 diabetes, particularly with patients taking sulphonylureas.

Hypoglycaemia

The symptoms of hypoglycaemia present acutely and progress rapidly as the level of sugar in the blood falls. The patient may begin with subtle behavioural changes, headache and excessive sweating of the hands and face. As the blood sugar falls below 3 mmol/l, the more obvious signs appear. These include:

- irritability
- intense hunger
- double vision
- shaking
- dizziness
- confusion
- difficulty speaking.

As the blood level continues to fall, severe hypoglycaemia develops. The patient may now experience fits, stroke-like symptoms and eventually coma.

Causes of hypoglycaemia

- Oral hypoglycaemic medication.
- Administering too much insulin without an increase in dietary intake.
- Insufficient or delayed dietary intake after insulin has been administered.
- Excessive exercise without taking extra food.
- Alcoholic binge
- Overaggressive treatment of hyperglycaemia.
- The 'honeymoon period'. This is where, after being commenced on insulin, the islet cells partially recover. This effect is short lasting but the extra new insulin may put the patient at risk.

Management of hypoglycaemia

Most people with diabetes become familiar with the warning signs, and they are taught how to test their own blood sugar level if they begin to suspect that it is falling. They are then able to prevent severe hypoglycaemia occurring by eating or taking glucose tablets. Some patients, however, do not have any warning of impending hypoglycaemia.

Severe hypoglycaemia is a medical emergency, which, if untreated, can result in permanent neurological damage. Accurate patient monitoring is therefore vital.

If the patient is still conscious and co-operative, 20 g of quick-acting carbohydrate should be given. This may be in the form of any food or drink with a high sugar content, such as dextrose tablets, chocolate or orange juice. This should be followed by more long-acting carbohydrate, such as a sandwich. If the patient is unable to eat or drink safely, glucagon 1 mg can be administered subcutaneously. If this fails to provide an appropriate response within 10 minutes, 30–50 ml of glucose 50% can be given intravenously.

If the patient has already become unconscious, the main priority is to maintain patient safety in terms of airway, breathing and circulation. Intravenous glucose should then be administered. If venous access is not available, 1 mg of intramuscular glucagon must be given.

Ketoacidosis

Diabetic ketoacidosis (DKA) is the result of absence or inadequate amounts of insulin. This results in disorders in the metabolism of fats, carbohydrates and proteins. DKA accounts for around 14% of all hospital diabetes-related admissions (Alexander et al. 2000).

The most common causes are:

- reduced or omitted insulin dose
- illness or infection
- undiagnosed diabetes.

Other causes include pregnancy and acute episodes such as myocardial infarct.

Blood tests will reveal the following:

- Raised blood glucose levels (between 16.6 and 44.4 mmol/l). The severity of the DKA is not necessarily related to the level of blood glucose. Some patients may have severe acidosis with blood levels as low as 5.5–11.1 mmol/l.
- Low pH (6.8–7.3).
- Low $P\text{co}_2$, reflecting respiratory compensation.

Pathophysiology of DKA

To care for a patient with DKA, it is important to understand how the signs and symptoms of the condition develop. The underlying pathophysiology of DKA is described below:

1. Glucose is unable to enter body cells without insulin. It accumulates in the blood causing hyperglycaemia.
2. Body cells are now unable to obtain glucose for metabolism and energy production.

3. The kidney cannot cope with absorbing the increased glucose from the glomerular filtrate, which results in glucose escaping into the urine (glycosuria).
4. Glucose is highly osmotic, i.e. it attracts water to itself. As more glucose is lost in the urine, large amounts of water are also lost with it (polyuria).
5. Passing excessive amounts of urine leads to symptoms of dehydration, which stimulates the thirst centre in the hypothalamus, causing the sensation of thirst (polydipsia).
6. The cellular requirement for energy is not being met. The body's response to this is to increase the secretion of glucagon and other stress hormones, in an attempt to increase glucose production. As a result, liver stores of glycogen are converted to glucose. Glucose is produced from the breakdown of body fat and protein (gluconeogenesis). Blood glucose now rises even further.
7. The body is now in a catabolic state, breaking down fat and protein.
8. Cell deprivation of glucose and excessive water loss cause electrolyte imbalance, resulting in muscle weakness.
9. As body fats are burnt for fuel, acids known as ketones are formed and begin to appear in the urine (ketonuria) and accumulate in the blood (ketonaemia). Additionally, acetone secreted by the lungs gives the breath a sweet 'pear drop' smell.
10. Ketone bodies are weak acids that release free hydrogen ions, causing a metabolic acidosis. In an attempt to compensate for this, the patient develops Kussmaul's breathing (deep sighing respirations), in an attempt to remove the hydrogen ions from the blood.
11. The biochemical changes may result in nausea and vomiting, and abdominal pain.
12. Uncontrolled lipolysis, gluconeogenesis and glycogenolysis continue as the starving cells attempt to produce glucose. This increases the blood glucose level, further increasing the osmotic diuresis, dehydration and acidosis to dangerous levels.

Nursing care for the patient in DKA
Effective care during the acute period demands that the nurse understands the cause and progression of DKA. The patient will be very ill, anxious and distressed, and may even be unconscious. The nurse needs to combine technical expertise with good communication skills to ensure both physical and psychological recovery.

Important aspects of care include:

- Assessment of the level of consciousness using the Glasgow Coma Scale.
- Maintainance the patient's airway.
- The unconscious patient will require a nasogastric tube to prevent aspira-

tion of stomach contents in the event of acute gastric paralysis and distension, a common occurrence in DKA. A urethral catheter may also be sited to enable accurate recording of fluid balance.

- Accurate hourly recording of the blood glucose level until the patient is eating and drinking again. Insulin will be administered on a sliding scale in accordance with the blood glucose levels.
- Cardiac monitoring may be required. Hyperkalaemia is common initially in DKA, which can give rise to cardiac arrhythmias. This should resolve as fluids and insulin are given, as this drives potassium back into the cells. Hypokalaemia may then follow, requiring the infusion of supplemental potassium.
- Record the BP, temperature, pulse and oxygen saturation levels hourly until stable. Supplemental oxygen may be required to maintain the saturation levels. A falling pulse, rising BP and increasing urine output indicate progress.
- Monitor the rate and depth of respirations. Respiration rate should return to normal as acidosis subsides.
- Monitor the urine output and test for the presence of ketones. These should disappear within 18–24 h. Appetite should return soon afterwards.
- Ensure that the intravenous infusion is administered as prescribed, via a suitable infusion device. The infusion solution may be changed according to the electrolyte and blood glucose levels.
- Accurate fluid balance is important in an acutely ill person with diabetes. High volumes of fluid (between 4 and 6 litres are usually required) are given to patients who may also have cardiac and renal problems because of the diabetes, and are therefore at risk if there is fluid overload.
- Observe the patient's hydration status (skin turgor, mucous membranes).
- Observe the cannula site for patency.
- Attend to physical comfort. Dehydration and hyperventilation necessitate good oral hygiene. Observe pressure areas regularly, particularly the heels.
- Give other prescribed medications. Intravenous antibiotics and low molecular-weight heparin may be prescribed.
- Address the patient's psychological needs. Give reassurance and explanations of all aspects of care to the patient and relatives.
- Keep accurate records of all aspects of nursing intervention.

When the patient is through the initial acute phase, the reason why the event occurred can be investigated and the opportunity taken to reinforce principles of good practice in relation to diabetes care and control. The patient's knowledge and understanding of the condition can be ascertained and the technique used in drawing up and injecting insulin and in recording blood sugar levels can also be checked. The patient may also benefit from referral to other members of the multidisciplinary team, such as the dietician or diabetes nurse specialist.

Education is an important aspect of the nurse's role. There are many support groups, websites and publications for people with diabetes, covering a wide range of issues relating to the condition. Information such as what patients should do if they become ill (Table 6.12) may be vital in preventing future admissions. It is therefore important that all nurses know how to access resources such as these, in order to give the most up-to-date research-based information.

Table 6.12 What to do when you become ill

- Never stop taking your insulin
- Blood sugar levels can rise even if you do not eat
- Try to maintain your carbohydrate intake with milk, sugar and snacks
- Try to maintain a high sugar-free fluid intake. Drinking fluid every hour helps to prevent dehydration.
- Check your blood sugar 2–4 hourly
- Adjust insulin only if you are confident about doing so
- Test your urine for ketones
- If blood sugar is less than 13 mmol/l, continue with your normal insulin dose
- Seek medical help if vomiting persists, conscious level changes or if breathing becomes rapid

---

Action point 5 – Case Scenario

Simon Grayson is 19. He has had type 1 diabetes for 8 months. He has been ill with vomiting and diarrhoea for the past 3 days and has not been eating much. Because of this, he felt it was best not to take his insulin. He has been admitted after being found in a semi-conscious state by his girlfriend.

- A diagnosis of diabetic ketoacidosis is made. His blood results are:
    glucose 32 mmol/l
    potassium 5.5 mmol/l
    bicarbonate 8 mmol/l
    $P\text{CO}_2$ 3.5 kPa
    $P\text{O}_2$ 12 kPa
    pH 7.05.

1. From what you have read, explain why the level of glucose in the blood continues to rise.
2. List your nursing priorities for the first 24 hours of the admission.
3. What education would you give to Simon to help him avoid similar episodes in the future?

The liver

Structure of the liver

The structure of the liver, together with its specialized blood supply, enable this organ to play a central role in metabolism while also protecting the body from micro-organisms and toxins absorbed via the digestive tract. The liver is the largest internal organ. It accounts for 5% of the neonate's body weight, but this proportion changes to 2% (approximately 1.4 kg) by adulthood. It is located in the abdominal cavity, under the right side of the diaphragm.

The liver is encapsulated within a fibrous coat, the Glisson capsule. It has four lobes: the large left and right lobes, and the smaller caudate and quadrate lobes. The liver's metabolic functions require a large blood supply, which comes from two sources. A quarter is provided via the hepatic artery. This arises from the aorta and thus carries oxygenated blood. The remaining three-quarters of blood is provided by the hepatic portal vein. This arises from the mesenteric and splenic veins, and thus carries blood that is deoxygenated but rich in nutrients absorbed from the gastrointestinal tract. The arterial and venous blood are mixed as they flow through specialized blood capillaries in the liver, called sinusoids. From these, blood flows via central veins through one of three hepatic veins into the inferior vena cava.

The lobes of the liver are made up of many microscopic lobules, which are the anatomical functional units of the liver. Each lobule is formed of hexagonal plates of hepatocytes, the functional cells of the liver. The hepatocytes are arranged so that they radiate out from a central vein, with sinusoids between the plates of cells. Sinusoids are lined with highly permeable endothelium, which enhances transport of nutrients from the blood into the hepatocytes, where metabolism occurs. The useful products of metabolism are secreted directly into the bloodstream. The sinusoids also contain Kupffer cells. These are cells of the reticuloendothelial system, which filter intestinal micro-organisms and old red blood cells from the passing blood and break them down by phagocytosis. The waste products of red blood cell breakdown are excreted into the bile ducts in the bile. Hepatocytes can regenerate if damaged or resected.

Functions of the liver

In addition to synthesis and excretion of bile, the liver has many metabolic, maintenance and storage functions. Metabolism involves the catabolism (breakdown) and synthesis (build-up) of substances.

The liver's role in fat metabolism starts when fat, which has been absorbed from the intestine in the form of triglycerides and fatty acids, enters the liver via the lymphatics. The liver converts triglycerides to many substances essential for body functioning and regulation. Fatty acids may be converted into prostaglandins or ketone bodies. Ketone bodies may be used to produce metabolic energy via the citric acid cycle within the cells. Lipoproteins, synthesized in the liver from carbohydrate and protein, are released into the bloodstream and then deposited as adipose cells for storage. Phospholipids and cholesterol, which are required for the production of plasma membrane components, bile, steroid hormones and vitamin D, are also manufactured in the liver.

The liver has a key role in carbohydrate metabolism. It regulates blood sugar levels by the conversion and storage of glycogen from glucose (glucogenesis), conversion of glucose to fat for storage, release of glucose during hypoglycaemia and take-up of glucose during hyperglycaemia. When glycogen stores have been used up, the liver converts amino acids (from protein) and glycerol (from fat) to glucose, a process called gluconeogenesis (formation of new sugar).

Protein metabolism is a further essential role of the liver. This organ breaks down amino acids to ammonia, a process called deamination. It then converts ammonia to urea, which is passed into the blood, carried to the kidneys and excreted in the urine. The liver also breaks down amino acids to ketoacids, such as pyruvic acid, which are then converted to fatty acids for fat synthesis or storage, or used for the production of metabolic energy for the liver cells via the citric acid cycle. The liver has a key role in: the maintenance of blood volume and plasma oncotic pressure via synthesis of albumin and other plasma proteins; haemostasis through the manufacture of most clotting factors, such as fibrinogen and prothrombin; and immunity via synthesis of most globulins. Synthesis of non-essential amino acids and serum enzymes also occurs in this organ.

Detoxification of drugs and dyes occurs in the liver. It alters endogenous substances such as steroids and hormones and exogenous substances (e.g. alcohol or barbiturates) to make them less harmful and less biologically active. This process is called metabolic detoxification or biotransformation. It prevents excessive accumulation and adverse effects by reducing the amount of the substance reabsorbed and promoting excretion from the intestine or the renal tubule.

The liver stores fat, glycogen, minerals such as iron and copper, and vitamins A, B_{12}, D, E and K for up to several years. The length of storage time depends on the vitamin.

Assessment of the patient with liver disease

In asymptomatic patients, discovery of liver disease may occur incidentally during routine tests. Examples of this include abnormal results of LFTs or coagulation screen, the discovery of an enlarged liver on clinical examination or positive hepatitis virus serology on blood donor screening.

Table 6.13 Symptoms of liver disease

- Jaundice
- Ascites
- Variceal haemorrhage
- Hepatic encephalopathy
- Hepatomegaly
- Splenomegaly
- Hand changes: finger clubbing due to arteriovenous shunting of blood in the lungs, white fingernails with transverse bands, Dupuytren's contracture or palmar erythema (a redness of hands and soles of feet attributed to endocrine and vitamin imbalances with a hyperdynamic circulation)
- Spider naevi: a central dilated arteriole with smaller vessels radiating from it found on the skin of the face, neck, arms, hands and upper part of the trunk. These are related to endocrine imbalance and may bleed profusely
- Gynaecomastia due to hormonal imbalances, including testicular atrophy and loss of body hair, breast enlargement or changes
- Asterixis or liver flap: when the patient is asked to hyperextend the wrist a tremor is seen with a flap at the metacarpophalangeal joints. It is a sign of hepatic encephalopathy and impaired cerebral metabolism, and therefore of severe liver disease

Patients may experience non-specific symptoms which do not directly indicate liver disease. These include lethargy, weakness, anorexia or nausea. However, patients with significant liver disease present with the symptoms listed in Table 6.13. The first four of these will be discussed in detail later.

These symptoms suggest liver disease, but do not indicate the diagnosis. This will be aided by information obtained from the clinical history (Table 6.14).

Investigations used to confirm diagnosis include: blood investigations such as LFTs and coagulation screen; ultrasound scan; endoscopy; ERCP; hepatic angiography; liver biopsy; and histology.

Chronic liver failure

Causes of chronic liver disease are listed in Table 6.15.

In chronic liver disease, hepatocytes are destroyed faster than they can be regenerated. This results in cirrhosis: the formation of macro- and micro-nodules, which affect the structure of the liver and its blood supply. These structural changes impede blood flow through the liver, causing portal hypertension: high pressure in the hepatic portal vein. To attempt to compensate for this increased pressure, collateral vessels are formed to divert blood from the high-pressure hepatic portal vein. However, this means that blood rich in gastrointestinal bacteria and toxins bypasses the mechanisms of

Table 6.14 Making a diagnosis from the clinical history in liver disease

Information from clinical history	May indicate
Recurrent jaundice	Gallstones, alcoholic liver disease, chronic hepatitis or (rarely) familial jaundice
Transfusion of blood products or intravenous drug abuse	Hepatitis B or C
Overseas travel to endemic areas	Viral hepatitis or parasitic infection (schistosomiasis or malaria)
Previous biliary surgery	Ascending cholangitis or liver abscess
Travel to countries with poor sanitation	Hepatitis A
Ingestion of toxic substances, e.g. anti-tuberculosis drugs, alternative remedies (e.g. Jamaican bush tea), *Amanita phalloides* mushrooms or a large dose of paracetamol (acetaminophen)	Acute liver failure

Table 6.15 Causes of chronic liver disease

- Viral hepatitis B, C, D
- Alcohol
- Metabolic causes, e.g. Wilson's disease, genetic haemochromatosis, alpha-1 antitrypsin deficiency,
- Biliary disease, e.g. extrahepatic biliary obstruction, primary biliary cirrhosis, primary sclerosing cholangitis, childhood biliary atresia
- Venous outflow obstruction, e.g. Budd–Chiari syndrome
- Drugs, toxins, e.g. methotrexate, amiodarone
- Immunological, e.g. autoimmune disease, graft-versus-host disease
- Other infections, e.g. syphilis, schistosomiasis

Adapted from Friedman and Keeffe (1998)

metabolism and detoxification that usually occur within the liver. This has several systemic effects:

- There is an increased risk of sepsis due to bacteria absorbed via the gut.
- Raised circulating levels of endogenous substances such as nitric oxide and prostaglandins result in a hyperdynamic circulation, thus exacerbating portal hypertension.
- Exogenous substances absorbed via the gut, such as proteins, are not deaminated by the liver but remain in the bloodstream without being

detoxified. This is termed portosystemic shunting. These amino acids may then cross the blood–brain barrier, resulting in hepatic encephalopathy. Portal hypertension also aids the formation of ascites, congestive splenomegaly and oesophageal varices.

Management of the patient with chronic liver disease involves treating the cause where possible, e.g. alcohol dependence. Second-line treatment involves symptom management when there is decompensation. This is when the diseased liver is unable to cope with excess requirements placed on it, e.g. during infection or following an alcoholic binge. When symptoms become unmanageable the patient may be considered for transplantation, although the criteria for transplant listing depend on the underlying cause of the chronic liver disease, and the patient may not survive the time spent waiting for an organ to become available.

Jaundice

Jaundice (icterus) is yellow discoloration of skin, sclera and mucous membranes caused by the accumulation of bilirubin. The cause may be haemolytic, hepatocellular or obstructive.

Haemolytic jaundice is not caused by liver failure, but is due to excess breakdown of red blood cells into bilirubin. Hepatocytes cannot conjugate this as rapidly as it is formed and so it enters the bloodstream and is deposited in the tissues. The blood contains unconjugated (fat-soluble) bilirubin, and the stools and urine are normal in colour. This may be termed pre-hepatic failure, and examples are neonatal jaundice and jaundice following massive blood transfusion.

Hepatocellular jaundice is caused by liver failure: damaged hepatocytes or obstructed intrahepatic bile ducts (bile canaliculi) result in the liver being unable to conjugate and excrete bilirubin. The blood contains unconjugated (fat-soluble) bilirubin. The stools may be normal or light in colour, and the urine will initially be normal in colour but will become dark once the renal threshold is reached. This may be termed intrahepatic failure, and an example is decompensation of alcoholic liver disease following alcoholic binge drinking.

In obstructive jaundice (cholestasis), hepatocytes conjugate bilirubin but the bile formed cannot pass via the normal route of excretion due to obstruction of the extrahepatic bile ducts. The blood contains conjugated bilirubin, the stools are pale or clay-coloured and urine is dark due to excretion of water-soluble bilirubin. This may be termed post-hepatic failure, and an example is duct stricture or pancreatic tumour.

The primary treatment for jaundice is to treat the cause, e.g. relief of biliary stricture. The second line of treatment is to alleviate symptoms, e.g.

pruritis. Pruritis causes much discomfort to patients, who suffer sleeplessness and skin excoriation due to scratching. The mechanism that causes pruritis is unknown, but treatment may include administration of bile salts such as ursodeoxycholic acid, which increase the proportion of conjugated (and therefore water-soluble) bile salts in the blood, thus aiding excretion via the kidneys.

Ascites

Ascites is the pathological accumulation of excess fluid in the abdominal cavity, which most commonly occurs due to chronic liver disease (cirrhosis accounts for approximately 81% of cases). It is usually a late sign, indicating severe liver disease. Ascites may also be caused by malignancy (10%), cardiac failure, tuberculosis, dialysis or acute liver failure.

There are several proposed mechanisms for ascites formation, but the initial step is believed to be portal hypertension, which causes formation of excess fluid within the congested hepatic sinusoids. This fluid is unable to drain via the hepatic lymphatics due to impairment and it sweeps across the liver surface and pools in the peritoneal cavity. This initial stage, and the presence of increased levels of endogenous substances such as renin, aldosterone, angiotensin and vasopressin, has resulted in several theoretical mechanisms for ascites formation being proposed.

The overflow theory posits that the damaged liver causes a direct rise in the amount of sodium retained via the kidneys, which in turn increases blood volume. The underfill theory suggests that portal hypertension and seepage of fluid into the abdomen cause a reduction in blood volume, with an accompanying increase in oncotic pressure within the blood. Additionally, portal hypertension results in decreased portal blood flow. These factors combine to cause a secondary increase in renal sodium retention as a compensatory mechanism. Neither of these theories adequately explains the mechanism involved and, recently, a modification of the underfill theory, the peripheral arterial vasodilatation theory, has been proposed. This theory recognizes that there is both a reduction in blood volume and arterial vasodilatation, resulting in effective underfilling of splanchnic arterial vessels. The cause of vasodilatation is unknown, but is thought to include mediators such as nitric oxide, prostaglandins and glucagon. These factors result in a secondary increase in renal sodium retention.

In addition, synthesis of albumin is disrupted in chronic liver failure. This is a plasma protein essential for maintaining blood colloid osmotic pressure and a reduced level can exacerbate ascites and peripheral oedema.

Ascites may develop slowly over several months or suddenly due to decompensation following an event that causes the failing liver no longer to cope with the requirement placed on it. Examples of decompensating events include alcoholic binges, infection and variceal haemorrhage.

Approximately 11% of patients with cirrhotic ascites develop spontaneous bacterial peritonitis (SBP). This complication is believed to occur due to translocation of bacteria through the intestinal wall or via the bloodstream. Symptoms of SBP include abdominal pain, pyrexia and hypotension. In two-thirds of patients who develop SBP, a recurrence will occur within a year, and this in part explains why, once a patient develops the symptom of ascites, the 2-year survival rate is 50%. Life-long antibiotics may be prescribed to prevent re-infection, although such prophylaxis has yet to be proven to reduce mortality and there are concerns about the potential emergence of multiresistant bacteria.

In ascites, although sodium is retained, the serum sodium level may be low owing to dilution caused by fluid retention. This underpins the first line of treatment, which is a low-sodium diet. In addition, the stimulation of aldosterone in ascites is countered by the use of spironolactone as the diuretic of choice. If ascites does not resolve quickly enough, furosemide may also be prescribed. Paracentesis may be used, although this may increase the risk of spontaneous bacterial peritonitis. Fast removal of fluid via paracentesis requires intravenous colloid fluid replacement, as there is a risk of dehydration with large-volume fluid removal. There are no agreed recommendations for the volume of ascites removed at one time, the length of time that the paracentesis catheter remains *in situ* and the volume of replacement fluid. Shunts, such as a transjugular intrahepatic portosystemic shunt (TIPS) or a peritoneal–venous shunt, may be used to treat refractory ascites. These work due to the pressure difference between the hepatic portal vein in the peritoneal cavity and the superior vena cava in the thoracic cavity. They have a valve to prevent backflow. Complications that may occur with shunts are blockage, increased risk of infection, hepatic encephalopathy and scarring, which would hinder future liver transplantation.

Variceal haemorrhage

As discussed above, cirrhosis results in the formation of collateral vessels to divert blood away from the high-pressure portal vein. The new vessels formed have little elastic tissue in their walls and continual high pressure results in them becoming distended and varicose. These varices are often formed at the junction of the oesophagus and stomach, where they are superficial and liable to rupture. Average mortality rate in patients with variceal haemorrhage is 30%, but this varies according to the degree of liver disease: 5% mortality rate with mild liver disease; 70% with severe liver disease because of associated coagulopathy, cardiovascular compromise due to ascites and increased risk of aspiration pneumonia in patients with encephalopathy.

Signs of variceal haemorrhage include haematemesis, melaena, tachycardia and hypotension. Initial management is focused on resuscitation:

maintenance of a clear airway; mechanical support of the patient's breathing if required; and fluid resuscitation to avoid hypovolaemic shock. Terlipressin may be given intravenously for selective vasoconstriction of splanchnic arterioles and therefore to reduce bleeding at source.

A Sengstaken–Blakemore or Minnesota balloon tamponade tube may also be inserted during variceal haemorrhage. These tubes have a number of lumina: one allows inflation of a balloon in the stomach to compress the site of bleeding at the oesophagogastric junction from below; the second is rarely needed, but allows inflation of a balloon in the oesophagus to compress the site of bleeding from above; the third allows aspiration of gastric contents to reduce blood entering the intestine, and therefore prevent encephalopathy; and the fourth allows aspiration of oesophageal contents to reduce aspiration of secretions into the lungs. A patient with a balloon tamponade tube will be transferred to a critical care unit for continual observation and monitoring, as movement of the tube may cause asphyxiation of the patient.

When the patient has stabilized oesophago-gastroduodenoscopy (OGD) may be performed to locate the site of bleeding. Once identified, the varices may be treated by endoscopic sclerotherapy or ligation. Sclerotherapy involves direct injection of a chemical agent into the varix to thrombose it. In ligation or banding, the varix is sucked into a chamber within the endoscope and a rubber band is fixed around the base of the varix. The varix gradually necroses, leaving a small ulcer. In addition, the patient may be prescribed low-dose beta blockers such as propranolol to reduce portal hypertension.

Hepatic encephalopathy

Hepatic encephalopathy may occur in chronic or acute liver failure. If patients with liver disease develop neurological or psychiatric symptoms, they should be assumed to be due to hepatic encephalopathy unless proved otherwise. The diagnosis of hepatic encephalopathy is clinical rather than based on blood ammonia levels, and may be missed in patients where liver disease has not yet been recognized.

There are two theoretical mechanisms proposed to explain hepatic encephalopathy. The first is that the dysfunctioning liver cannot produce substances that usually maintain central nervous system (CNS) function. The second is that inadequately functioning hepatocytes and portosystemic shunting allow gut-derived toxic substances to remain in the systemic bloodstream. These are believed to cross the blood–brain barrier and hence cause irritation or suppression of the CNS. Substances that may be implicated include ammonia, gamma-aminobutyric acid (GABA), mercaptans, serotonin and endogenously occurring benzodiazepines. It is likely that more than one substance may be involved, and that the mechanism differs in chronic and acute liver failure.

Trey and Davidson (1970) developed a commonly used classification tool for assessment of brain function deterioration (Table 6.16).

Table 6.16 Classification tool for assessment of brain function deterioration

---

Grade 1
Mild or episodic drowsiness, impaired intellect, concentration and psychomotor function, but rousable and coherent
Grade 2
Increased drowsiness with confusion and disorientation, rousable and conversant
Grade 3
Very drowsy, disorientated, responds to simple verbal commands, often agitated and aggressive
Grade 4
Unresponsive, except to painful stimuli. May be complicated by evidence of cerebral oedema

---

In chronic liver dysfunction encephalopathy may occur as a single event, on a recurrent basis or be subclinical. This is where a patient appears to be functioning normally but one of the following neurological tests shows a deficit to be present: Reitan trail A or B; Digit Symbol; Block Design; or Purdue Peg Board. When assessed in this way, subclinical hepatic encephalopathy may be found in 60–70% of cirrhotic patients, even if their disease is compensated. The progress of hepatic encephalopathy appears to be closely linked to worsening liver function.

Patients with hepatic encephalopathy are managed initially by ruling out other causes of encephalopathy. These include sepsis, acidosis, uraemia, withdrawal from addictive substances such as alcohol, hypoxia and intracerebral haemorrhage.

Precipitating causes are then treated. These are factors that exacerbate hepatic encephalopathy by increasing production or absorption of substances from the gut, or by less identifiable means. They include:

- sepsis
- constipation
- dehydration
- hypokalaemia
- alkalosis
- dietary protein overload
- poor compliance with lactulose therapy.

Finally, therapy is given, although this is based on practical experience rather than scientific proof, as the mechanisms causing encephalopathy in both chronic and acute liver disease are yet to be confirmed. Lactulose is given orally or nasogastrically to ensure that two to three loose bowel movements are passed daily. Gut cleansing with enemas may also be used.

If these treatments fail, second-line treatment includes giving a low-protein diet. However, this is controversial, as many patients with chronic liver disease are malnourished. To counter this, a diet rich in vegetable proteins or branched-chain amino acids may be given as this is less likely to result in hepatic encephalopathy. Antibiotics such as neomycin, metronidazole or vancomycin may be given, as may the short-acting benzodiazepine antagonist flumazenil.

Acute liver failure

Trey and Davidson (1970) defined acute liver failure as acute onset of liver disease with coagulopathy but no previous evidence of liver disease. There is also development of hepatic encephalopathy within 8 weeks of the onset of illness. This may also be termed fulminant hepatic failure. The causes of acute liver disease are listed in Table 6.17.

Table 6.17 Causes of acute liver disease

- Viral hepatitis A, B, C, D, E
- Cytomegalovirus
- Herpes viruses 1, 2 and 6
- Epstein–Barr virus
- Drug induced, e.g. paracetamol (acetaminophen)
- Toxins, e.g. *Amanita phalloides* mushrooms, organic solvents
- Acute fatty liver of pregnancy
- Vascular, e.g. Budd–Chiari syndrome, heatstroke
- Other causes, e.g. Wilson's disease, autoimmune hepatitis, liver tumour

---

Adapted from Friedman and Keeffe (1998).

Complications of acute liver failure include hepatic encephalopathy, cerebral oedema, coagulopathy, renal failure, hypoglycaemia, metabolic acidosis or alkalosis, and sepsis. The effect that liver failure has on other organs means that these patients require monitoring in an ICU.

Management involves supporting the patient by treating symptoms until the liver recovers or liver transplantation can take place. Following paracetamol overdose, N-acetylcysteine is administered to restore glutathione stores.

Patients who have hepatic encephalopathy due to acute liver failure require all the therapies described for chronic liver failure, as well as treatment for the life-threatening complication of cerebral oedema. This occurs in over 75% of patients with grade 4 encephalopathy associated with acute liver failure, particularly where the onset of liver dysfunction has been rapid. If the patient is nursed in an ICU, intracranial pressure or jugular venous saturation can be monitored. These will indicate changes caused by increased swelling within the cranium, which will impair cerebral blood flow and could result in irreversible brain damage or death. Treatment includes: raising the bed head to promote drainage of fluid; avoiding hypotension, hypoxia or hypercapnia; and administration of the osmotic diuretic mannitol.

Experimental therapies such as high-flow haemofiltration and extracorporeal liver assist devices are currently being developed, but long-term studies have yet to be undertaken to prove their effectiveness.

If supportive measures are inadequate then liver transplantation may be appropriate. O'Grady et al. (1989) have identified criteria for transplantation in acute liver failure (Table 6.18).

Friedman and Keeffe (1998) cite 5-year survival rates following liver transplantation as 80–85%. Developments in immunosuppression therapy, surgical technique, anaesthesia and patient selection have all improved survival.

Table 6.18 Criteria for transplantation in acute liver failure

---

- Acute liver failure due to paracetamol overdose
  pH < 7.30 *or* prothrombin time > 100 s (= INR of 6.5) *and* creatinine > 300 µmol/l
- Acute liver failure due to other causes, e.g. viral hepatitis
  Prothrombin time > 100 s (= INR of 6.5) *or any three of the following*:
  - – age < 10 or > 40 years
  - – duration of jaundice before encephalopathy > 7days
  - – serum bilirubin > 300 µmol/l
  - – prothrombin time > 50 s (= INR of 3.5)

INR, international normalized ratio.

Immediate postoperative care is in an ICU. The most common postoperative complications occur as a result of infection or rejection. Suspected cytomegalovirus is treated with ganciclovir as there is high mortality if it is left untreated.

Rejection is a common problem. Acute rejection may occur between 1 and 4 weeks post-transplantation, and chronic rejection may occur at 4–6 months. Treatment is with steroids and immunosuppressive drugs, including tacrolimus, cyclosporin and azathioprine. Psychosocial factors play an important role in long-term success following liver transplantation because of the side effects of the drugs and the lifestyle adjustments required. These include: strict drug regimen; weight gain due to steroid therapy; infections; and increased body hair growth due to immunosuppressive drugs.

Summary

The nurse caring for a patient with a metabolic condition (in common with all other areas of specialized nursing) plays a vitally important role. This chapter covers the areas of anatomy, physiology and pharmacology relating to the care of these patients. All of these factors must be considered to ensure we give our patients the very best care we can. The nurse makes numerous decisions each day and it is important that those decisions are as safe and fully informed as possible.

References and further reading

Alexander MF, Fawcett JN, Runciman PJ (2000) Nursing Practice: hospital and home. The adult, 2nd edn. Edinburgh: Churchill Livingstone.

Bass M (1998) Fluid and electrolyte management of ascites in patients with cirrhosis. Critical Care Nursing Clinics of North America 10(4): 459–467.

Bassett C, Makin L (2000) Caring for the Seriously Ill Patient. London: Arnold.

Beckingham IJ (2001) ABC of diseases of liver, pancreas and biliary system. Gallstone disease. British Medical Journal 322: 91–94.

Campbell J (1999) Nursing care for jaundice. Nursing Times 95(4): 53–55.

Coad NR (1999) The management of acute severe pancreatitis. British Journal of Intensive Care 8: 38–45.

Diabetes UK (the new name for the British Diabetic Association) website (www.diabetes.org.uk).

eGuidelines website (www.eguidelines.co.uk).

Friedman LS, Keeffe EB (1998) Handbook of Liver Disease. Edinburgh: Churchill Livingstone.

Glazer G, Mann DV (1998) United Kingdom guidelines for the management of acute pancreatitis. Gut 42(Supplement 2): S1–S13.

Habeeb KS, Herrera JL (1997) Management of ascites: paracentesis as a guide, Postgraduate Medicine 101(1): 191–200.

Hawker F (1993) The Liver: critical care management. Saunders: London.

Heaton ND (1997) Liver transplantation in children. Care of the Critically Ill 13(3): 90–95.

Higgins A (2000) Understanding Laboratory Investigations. Oxford: Blackwell Science.

Hirsch IB (1996) Surveillance for complications of diabetes. Don't wait for symptoms before intervening. Postgraduate Medicine 99(3): 147–162.

Huether SE, McCance KL (1996) Understanding Pathophysiology. St Louis, MO: Mosby.

Johnson CD (1998) Severe acute pancreatitis: a continuing challenge for the intensive care team. British Journal of Intensive Care 12: 130–137.

Krentz AJ (2000) Diabetes. London: Churchill Livingstone.

Lazarus JH (1997) Hyperthyroidism. The Lancet 349: 339–343.

Marieb EN (1998) Human Anatomy and Physiology. California: Benjamin Cummings..

McCaffrey P (1991) Making sense of the Sengstaken tube. Nursing Times 87(36): 40–42.

Mergener K, Baillie J (1998) Acute pancreatitis. British Medical Journal 316: 44–48.

Metheny NM (2000) Fluid and Electrolyte Balance, 4th edn. Philadelphia, PA: Lippincott.

Mills PR (1998) Clinical assessment of liver disease. Medicine 26(12): 1–5.

Mowat AP (1994) Liver Disorders in Childhood. Oxford: Butterworth-Heinemann.

National Diabetes Education Initiative website (www.ndei.org).

National Service Framework for Diabetes (2001) www.doh.gov.uk/nsf/diabetes

O'Grady JG, Alexander GJM, Hayllar KM, Williams R (1989) Early indicators of prognosis in fulminant hepatic failure. Gastroenterology 97: 439–445.

Raiford DS (1995) Pruritis of chronic cholestasis. Quarterly Journal of Medicine 88: 603–607.

Runyon BA (1998) Management of adult patients with ascites caused by cirrhosis. Hepatology 27(1): 264–272.

Salter M (1997) Altered Body Image. London: Baillière Tindall.

Springings D, Chambers J (2001) Acute Medicine. A practical guide to the management of medical emergencies. London: Blackwell Science.

Torrance C, Serginson E (1999) Surgical Nursing. Kent: Baillière Tindall.

Tortora GJ, Grabowski SR (2000) Principles of Anatomy and Physiology, 9th edn. New York: John Wiley.

Trey C, Davidson CS (1970) The management of fulminant hepatic failure. In Popper B, Schaffner F (eds) Progress in Liver Diseases. New York: Grune & Stratton.

UKPDS (1998) Tight glycaemic control with diet, sulphonylureas, metformin or insulin in patients with type 2 diabetes. Journal of the American Medical Association 281(21:) 2005–2012.

CHAPTER SEVEN

Pain

JANE BASSETT AND CHRIS BASSETT

Introduction

Pain is a sensation that we all experience at some time. In some ways, pain may be thought of as a curse that we could well do without; it is, however, a blessing that protects us from serious and potentially debilitating injury. The statement above, 'we all experience pain at some time' is not entirely true, as there are people, mercifully few in number, who for one reason or another (injury or disease) cannot experience the sensation of pain. They are often very seriously handicapped and unable to function in a normal or safe way in their daily life. This chapter introduces the sometimes complex subject of pain. It describes the mechanism of pain, considers the many factors that influence how we interpret pain, and outlines assessment and treatment. It will ultimately prepare readers to make informed and effective decisions regarding pain in patients and clients.

All nurses are accountable to their patients and clients and it is their duty to prepare themselves to give the very best and most up-to-date advice and care. The nurse is a key person in the eyes of the patient, being very often the only constant in the patient's world. The nurse in the ward or care setting is there 24 hours a day, whereas the doctor is in attendance sometimes for as little as 20 minutes throughout the whole day.

It is the nurse who must be aware and constantly observe for signs of pain. The patient or client may express pain in a very clear way ('Nurse, I have terrible pain in my back'). However, this is not always the case, and nurses must look for other signs of pain, including behavioural or biological changes in the patient. Nurses are taking much more of a high profile in terms of study, and are becoming true specialists in pain control. Many are undertaking diplomas and degrees, and are carrying out research into the science of pain control. This chapter provides the basis of knowledge from which will come a broader understanding of pain. Reflective questions in the form of action points are included throughout to help underpin your learning.

A short history of pain

It can be very useful to consider how people before us have tried to make sense of the pain experience. It provides us with an insight into how the theories of pain came about and can help us to understand pain more fully. In the early accounts of pain, there is a belief that pain was a punishment inflicted on the sufferer by an angry spirit. The Greek philosopher Plato considered pain as being purely an emotional sensation; he believed that the heart was the centre responsible for interpretation and generation of pain. This belief persisted until the second century, when the Roman doctor Galen correctly identified the brain as the centre of sensation and, indeed, pain. He also identified that there was a separate set of nerves for each of the different senses. We can trace back the roots of many of our beliefs and sayings, such as 'feeling with the heart' or suffering a 'broken heart', to the very earliest attempts at understanding pain. It is important to consider the patient as having an affective and physical aspect to pain, and we should thank the early thinkers for aiding our perception of pain today.

What is pain?

Pain is an experience of the whole individual, both mind and body. This concept is central to all writers who discuss and describe pain.

> All pain is real, regardless of its cause. Almost all pain has both physical and psychological components.
>
> McCaffery and Beebe (1989)

Some pain is made up entirely of psychological components; indeed, the phrase 'it is all in the mind' can be true. However, it should be remembered that we as nurses are not there to act as judges in considering whether pain really exists or not. We must record, measure and understand the pain, be it psychological, physical or a combination of the two. Pain is of great importance to us and as McCaffery (1972) points out: 'Pain is whatever the experiencing person says it is and exists whenever he says it does.'

It is important that we enshrine this statement in our practice as nurses.

Defining pain

It is essential at this stage to pause to reflect on what pain actually is and how it affects our lives.

Action point 1

How would you define pain? When did you last feel severe pain. How did it affect you?

There is a difficulty in describing pain, which underlines one of the key problems that nurses face when trying to measure pain: if it is difficult for the individual experiencing the sensation of pain to explain what and how much of it they are feeling, then how can we do so? The problem of pain measurement and its assessment is explored later in this chapter.

Why do we feel pain?

Pain is a physiological safety feature; it is designed to protect our delicate bodies from damage and harm. Those unfortunate people mentioned above who cannot feel pain are in constant danger of physical damage, sometimes severe in nature. How do you know when, for instance, you have damaged a joint? If you are unaware that injury has taken place, you will continue to walk around and may cause irreparable damage to the injured joint. If you cannot feel the pain associated with an infected and inflamed appendix, it may perforate, causing possible peritonitis and, ultimately, death.

These examples show how pain is an essential part of our life protecting us constantly from harm.

Types of pain

Pain may be described as being chronic or acute. Acute pain is sudden in onset and short lasting in nature (measured in days rather than months). Acute pain may be felt following an operation, and will also be felt in other conditions, such as renal colic, acute pancreatitis, myocardial infarction and trauma. A typical acute pain that most of us will have experienced is one caused by a twisted ankle or as a result of hitting our finger with a heavy object such as a hammer. The pain is severe and usually localized, and will reduce if the area is kept still and allowed to heal. Eventually, when the injury has recovered, the pain will subside and disappear, having outlived its usefulness.

Chronic pain by definition is long lasting and may be the result of an underlying injury that does not heal rapidly, such as an injured back, or it may be a symptom of a malignant disease like some, but not all, cancers. Chronic pain can persist for months, years or throughout the sufferer's entire lifetime and is, by its very nature, clearly handicapping; it can cause the sufferer to become less able to function fully in their everyday life and can ruin their quality of life. The key question must be, how can you, as a nurse, help to reduce the pain or help the patient to devise ways of reducing the negative effects of the pain, thus improving their lives?

Action point 2

If you have had quite severe pain in the past, try to remember how it made you feel.

Pain can cause depression and increasing withdrawal into a world of isolation from family, friends, happiness or satisfaction. It is impossible to share one's pain, even with a loved one, and the description of pain often does not fully express its extent or depth, and exactly what it means to the sufferer. The nurse, too, is outside what has been described as the patient's 'interior landscape of pain' (Fordham and Dunn 1994). The nurse must seek ways of getting closer to the person, and in so doing be better placed to help them cope more fully with their experience.

Action point 3

What can you do to help the patient who is in pain? What do you need to find out?

Nurses, at whatever level, has begun to gather skills and attributes that can give them certain advantages. They have undergone training specifically designed to enable them to understand the patient better. They have knowledge and skills of communication, anatomy, physiology and psychology, and, via the doctor, have access to pharmacological and complementary methods of pain control.

Action point 4

What are the nurse's responsibilities towards the patient in pain?

As a nurse, it is essential that you work with the best interests of the patient in mind at all times. Clearly, as your knowledge and understanding of care improve, so does your ability to provide that care. It is of course essential that the patient or client in pain is given adequate and timely pain control. Each registered nurse, midwife and health visitor shall:

> Act in such a way as to promote and safeguard the well-being and interests of patients and clients.
>
> Clause 1 UKCC Code of Conduct (1986)

Biophysical explanation of pain

There are currently four main theories that attempt to explain pain. These have been devised by observing patients and by carrying out research in the laboratory setting. The four theories are as follows:

1. Pattern theory: a summation of nerve impulses occurs over time and (or) space in non-specific nerves.
2. Specificity theory: there is a direct, dedicated nerve 'hotline', from the site of injury to the brain.
3. Gate control theory: a modifiable opening and closing mechanism exists in the nervous system.
4. Post-gate control theories: a continuously active nervous system modifies input, output, reception and response.

The anatomy and physiology of pain

Whichever theory of pain is favoured, all four rely on the transmission of impulses (the pain message) by nerves across the synapse from the site of the pain to the higher centres of the brain. The major parts of the nervous system involved in the 'pain process' are:

- the receptors of the skin and tissues
- the peripheral nerves
- neuronal aggregates in the spinal cord and associated fibres
- the brain stem and thalamus
- the limbic system
- the cerebral cortex.

Nociceptors

Pain receptors, or nociceptors, are situated throughout the skin and subcutaneous tissues. There is a variety of types of nociceptor: some are
associated with touch, pressure sensation and stretching, others with transmitting the sensations of hot and cold. The nociceptors are further
subdivided into specialist receptors. Some transmit chemical irritation, such
as insect and nettle stings, others mechanical injury, trauma and damage.

The nociceptors are denser in some areas of the body than others, for
instance the hands are particularly well supplied with them. Nociceptors are
also sensitive to the inflammatory processes. Histamine, bradykinine and
serotonin produced in the inflammatory response will all trigger the nociceptors. The way a nociceptor responds is similar to the way in which other
nerve impulses are transmitted in the nervous system. For example, if you
prick your finger with a needle, positive sodium ions (Na^+) from outside the
cell will flow into the cell, reversing the potential of the cell and generating
an action potential. This action potential spreads to the next associated
nerve fibre in the chain, thus spreading the sensation of pain from the pain
site to the brain.

Pain fibres

Pain fibres are the next structure that must be considered. The needle-prick
injury, having been identified and sent on its way, now travels along the pain
fibres. These fibres comprise the myelinated A beta fibres and the unmyeli-
nated C fibres. The speed of impulse is faster in the A beta fibres than in the
C fibres. Even a minor pain will not be transferred by a single fibre, but will
instead be carried by several fibres. Therefore, even a needle prick will result
in a complex series of sensations, both painful and non-painful, due to the
involvement of a number of mixed fibres. When the needle prick occurs, there
is firing of the A beta and C fibres. The rapidly transmitting A beta fibres give
rise to the well-experienced sharp, sudden pain (ouch!), which is followed by
the pain carried by the slower-transmitting C fibres. It is now generally believed
that the C fibres are responsible for the slower, prolonged pain following a sudden injury. The longer effect of the C-fibre activity transmitting the aching, dull
pain is thought to be due to the release of such inflammatory chemicals as histamine, serotonin and other active substances found in the injured tissue.

Pain pathways in the spinal cord

The nociceptors and sensory fibres have their cell bodies within the dorsal
root ganglia, which enter the spinal cord at the dorsal horn of the grey mat-

ter. It is at this point in the dorsal horn that the pain impulses are organized, sorted and then transmitted to the brain via specialized tracks.

Pain transmission to higher centres

The fibres responsible for pain transmission make highly complex connections within the brain. These include areas such as the hypothalamus, the thalamus, the limbic system and the grey matter of the midbrain. The function of the brain in modulating and recognizing pain is extremely complex and not fully understood. However, theories (mentioned earlier) have been developed to explain many of the anomalies that exist in the study of pain. The most prominent theory remains the 'gate theory', proposed by Melzack and Wall (1965). There are no theories that account for all the multitudes of pain and perceptions. Melzack and Wall's proposed theory is perhaps the most comprehensive; they stated that the substantia gelatinosa of the dorsal horn acted as a 'pain gate'. This gate, it was stated, exerted a variable degree of pain inhibition on the transmission of impulses from the nociceptors

The theory states that an increase in the sensory input by the larger A beta fibres tends to close the gate to pain impulses, whereas an increase in small A delta fibres and C fibre activity tends to open it. A balance of the relative activity between the large and small fibres determines the pain level actually experienced.

The pain gate

Melzack and Wall further stated that a pain bypass exists, involving the A beta fibres. These fibres generate descending impulses from the conscious brain to the substantia gelatinosa, which then closes the gate and reduces the pain. These descending impulses can also affect the perception of pain. This mechanism may explain how the influences of culture, society, personality and training modify the pain that is felt. We will return to these important factors later in the chapter to explore more fully the cultural and social influences on pain.

Endogenous (inbuilt) means of reducing pain

The study of opiate drugs led to the discovery that the body, in response to certain stimuli, releases substances that moderate the level of pain experienced by an individual. Once released, these substances are known to bind to receptors and, in doing so, their analgesic properties reduce the sensation of pain. These endogenous substances are the endorphins and their subgroup the enkephalins. They can be found in all parts of the nervous system.

Endorphins are released as a response to physical and psychological stimuli. They then pass into the bloodstream and are carried through to the opiate receptors, which are located throughout the nervous system.

The existence of a natural substance whose action is to reduce pain makes great biological sense, inasmuch as it helps us to remain effective when injury or stress has occurred.

Summary

It is clear that pain is not simply a stimulus-and-response mechanism. Variations in causes and types of pain indicate that there are other factors at play in the transmission of pain. Pain modulation is a dynamic process operating continuously to protect the person from damage.

Culture and pain

Do people from different cultures feel pain differently? If so, how will this affect the way that we care for our patients or clients?

Action point 5

We practise in a multicultural society. Do you think that culture affects pain perception?

There is evidence to show that cultural and ethnic origin influence the way that we experience pain and our acceptance of it. It is not just the type, site or extent of the injury or disease that dictates the patient's pain level. Burns (1988) suggests that culture and even associated religious upbringing can significantly affect the level of pain tolerated by an individual. Many examples exist of how people can tolerate high levels of pain. Ritualistic self-mutilation and fire walking are practised in certain religious cults in India, for example. The nurse must understand the part played by an individual's ethnic and cultural background as it will affect the care and pain assessment and will certainly affect the pain behaviour.

Different cultures may have markedly contrasting ways. This is underlined by the classic work carried out by Zborowski (1952), who observed that ethnic origins influence the ways that individual groups react to pain. He identified that what he described as a 'future orientation' and a 'present orientation' existed in the way that two groups reacted to a similar pain stimulus. He studied Italian and Jewish groups in the USA. People from the

Italian community manifested a reaction to pain by overt expressions of grief and crying and seeking 'present-orientated' sympathy. The Jewish community tended to be less expressive with their reaction to the pain, but would worry about the future of their pain. They continued to complain despite the removal of the pain stimulus. This was in contrast to the Italian group, who ceased complaining as soon as the stimulus was removed. It is clear that the nurse must understand these considerations in whichever area he or she works. We are beginning now to see how difficult it can be to care for our patients who are in pain.

Assessing the patient's pain

Action point 6

What factors need to be taken into consideration so that we can look after those we care for?

When we can assess the patient's pain accurately, we can treat it more effectively. Truly effective treatment of pain is not possible until the nurse has made an accurate and careful assessment of the patient. As mentioned earlier in the chapter, the nature of pain is unique to the patient.

Action point 7

Think of the ways you have seen patients or clients react to pain.

Every person will perceive, react and describe their pain differently. This requires the nurse to be methodical, painstaking and persistent when assessing pain. Once you have a brief understanding of assessment and a grasp of how pain mechanisms work, you can adapt what you know to many different care situations

Taking the history

It is important for the nurse to be thorough and methodical when assessing a patient, just as it is for the physician assessing the patient. This information gives the nurse invaluable information to use later as an aid to decision making.

Description of the pain

> **Action point 8**
>
> What words have you heard used to describe a patient's pain?

It is vital to listen to the patient when he describes his pain. 'Burning' may indicate nerve involvement. A 'nagging ache' may suggest visceral pain. A 'sharp, stabbing' pain could indicate a loose bone fragment in the tissues of a joint. Other words used may include:

- pulsating
- drilling
- cutting
- gnawing
- rasping
- heavy
- searing
- exhausting
- sickening
- killing
- hot
- cold
- blinding
- wretched.

Position of the pain

This location of the pain is important, too, and a body chart that is filled out by the patient, indicating site and extent of pain, is helpful. These are simple and easy to fill out even for the young or disabled, or they can be filled out by the nurse if the patient is too debilitated. They can give an excellent running record of how pain treatment is progressing and are important when evaluating nursing care.

Onset of the pain

A history of the onset of the pain may give important clues as to its source. Sometimes the patient's pain may be attributed to an unrelated event. This might have important implications in planning treatment. It may also lead to the patient misunderstanding the origin of his pain.

Factors affecting pain

These factors are clearly very important when taking a pain assessment. Questions such as: 'What brings on the pain?' and 'Is it associated with food activity, stress, anxiety or other activities of living?' will also provide important information.

Assessing acute pain

- Intensity, position, description
- Can the patient bear the pain?
- Are there factors affecting the pain, such as anxiety, stress or activity?
- Does the patient understand the pain? What can you tell them?

Assessing chronic pain

- Consider the use of a pain diary to record the pain
- Look for factors that worsen the pain
- Check for the effectiveness of current pain control
- Assess the patient's mental state: fear, anxiety or depression
- Assess the patient's family. Can they cope?
- How does the patient cope with the pain? The nurse must learn from him and his carers
- Discuss pain-reducing strategies

Action point 9

Can you think of other adult patients whom you may deal with in practice and who may have particular problems expressing and explaining their pain?

The person with learning disabilities in pain

It may be argued that many of the techniques used to assess children can be transferred to the patient with a learning disability. The description 'learning disability' is fraught with problems, because the patient may suffer from a wide variety of inextricably intertwined physical, psychological and social problems. These may present as a wide variety of behaviour and expressions of pain. It is important to have a clear and non-judgemental attitude towards the client and, in common with all types of nursing, a clear and detailed assessment of the patient's general condition and lifestyle is needed to plan all aspects of care that may be needed.

The primary condition that has caused the learning disability may be important, and it may well be causing the actual pain. There may also be secondary problems, such as epilepsy, which must be considered, especially when deciding on the use of analgesics. Disorders of circulation, both centrally (congenital heart defects) and peripherally, may create abnormal blood pressure readings. This in turn can make it harder to use the biophysical aspects of pain sensation as a measure of pain. With clients who are destructive and exhibit behavioural problems, it can be difficult to manage their treatment and pain. The nurse must include the individual's carers in the management of care. This co-operation must be maintained throughout the time the client is in pain and will underpin the nursing care that can be offered.

Mental illness and pain

Pain is perhaps the most common of all symptoms in medicine. It is also very common in psychiatry. Pain disorder is referred to in the *Diagnostic and Statistical Manual of Mental Disorders*, published by the American Psychiatric Association. Pain itself may cause psychological distress, or it may be caused by psychological disorders. Pain may be a feature of many psychological conditions, such as depression, hysteria and schizophrenia. It is also often a clear feature in patients suffering from hypochondria, which is the belief that they are suffering from a physical illness. In this case, the pain is often continuous, does not respond to analgesia or other means of pain relief, and does not wake the person from sleep. The pain, when described by the client, is often associated with emotional stress or trauma. It is clear that, as nurses, we need to be very careful not to dismiss any patient or client we think is suffering from a psychiatric disorder that is causing them to believe they have pain. We know that there is no definitive test that measures pain. Who is to say that the pain is not real, and a sign of illness or trauma? Complaints of pain must be taken seriously and medical help must be summoned to assess the patient. As nurses, we are accountable to our patients and must take great care when assessing them. We must always act on the safe side. Treatment for the patient for whom a physical cause cannot be found can be difficult, but antidepressant drugs have been used with some success, and behavioural treatment has also been of use for this type of patient.

General approaches to assessment

There are many approaches that will help to give as full a picture as possible of the patient's level and type of pain, which will help the nurse to help the patient overcome or come to terms with pain. The most common way of measuring pain is the visual analogue scale (Figure 7.1). The numerical rating scale and the verbal rating scale are also useful. Wherever possible, these rating scales should be used with other modes of assessment. There are also physical signs of pain that can be measured and do not require verbal assessment.

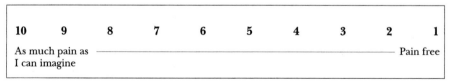

Figure 7.1 A simple visual analogue scale assessment tool.

Physiological changes

Pain stimulates the cardiovascular system and causes relative changes in blood pressure. Blood pressure rises when a person is in pain. This may be accompanied by raised pulse and respiratory rates, and there will be an increase in diaphoresis (sweating). In a young, fit person, this does not represent too much of a problem. However, if the patient is old or unwell, then this can cause extra physiological problems. There may also be a pallor of the skin tone, another sign of pain. Pain can cause disturbances of the endocrine system releasing cortisol, a hormone that can reduce the natural and beneficial inflammatory process, thus reducing the healing and repair of the patient's tissues.

Physical changes

In chronic pain, there may be wasting of the limb or area affected, because of a reluctance to use that area of the body. Reduced lymphatic drainage, again as a result of a reluctance to move the limb or area of the body, may lead to swelling. A body chart filled in by the patient may aid in assessment. It can help both the patient and the nurse to gauge the extent and coverage of the pain, and it will also provide a measure of success of the treatment, making it an essential part of the nursing care plan.

Treating pain

When the nurse has assessed the patient fully, she will then be in a position to provide help for that patient. Information about and understanding of pain are a key part of caring for the patient. It is also very important that nurses have knowledge of and understand the variety of treatments available.

Nurses are becoming increasingly specialized in all areas of practice. This is certainly true in the field of pain control, and innovative pain control teams made up of clinical nurse specialists, doctors, physiotherapists and other healthcare professionals are being created across the country. All these practitioners have great experience in pain control and a desire to help alleviate their patients' pain. There have also been great advances in the number and diversity of treatments available. In short, it is an exciting time for nurses who wish to expand their role in helping patients and clients who are in pain.

Action point 10

In what ways can we provide pain relief for our patients?

Analgesic drugs

Not surprisingly, some of the earliest medications discovered and used by humans were those aimed at reducing or removing pain. There are now many types of medication used to control pain, and nurses must be aware of the following factors when using drugs with their patients:

- safety
- efficiency
- effectiveness.

The nurse needs to be aware of the patient's analgesic history, and must ask the following questions:

- What drugs have you used in the past that have been particularly effective?
- Have you had any adverse reactions to any analgesia or sedatives?

These questions serve an important purpose when determining future treatment. The patient may also have firm opinions about the use of analgesia, especially the strong opiates, which may hold a particular negative significance.

The nurse must find out as much as possible about the patient's feelings and beliefs about drug therapy, and must also take the following areas into consideration:

- Body weight: this is essential to help the doctor estimate the dosage of the analgesia required.

- Age: this is also important when considering dosage. The very old or very young will not be able to cope with high doses of certain drugs.
- Respiratory function: certain types of analgesics and their dosage may have an effect on respiratory function, which could result in respiratory depression.
- Renal and liver function: if the patient's kidneys or liver are not functioning properly, the body may have a reduced ability to rid itself of the drugs, leading to potential toxicity.
- The patient's ability to ingest or digest drugs: the most common route of drug administration is via the oral route. Clearly, if the patient is unable to swallow or digest the drug then it would be pointless to give the drug by mouth. An alternative route of administration must then be considered.
- Other drugs: if, as is often the case, the patient is on other medication, it is essential that the prescribing doctor knows what that medication is, in order not to prescribe drugs that may react in a dangerous way or that may be rendered ineffective when mixed with the other drug(s).

The role of the nurse in drug administration

It is usually the nurse who handles and administers drugs, and you must remember that safety is essential. Clear records must be kept of the drugs administered, for the sake of both the patient and the nurse. The nurse also has a major responsibility to ensure that patients know what drugs they are taking, their side effects, and any special requirements to ensure safe and effective administration. Nurses are teachers too, and must educate patients, their families and carers in the administration of analgesic drugs.

We will now examine some of the more commonly used analgesics.

Pharmaceutical treatment of pain

Analgesics and related drug therapies are being developed and improved constantly. It is important for the nurse to keep abreast of these changes. The drugs used to treat pain fall into the following broad categories:

- simple analgesics
- opiate analgesics
- non-steroidal anti-inflammatory drugs (NSAIDs)
- corticosteroids.

Simple analgesics

Aspirin

Aspirin is a widely used analgesic that also has a useful anti-inflammatory action. It is available in tablet, soluble, slow-release, enteric-coated and suppository forms. It is particularly useful in low-to-moderate visceral pain. It is also used in rheumatoid arthritis because of its anti-inflammatory effects on the joints.

Side effects may include gastric inflammation, nausea, vomiting, iron deficiency anaemia (in long-term usage) and tinnitus. Reye's syndrome in children has been associated with aspirin, so it is not recommended for use in children.

Paracetamol

Paracetamol is another extremely widely used drug and has similar effects to aspirin. It does not, however, have an anti-inflammatory effect. It is available in tablet, soluble and elixir form.

It has few side effects, and is a very safe drug if used with care. However, when dosage is exceeded, severe liver damage can occur, and this can be fatal if not treated in time.

Opiate analgesics

When a milder analgesic has failed to control the pain, the use of opiates may be considered. This group of drugs acts centrally, reducing the perception of pain in the brain. It also causes euphoria and a reduction in anxiety. This group of drugs can be subdivided into:

- opiate agonists, which stimulate the opiate receptors
- opiate agonist antagonists, which stimulate the opiate receptors but then block them when used with other agonist analgesic drugs. The nurse must remember that, when drugs are mixed together, pain reduction may be difficult to achieve.

Opiate agonists (moderate-to-severe visceral pain)

Codeine phosphate
This is a useful drug that is often used to relieve pain in people with head injury, because it does not depress the respiratory centre of the brain. It is available in tablet, elixir or injection form.

Side effects include nausea, vomiting and constipation.

Dihydrocodeine
This is slightly stronger than codeine, and has the same side effects.

Compound analgesics
These consist of drugs that, used together, enhance the analgesic effects. To be aware of the side effects, one needs to be aware of the component drugs used in the compound and their side effects.

Common compound analgesics include:

- co-codamol – codeine and paracetamol
- co-dydramol – dihydrocodeine and paracetamol
- co-codaprin – codeine and aspirin.

Opiate agonists (severe visceral pain)

These are all controlled drugs.

Diamorphine
Diamorphine is a strong and effective analgesic that is highly soluble and therefore easier to reduce into injectible form. It is available in tablets, elixir and injection.

Side effects include constipation, nausea, respiratory depression and dependence.

Morphine
Morphine is a strong and effective analgesic usually considered a first line of treatment for severe visceral pain. It is available in tablet, sustained-release, elixir, injection or suppository form.

It has the same side effects as diamorphine.

Pethidine
Pethidine is a fast-acting, short-lasting analgesic that is not as strong as morphine. It is used in acute pain, such as postoperative pain.

Side effects include nausea, vomiting, respiratory depression and dry mouth.

Papaveretum
This has similar uses to pethidine, with some muscle relaxant properties. It is available in tablet and injection form.

Opiate agonist antagonists

Opiate agonist antagonists are used for the relief of moderate to severe pain.

Buprenorphine

This is a widely used and long-acting drug. It is especially useful because it can be given sublingually. It is available in tablet and injection form.

Side effects include nausea and vomiting, and occasionally confusion.

Non-steroidal anti-inflammatory drugs

NSAIDs are an extremely valuable addition to the straightforward analgesic drugs available. They are particularly useful for treating the pain caused by arthritis or bony secondary metastases, conditions characterized by the excessive release of prostaglandins. NSAIDs inhibit the release of these substances.

The general side effects of these drugs are similar to the side effects of aspirin, but are generally less frequent and milder.

Indomethacin

This is used in bone pain. It is available as a capsule, slow-release, injection or suppository.

Ibuprofen

As above. Available in tablet or elixir form.

Diclofenac sodium

Available in tablet, slow-release or injection form.

Corticosteroids

Corticosteroids can be effective for pain caused by lymphoedema, compressed nerves, intestinal obstruction and headache caused by raised intracranial pressure. The corticosteroid reduces pressure on the organ by reducing oedema. This reduces the inflammation and therefore the pressure. They are also very effective in reducing pain in inflammatory conditions, such as rheumatoid disease in the joints, or soft tissue injury, such as caused by stress injury, tendonitis or torn muscles.

Side effects include fluid retention, diabetes and gastric irritation, especially if the treatment is long term. As with all drugs, it is the nurse's responsibility to monitor patients for side effects. It is also vital that patients know how to monitor themselves and how to observe for side effects.

Dexamethasone

This is sometimes useful in malignant conditions as it reduces the effect of acute exacerbations of pain and discomfort. It is available in oral or injectable preparations.

Prednisolone

This is a commonly used drug, often in conjunction with NSAIDs. It is available in tablet, soluble, enteric-coated or enema form.

Hydrocortisone acetate

This corticosteroid is injected into the joint or soft tissue and has a direct effect on the pain in the local area. It can be very effective when injected carefully by the doctor.

Delivery of pain-relieving drugs

Action point 11

What routes of drug administration do you know of?

In addition to the more obvious routes – oral, sublingual, per rectum, etc. – there are other ways of giving pain-relieving agents, and it is important to understand specific methods of drug delivery in pain control.

The syringe driver

This is a relatively new innovation in the armoury of pain control and is becoming well established. It is a battery pump that delivers a constant measured dose of analgesic drug (usually an opiate). All the nurse needs to do is explain the pump to the patient or carer, and ensure that the syringe is filled on time and that the infusion site is not infected or inflamed. This type of pain control is particularly useful for those who are suffering with a terminal illness and are in severe pain. It can allow them to lead a much more full and active life. It may also help to prevent breakthrough pain, which can be extremely demoralizing for the patient, by maintaining effective levels of analgesia. This method can also be used for patients who cannot take drugs via the alimentary tract.

Patient-controlled analgesia

This method of pain control is of great use, particularly following surgery. It allows patients to administer and control (within limits) their own analgesia. Patient-controlled analgesia can deliver an infusion of the analgesic in several different ways. The patient can operate a button, which releases a programmed dose of drug. The pump can then be programmed to lock out for a period of time, thus preventing overdosing. The pump can also deliver a constant trickle of drug in a very similar way to the syringe driver; or it can deliver a combination of the two – a constant trickle, with the availability of metered bolus doses.

Epidural analgesia

This technique delivers analgesics or anti-inflammatory drugs into the epidural space in the spine, between the spinal dura and the ligamentum flavum. This method of pain control is widely used in childbirth, but is a serious consideration for use when other methods of pain control have not been successful. In this case, opiate drugs may be used as a bolus or an infusion into the epidural space, and they then act centrally by attaching to the opiate receptors. Local anaesthetic agents block the conduction of painful stimuli. This method of treatment can be difficult and complex to insert, and it needs a close level of supervision by the nurse to observe for side effects.

Anaesthetic agents may cause severe hypotension, which can be very sudden and is caused by vasodilatation. It is treated with intravenous fluid therapy to make up fluid volume. Opiate epidurals can have a similar effect to oral opiates, in that they may cause respiratory depression and a reduced gag reflex.

Entonox

Entonox is a gas, which, when inhaled, acts as an analgesic. It consists of 50% oxygen and 50% nitrous oxide. It is used most widely in childbirth but is also useful in many situations such as:

• dressing changes
• dressing burns
• invasive procedures
• following myocardial infarction
• trauma
• during painful physiotherapy procedures, etc.

Entonox is designed to be patient controlled and is delivered via a mask that the patient holds over the nose. The patient operates a demand valve to release the Entonox. In this way it is impossible to overdose, because when the sedative effects of the drug take hold the patient will relax the grip on the mask.

The use of various drugs and gases introduced into the body is still the most common way to control pain, and it is essential that the nurse is aware of all aspects of pharmaceutical analgesia. He or she is responsible for the patient's safety and the education of the patient and carer. However, there are many effective alternatives to drugs for relieving and reducing pain.

Complementary methods of pain control

It is not that long ago that so-called complementary methods of pain treatment were considered by nursing and medicine as strange or misguided. This view has changed radically in the past few years. Those involved in pain control have taken many of these alternative therapies and begun to use them with increasing effect. These therapies help us to enable our patients to overcome their pain, be it acute or chronic, postoperative or associated with a terminal illness. All nurses must be open-minded when considering alternative methods of pain relief. We are accountable to our patients, and part of that accountability includes a duty to keep up to date, so we must evaluate all new treatments that may benefit our patients.

Let us now look at some of the more popular complementary methods of pain relief.

Transcutaneous electrical nerve stimulation (TENS)

This, along with acupuncture, has become quite mainstream and is arguably no longer classed as a complementary therapy. It is a non-invasive method of pain relief that works by an electrical current being passed through the skin into the tissues via electrodes attached to the skin. When TENS is applied, the patient usually notices a tingling sensation. The machine must be adjusted to prevent either pain in the electrode area or movement in the skeletal muscles. Most machines are very compact and can be carried around, enabling the patient to achieve a more normal lifestyle. This treatment is becoming more widespread and an increasing number of TENS machines are available for use free from the NHS. Treatment using a TENS machine may need a doctor's prescription but is usually applied and managed by nurses. It is not fully understood how TENS works, but it is thought that it releases the body's own endorphins and enkephalins – the substances that block pain at the receptor sites at the afferent neurons. TENS is most often used to treat muscular pain, during painful procedures, during labour and for recurrent acute pains such as dysmenorrhoea and headaches (McCaffery and Beebe 1989). It is a still a relatively new therapy compared with many of the other alternative therapies, some of which may have been used for thousands of years.

Acupuncture

This ancient Chinese therapy uses thin needles, which are inserted into the body. The Chinese believe that there are energy points and channels throughout the body, which, when needles are inserted into them, can affect the sensation of pain and modulate unpleasant sensations. Many conventionally trained European doctors and nurses currently use this method with great success; some even use acupuncture to prevent pain in patients having even quite major operations that normally require a general anaesthetic.

Relaxation

This method of relieving pain works by concentrating the mind on a specific function, such as visualization and slow breathing. With practice, patients can learn to distract themselves from the pain. Specialized relaxation tapes with music and calming messages are widely available. The relaxation should be carried out with the patient in a comfortable reclined position. The technique can be difficult to master, but, once learnt, can be extremely useful.

Guided imagery

This is related to relaxation, but the patient is encouraged to imagine he is going on a journey to a place that he may have been to before or that he can imagine, such as a beach or a desert island. The key factor in this therapy is that the patient has left the pain behind. Various props, such as evocative music, sounds, smells or photographs, can be used to aid in the imaginary journey. This technique is often used with relaxation

Massage

Massage has particular benefits for the person in pain. It can provide deep heat and stimulation to an injured area, providing increased healing and reduced effects of inflammation. It also provides the close human contact so important to all of us. Nurses can learn massage skills and become trained massage therapists. It can also be used safely in a way that allows even a junior nurse to deliver specific limited treatments. The nurse must be sensitive to the patient's wishes and apply massage in an appropriate and careful way. Some patients benefit from a firm massage, while others need only a light and gentle touch. Massage can provide relaxation, aid sleep and generally make the patient feel less anxious, helping to break the cycle of pain. Massage oil, baby oil, talcum powder or soapy water may be used for this therapy.

Aromatherapy

Aromatherapy is popular with many people today, not just those who are ill or in pain. In hospital and health settings, it is generally nurses who are pioneering its use. Aromatherapy is a particularly pleasant way to help people overcome their stress, anxiety, depression and pain, and the use of essential oils distilled from naturally occurring plants, flowers and herbs has been used for many centuries. These oils are usually readily available from high street shops. The oils and massage have a relaxing effect and if the right oils are used as props in guided imagery they can prompt memories of a relaxed state. They are dropped on a little water, which is gently heated on a lamp to give a vaporized perfume in the air. If the oils are too concentrated they could present a danger to the patient. The people most susceptible are pregnant women and those suffering from diseases such as hypertension or other chronic health problems.

Many books on aromatherapy are available, but, in common with all complementary therapies, it should be remembered that a good level of knowledge and training is essential before practising this treatment.

Reflexology

This is another therapy based on an ancient belief. Practitioners believe every part of the body is related to a zone on the sole of the foot. Therefore by massaging the relevant area of the foot, the person's pain may be reduced. This is a very specialist skill but, given time, can be learnt by a nurse.

The future of complementary therapy for pain control

There is little doubt that not enough credence has been given to these alternative therapies in the past by both the general public and the medical profession. Recently, however, the British Medical Association has changed its stance somewhat and taken some of these therapies more seriously. As we learn more about these practices, we can use them to complement the care we already provide and continue to enhance the wellbeing of our patients.

Psychological approaches to pain control

We know that pain has both physical and psychological components and, as mentioned above, nurses must be prepared to treat their patients with pharmaceutical preparations, psychological approaches and complementary therapies. Often, a combination of all three approaches is required to help relieve pain. The psychological aspects of nursing care are explored more fully in Chapter 8.

> **Action point 1**
>
> Think of a patient you have cared for who was in pain. In light of your new knowledge, consider how you might care for similar patients in future.

Summary

Arguably, the relationship that the nurse enjoys with the patient is the key to effective nursing care. Communication between the nurse and the patient is essential, as is an in-depth knowledge of sociology, psychology, anatomy, physiology and pharmacology. All of these factors must be used to ensure that we give our patients the very best care we can. Pain management in nursing is developing rapidly, and nurses are becoming more and more involved in developing this vital service for patients.

References and further reading

Bonica JJ (1990) The Management of Pain, 2nd edn. London: Lea & Febinger.

British Medical Association (1993) Report on Complementary Therapies. London: BMA.

Burns RB (1988) Essential Psychology. Lancaster: MTP Press.

Carrol D (1993) Pain Management and Nursing Care. London: Butterworth-Heinemann.

Coderre TJ (1993) Contribution of central neuroplasticity to pathological pain. Pain 52: 258–285.

Cousins MJ, Bridenbaugh PO (1998) Neural Blockade in Clinical Anaesthesia and Management of Pain. New York: Lippincott.

Dahl JB, Kehlet H (1993) The value of pre-emptive analgesia in the treatment of post-operative pain. British Journal of Anaesthesia 70: 434–439.

Degenarr R (1979) Some philosophical considerations on pain. Pain 17: 281–304.

Fordham M, Dunn A (1994) Alongside the Patient in Pain. London: Baillière Tindall.

Lundberg T (1984) Electrical stimulation in the relief of pain. Physiotherapy 21: 12–16.

McClure JH, Wildsmith JA (1985) Conduction Blockade for Postoperative Analgesia. London: Edward Arnold.

McCaffery M (1972) Nursing Management of the Patient in Pain. Philadelphia, PA: Lippincott.

McCaffery M, Beebe A (1989) Pain. St Louis, MO: Mosby.

Melzack R, Wall PD (1965) Pain mechanisms: a new theory. Science 50: 971–979.

Ray C (1982) The concept of coping. Psychological Medicine 12: 385–395.

UKCC (1986) Code of Professional Conduct. London: UKCC.

Wall P, Melzack R (1994) Textbook of Pain. Edinburgh: Churchill Livingstone.

Zborowski F (1952) Cultural components in responses to pain. Journal of Social Issues 8: 16–30.

CHAPTER EIGHT

Psychological needs

JILL JESPER

Introduction

This chapter identifies psychological needs, their influences and expression, and explores ways in which nurses can attempt to meet these needs in hospitalized patients. The contents and guidelines can be applied to all patients who need psychological support during their treatment in hospital.

The emphasis is on raised awareness of factors that may compromise psychological wellbeing in patients, with a view to addressing these factors in a proactive manner. Psychological theories are addressed briefly, to clarify perspectives on approaches to helping.

Psychological care is viewed as a whole way of being rather than solely as theoretical insight and a range of communication skills. It encompasses a range of roles and responsibilities, including: educative, informative and supportive interventions; empowering strategies; and therapeutic activities. It can help the patient to maintain a sense of 'self', an element of control, a feeling that care provision is a shared and negotiated activity, not an imposition of protocol. It can be a valuing experience, based on the acknowledgement and respect of human need.

What are psychological needs?

Action point 1

Why do we need to worry about psychological needs when caring for our patients? Make a list of the things that may upset your patient, then read on and consider ways that you might help your patient to feel more comfortable.

Psychological needs are those that we all know something about. Maslow (1968) suggests that humans share common yet individual needs. These range from the basic to the more complex, and within this range are the need for safety, belonging, acceptance, cognition, aesthetic appreciation, self-fulfilment and realization of potential.

The concept will probably be familiar, even if the terms used are not. For example, there are times when we feel emotionally vulnerable or afraid, times when we need the security of home and of those we love. Safety in this case is not just a physical need. Consider the experience of feeling rejected by peers, and the relief we feel when accepted by a new group of colleagues at work. This illustrates the importance of belonging.

Maslow's view of human need incorporates a hierarchy, with self-actualization at the top. Self-actualization is about personal fulfilment, and in Maslow's view, this cannot be achieved until needs at the lower level of the hierarchy have been met. Meeting these needs can be complex. For example, the achievement of cognitive potential is dependent on the ability to know, understand and problem solve. These tasks are complicated by human emotion and by changing personal circumstances and experiences. We all experience confusion and dependency from time to time and we all experience negative pressures, such as different forms of loss, insecurity, difficulties in problem solving and frustration. On the other hand, we could probably all identify with psychological wellbeing, when we do cope with difficult situations, control our behaviour and use logic to help to clarify possible solutions to problems.

Theories of psychological needs

There may be a tendency to assume that as nurses, because we generally possess reasonable assessment and care-planning skills, we can assess and meet the psychological needs of those in our care. This is not always the case. Perhaps one of the reasons for this is that, as individuals, we all have different perceptions of our world; we see things in different ways.

Different psychological theorists offer their ideas about the origins and manifestation of human thoughts, feelings and behaviours. They help to illustrate how people develop their perceptions, adopt certain attitudes and behaviours, and experience certain feelings. Some of these theories are outlined briefly below.

Cognitive theory

Cognitive theory includes individual perception. Perceptions vary considerably and are dependent on many factors. Previous life experience will play some significance in how we 'see' a situation. We may have experienced that situation before, and thus we may have useful information stored in our memory, which can be utilized. Sophisticated mental processes ensure that this information is retrieved, but the way in which it is utilized may also be dependent on the positive or negative feelings associated with those perceptions. The process of knowing and understanding involves attention to and retention of information derived from a variety of sources. This knowledge and understanding may then be influenced by positive or negative emotions and the result will be the consequent action.

Essentially, cognitive approaches are about conscious processes, those that gather and organize relevant information with the intention of taking a specific course of action. Factors that compromise cognitive ability include:

• limitations in prior experience (of that situation)
• high levels of emotion
• lack of motivation towards problem solving
• difficulties in information storage and retrieval
• intellectual ability and capacity
• neurological changes or traumatic damage.

Think about how many of these factors may influence the patients in our care. Think about patients who are anxious, unclear about their diagnosis and prognosis, those who have difficulties in independent decision making, those who are depressed or have organic neurological changes that render cognitive processes difficult.

Behavioural theory

The behavioural view is based on the principle of observable action, factors that predispose to it and consequences of it. It is argued by the behaviourists that, because one cannot see the workings of the mind, the only scientific data is human behaviour, which is measurable and modifiable. The impact of conditioning is recognized as a powerful force in the learning process. This also includes learned negative behaviours such as phobias and anxieties.

Behaviourism, therefore, helps us to understand how positive and negative behaviour can be reinforced or strengthened – in effect, how the response gained as a result of personal actions will determine whether that action is more or less likely to happen again in the future.

Perhaps one example of this is the positive effect of praise, a social reinforcer, which can be extremely powerful in increasing the likelihood of approved behaviour. Equally, we can see how inappropriate behaviour can increase if attention is given to this action. An example of this might be the attention we give to someone who self-injures; this is a behaviour that is harmful to the individual and therefore could be seen as inappropriate, but at the same time, from a 'duty to care perspective', it is very difficult to ignore.

Behavioural approaches can provide a logical means of teaching new skills and actions. In recent years, there has been an integration of cognitive and behavioural approaches. These techniques have included the behavioural approach to goal attainment, i.e. breaking complex tasks into simple, attainable stages and clarifying factors that assist in the maintenance of learned behaviour, along with cognitive techniques that clarify personal perceptions and establish strategies for self-regulation. The personal ownership of problem-solving techniques encouraged by cognitive approaches has enabled behaviourism to become a rigorous yet ethically justified approach, which does not impose standards on the individual, but supports them in achieving personal goals. Such developments have enabled the fundamental principles of humanism to be more easily addressed in nursing practice.

Humanistic theory

Humanistic theory is a concept familiar to nursing philosophy. This theory is based on the concept of a congruent self, with a desire for personal growth, autonomy and responsibility. The emphasis is on the self as a whole, with equal value placed on biological, psychological, social and spiritual components. The person-centred orientation associated with this theory enables the uniqueness of human beings to be celebrated and challenges the power base within the nurse–patient relationship (Rogers 1961). The conditions of that relationship are based on a fundamental way of being, which includes genuine and mutual respect, empathy, trust, positive regard and human warmth (Egan 1990). Maslow's developmental theory is fundamentally based on the humanistic approach. In terms of need fulfilment, Maslow (1968) believed that we all have potential to self-actualize. We are equipped with sometimes surprising resources and the capacity to exert some control over our lives and to realize opportunities for growth and development. In some situations we may need help and, in this case, the humanistic theory offers nurses facilitative strategies that can help the individual to return as far as possible to a state of independence and wellbeing. These strategies are addressed more in the section on 'Helping the patient and embracing your own personality', page 303.

Psychoanalytic theory

Pychoanalytic theory is concerned more with the unconscious mind and the way in which our developing personality is influenced by conflicts between its components – the id (basic drive), ego (reality principle) and superego (moral conscience) – and satisfactory attainment of the psychosexual stages.

The emphasis is on conflict resolution and how satisfactorily the psychosexual stages of early life have been attained. It is believed that fixation in any of these stages (as a result of ineffective gratification in childhood) can lead to regression to that stage in later experiences of stress. Stress responses can become neurotic, in that unrealistic fears may become apparent, or there may be examples of repressed emotion or behaviour.

The psychoanalytic perspective may not be easy to exemplify in the general care of the sick patient. However, one aspect of psychoanalytic theory that is commonly observed is the expression of mental defence mechanisms.

Mental defence mechanisms are unconscious processes that exist as short-term strategies to cope with traumatic or uncomfortable experiences. Examples of these can include denial of a painful loss in bereavement, or projection, which can be shown when we are unable, or unwilling, to take responsibility for the aspects of our 'self' that we either dislike or prefer not to acknowledge. We may also hear examples of 'intellectualization', when people attempt to separate emotion from situations that may have a traumatic impact. An example of this might be the use of jargon in sensitive circumstances. Mental defence mechanisms are normal processes. It is only when they become long-term coping strategies that they begin to have a pathological effect. This effect might be manifested in the individual's increasing reluctance to confront difficulties in his life, or in his continual denial of the reality of a situation.

Stress and its demands

Action point 2

Patients often become anxious or uncomfortable in hospital. In what ways have patients exhibited this stress? Make a short list.

It is apparent that one factor that has an effect on psychological wellbeing is the way in which we cope with stress. There is no simple definition of stress, as we all respond to stimuli in unique ways. However, there are common stressors, such as serious illness or injury, which we can anticipate may create difficulties in coping. There are many different coping strategies, and some of these will be addressed later in this chapter from the perspective of the helping relationship.

Stress can vary in intensity; it can also develop slowly over a period of time. Prolonged stress can lead to anxiety. Other views on stress include the 'general response of the body to any demand (pleasant or unpleasant) that is made upon it'. Therefore, stress can be perceived as a positive or negative state of arousal. The response to the stressor is immediate and rapid; automatic responses enable our body to prepare for fight or flight (the difference between life or death). Selye (1956) suggests that stress is a 'non-specific' concept that represents change and the way in which individuals respond to it. He proposes that the initial symptoms of almost any disease or trauma are virtually identical, i.e. the body responds in the same way to any stressor, whether it is external and environmental or whether it arises from within the body itself. He had defined stress as 'the individual's psycho/physiological response, mediated largely by the autonomic nervous system and the endocrine system, to any demands made upon the individual...'. He refers to the response process as the General Adaptation Syndrome, which occurs in three stages:

1. Alarm reaction – these are the physiological changes associated with emotion. There is activation of the sympathetic nervous system, increased production of adrenaline and noradrenaline, increased production of blood sugar and preparation of the body for fight/flight.
2. Resistance – if the stressor is not removed, the body begins to recover a little and there is subsequently a decrease in sympathetic activity.
3. Exhaustion – this is when the body begins to return to normal and there is a subsequent depletion of physical resources.

When stress is perpetuated, the continuous physical demands made on the body can extend the exhaustion phase. The body will then take longer to recover and there may be an increased susceptibility to illness. The body's own natural defences are compromised, as lymphocyte production can be reduced. Hypertension may occur and the individual becomes more susceptible to cardiovascular disease. Anxiety begins to increase as stress is perpetuated. The inability to cope with stress as a result of compromised resources or physical illness is a common experience for patients in hospital.

Factors that contribute to stress in hospitalized patients include complex emotions such as anger, fear, pain and impatience. Major life events such as birth, death, separation and role change can produce insecurities and difficulties in adaptation. Internal conflicts such as the decision to undergo major surgery or chemotherapy, and to deal with the consequences of these invasive experiences, are often difficult to resolve, as they are very personal and responsible decisions. The diagnosis and prognosis of illness may take time. The individual may be so fearful of this that he avoids consulting medical practitioners until the symptoms of illness can no longer be ignored.

Loss and bereavement

> **Action point 3**
>
> Loss or bereavement is something that nurses often find difficult to cope with. In what ways have you seen this dealt with by nurses?

If we take the example of major life events, we can easily identify with the stress they often cause. In some cases, this stress is exacerbated by a profound sense of loss. Loss is a common, yet very individual concept. We all experience loss in one way or another, but the way in which we respond to it will vary according to our own coping strategies, our own perceptions and the actual circumstances surrounding the loss.

Loss may be experienced in different forms. It may be the loss of someone important to us, through death, serious illness, divorce or role transition (for example, children moving away from home, adults having their first child). Loss may also be related to changes in body image, as a result of traumatic injury, surgery or progressive illness. Grieving, the way in which we react to loss, can be manifested in complex ways. Many theorists refer to a 'grieving process', a natural process that takes us through a range of emotions and leads eventually to some degree of acceptance or resolution. Theorists such as Kubler-Ross (1970) and Ramsey and DeGroot (1977) agree to some common manifestations of bereavement including shock and denial ('it's not true!'), followed by anger, rage and resentment, extreme anxiety and disorganization. There may be a degree of bargaining ('What if I do this...?') and, later, perhaps a period of depression.

It is important, as nurses, to recognize the stages of grieving as normal and to accept that individuals do not necessarily reach a certain stage within a specified time. Indeed, individual emotions may swing back and forth. They may also repress certain emotions, either because they prefer not to disclose their emotional pain to others, or perhaps as a result of preferred religious or cultural practices of grieving.

Worden (1991) recognizes that there are various 'tasks of mourning'. These include 'acceptance of the reality of the loss', 'working through the pain of grieving', 'adjustment to the (new) environment' and 'emotional relocation' (moving on). He also recognizes that individuals may suffer 'complicated grieving', for example when they are unable to accept the loss and overcome the pain, and suffer pathological effects as a consequence.

Some of the patients for whom you will be caring may have experienced loss and may be experiencing grief. They may include people who have been given a terminal diagnosis, had a mastectomy, a colostomy, become immobile or suffered organic neurological changes. Care may also need to embrace the needs of the relatives and closest friends of such individuals and, significantly, the loved ones of those who have died. Nurses may sometimes experience frustration when unable to ease the pain of those who are grieving, as often it is difficult to invest the time required. This is when other disciplines can help to provide a co-ordinated effort; thus the liaison nurse, the psychologist, the counsellor and the support group, among others, may be of help. Nurses may also need to acknowledge their own experiences of loss and gain personal support; nursing can be a very emotional experience. The example of changing body image was previously mentioned as a source of stress and may indeed contribute to the experience of loss. Body image changes, either internal or external, can have a major impact on the concept of self and thus provoke anxiety. This particular example will now be explored in a little more detail.

Action point 4 – case scenario

Joan is 43 years of age. She has recently been diagnosed as having a bowel tumour. This necessitated major surgery to remove the tumour, and Joan now has a colostomy and requires chemotherapy. She is extremely distressed. She cannot bear to look at the colostomy, feels it is not part of her, and that she will never be able to handle this 'abnormality'. She also feels she cannot face the future; she has heard 'all sorts of things' about chemotherapy, fears pain and hair loss, and a total loss of independence.

Joan's family visit her as often as possible. They are so relieved that she is alive; her children simply want their mum to come home.

Issues to consider:
• What are Joan's psychological needs?
• Might she be experiencing loss and bereavement? How is this manifested?
• What might the impact of such major body changes be on her self-concept?
• What could I begin to do to help?

Body image and self-concept

Body image combines the outward self, that which is presented to others, and the inner self, which includes the physical functions of the body and the self-concept. Any alteration to physical functioning can have an effect on the way we see and feel about ourselves. The nature of the illness and its prognosis, along with the visibility of the change, can have a powerful effect on individual coping and motivation. The change may be slow or rapid, may involve boundaries and limitations, may have an impact on future lifestyle and may significantly change one's self-concept. It is commonly believed that body image has three essential components – body reality, body ideal and body presentation (Price 1990). It is the balance of these components that can become compromised when change occurs. Social influence can have a major impact on body presentation; the stereotypical 'beautiful body' often produces unattainable goals for individuals and it is this inability to achieve the body ideal that contributes to a negative self-concept. For a person who is ill, the changes could enhance their quality of life, for example in the person who has surgery to remove a tumour and is rewarded with full recovery. However, the changes could also be perceived very negatively, depending on the visibility of the change. For example, amputation may be necessary to save life, but may significantly alter individual lifestyle, mobility, activity and personal potential. One of the difficulties encountered with adapting to altered body image is the fragility of the self-concept.

Self-concept is generally viewed as having three components – the self-image, the self-esteem and the ideal self. The self-image is generally taken to mean the way in which we see ourselves, i.e. the social roles and the personality traits we possess. In describing their self-image, individuals often also describe their physical self, i.e. their height, weight, colour, etc. These aspects specifically are part of the body image. The self-esteem is more evaluative than descriptive, as it indicates the value we place on our self. This tends to vary according to the response of others to us and according to how much our real self differs from our ideal self. The ideal self, therefore, is that which we strive towards and it is perhaps this component that causes the greatest frustration – the further we are from achieving our ideal self, the more critical we are likely to be of our real self. It is these, among other issues, that become important in providing individualized care for those experiencing hospitalization.

What does becoming a hospitalized patient mean?

The process of hospitalization is a means by which symptoms of ill health may be identified, investigated and monitored, leading to diagnosis and, in many cases, medical treatment and nursing intervention. The process may also provide intensive or rehabilitative care. Care generally extends beyond the patient, to family, partners and friends.

Ideally, the experience of hospitalization should be a positive one. A desirable goal would be to ensure that the patient returns to normal functioning as quickly as possible, with a greater sense of general wellbeing and improved health. In this positive context, hospitalization can validate or alleviate symptoms, enable the patient to be better informed about the condition and become better equipped, emotionally, intellectually and physically, to deal with the situation.

Experience of the nurse–patient relationship should be mutually validating and respectful, with a sharing of resources and a realization of opportunities to facilitate adaptation and/or recovery. The patient has a responsibility within this relationship, and the nurse has a responsibility to work towards acting 'in the best interests of the patient' (UKCC 1992), to demonstrate effective interpersonal skills, to promote trust by demonstrating competence, and to acknowledge fundamental human rights and how they might be fulfilled.

Negative aspects of hospitalization include those that Goffman (1968) describes within the process of 'deindividuation'. Deindividuation is the process of becoming a hospitalized patient. Negative perceptions of the role of patient include the view of the 'passive recipient' of care, the anonymous individual who becomes a 'case', a subject of investigation, a 'condition' to be treated and a compliant subject whose ability to monitor, regulate or control the environment and events occurring within that environment is compromised. There may be feelings of disempowerment, and a sense of well-intentioned, but essentially paternalistic, control. There may be a perception of emotional detachment and a focus on rituals, policies, procedures and clinical jargon.

Socialization into this role can be subtle but rapid. The impact can be learned helplessness; individuals become deskilled and dependent on others; they may respond passively, in a compliant manner, even if they do not agree to the actions being taken. There is a greater sense of vulnerability, and a potentially heightened emotional sensitivity and state of arousal. Much of this encapsulates the negatively perceived role of the patient.

Deviation from the expected role of patient can result in 'punishment' by nurses, through alienation (negative reinforcement), negative labelling and stigmatizing attitudes (negative stereotypical or discriminatory thoughts). Examples include ignoring the demanding patient, using depersonalizing labels to describe individuals, or making assumptions that people with a similar condition will have exactly the same needs and requirements. The patient may in turn show an increase in defensive behaviour, such as verbal or physical aggression, hostility or reluctance to disclose information. There may be feelings of anxiety related to separation and detachment from normal roles, relationships and positive self-concept. This may be manifested in impatience, constant questioning and the need for reassurance. There may even be experiences in which the individual feels devalued, such as those procedures that compromise human dignity, respect and self-esteem.

> **Action point 5 – Case scenario**
>
> Edward is 70 years of age. He is recovering from a myocardial infarction. His care involves gradual rehabilitation. Edward has never been so ill. He has suffered only from minor ailments and has maintained an active life at home. His wife died several years ago, he still misses her but has adapted very well, establishing a positive social life. He has taken care of himself very well, maintaining his home, shopping and cooking himself at least 'one good meal a day'. Since hospitalization, however, his motivation has significantly declined. He seems listless and passive; he is reluctant to exercise and feels he is not going to be able to manage at home. He can't understand why this 'heart attack' occurred; he has 'always been fit and taken care of himself'. He has become quite dependent on the nursing team.
>
> Issues to consider
> • What are the major concerns regarding Edward's situation?
> • What does his current behaviour suggest?
> • What can nurses do to engage him constructively in the rehabilitation process?

Role theory

Many nurse–patient relationship issues are related to role perceptions, i.e. how we see ourselves in a given situation. Roles are the 'parts' we play, the identities we take on within different aspects of our life.

From a sociological perspective, we can perhaps appreciate the significance of primary and secondary socialization as a means of role acquisition, i.e. the ways in which parents, peers and other elements of society teach us what to do in certain circumstances. We can also appreciate that, in terms of ascribed role, some aspects of behaviour may be predetermined, i.e. individuals born into a specific set of circumstances. From a psychological perspective, we can perhaps identify with examples of conditioning, where people have been manipulated into specific roles and behaviours gradually through the consistent application of reinforcement techniques. Considering examples used previously in this chapter, we can also identify with the patient whose 'appropriate' behaviour is rewarded in various ways, reinforcing the image of the 'model patient'.

There are opportunities for the patient to manipulate situations to maximize the potential around them. For example, the patient who uses the sick role to validate exemption from responsibilities and becomes dependent on others; or, alternatively and perhaps more positively, engages diverse resources to facilitate recovery.

Gibson (1950) suggests that many patients know what changes are required to facilitate their own recovery but lack the skills and resources to do so. This is perhaps where the nurse can actively facilitate opportunities for personal growth and enhanced personal autonomy by making her own knowledge and skills accessible to the patient, by mobilizing resources, by demonstrating effective interpersonal skills and by acknowledging individual rights and responsibilities.

Assessing psychological needs

It is not the intention of this chapter to propose that nurses conduct psychological assessment; clearly this specialist skill remains the remit of the clinical psychologist. However, it is proposed that nurses should identify and acknowledge specific psychological needs in order to enhance the potential of holistic assessment. It is essential that the assessment process gathers significant information: that which facilitates intervention, but ensures that the individual is acknowledged as unique and treated as a person. Equally, the assessment should not be viewed as something the nurse does to the patient; it should become a shared activity in which both nurse and patient participate. Patients may not have had training in how to interpret and document relevant information, but they know more about their own symptoms and lifestyle. The nurse, on the other hand, possesses specific skills that help to extract information from the patient, and has some propositions about how this information will be used to determine intervention. But the nurse cannot be sure what information patients require, and at what level, or what support patients require and how they would like this to be offered. It takes time to establish the level of trust that enables disclosure of often significant, but very intimate, information, and many patients will make their own informal assessment of the nurse in order to determine how and what to disclose.

To facilitate comprehensive and holistic assessment, the following issues are worthy of exploration:

• Consider the patient's knowledge and understanding about the current situation. What does he already know about the illness; what does it mean in respect of personal perceptions, self-concept, lifestyle, general feelings and behaviours? What level of support does the patient feel is needed, and from whom? Consider how this might be provided.
• Observe and discuss any defensive behaviour exhibited by the patient. Acknowledge and discuss any stressors that exist and identify those responses that are normal and those that may indicate inability to cope.

- Clarify roles and responsibilities of those involved in care delivery; check the patient's understanding of this. Offer therapeutic options and consider their understanding and response to these.
- Identify any factors that might impede information processing or retention. These may include neurological changes, trauma, cognitive deterioration, complex and confusing emotions, presence of mental illness and any evidence of disrupted development (physical, cognitive, emotional, behavioural).
- Consider the presence and perception of pain; identify the range of basic to more complex physical needs and how these can best be met.
- Identify any normal routines that could be maintained during the process of hospitalization. Identify communication strategies that will facilitate effective interaction.

It could be argued that effective assessment also incorporates self-appraisal from the perspective of the nurse.

- Consider, for example, personal knowledge, skills and resources, and determine any deficits that need to be addressed in order to assess and deliver care effectively.
- Identify and acknowledge any personal prejudices or stigmatizing attitudes that might compromise individualized care.
- Identify and address personal stressors in order to avoid their projection towards the patient.
- Consider examples of punitive or potentially negligent behaviour towards patients and acknowledge means by which these can be avoided.
- Consider ways in which action can be proactive rather than reactive.
- Explore personal potential for creativity with resources and utilize diverse methods of assessment to gather a wider range and possibly greater depth of information.
- Acknowledge your own limitations, psychological, social and behavioural, and learn to celebrate your own individuality and potential.

Assessment is more than data gathering; it is an essential component of relationship building. This is often what the patient remembers most when they reflect on their experience of hospitalization.

Helping the patient and embracing your own personality

The ways in which patients are helped during their stay in hospital may be dependent on a wide range of factors. These include models and philosophies of care, policies and protocols, health policy guidelines, availability of resources, and knowledge, skills and potential of the care-giving team. The impact of these factors makes it impossible to determine a prescriptive strategy for helping the patient. It would in fact be inappropriate to do so, as patient care will inevitably vary according to individual circumstances and according to the individuals involved in care delivery. To show how strategies might be individually tailored, an approach using Maslow's hierarchy is explored briefly at the end of this section. Before this, and to emphasize the importance of interpersonal skills in delivering psychological care, more personalized aspects of helping are now explored.

As individuals, nurses will be guided by their own personal philosophies, their own values and beliefs about what could be and should be achieved through their interaction with the patient. This approach may incorporate a particular psychological orientation to one or more of the theories outlined earlier. This can help when specific skills need to be taught, when individual perceptions need to be clarified or addressed, or when individual actions need to be more clearly understood.

In general, a range of qualities is essential for the helping relationship. The following guidelines indicate those that embrace not only the concept of human caring, but also the potential to incorporate aspects of the personality that make a nurse unique.

Listening and responding is vital

Listen to the patient. Employ the skills of active and passive listening in accordance with the situation. If you need to know more, use open questions. If you need to acknowledge the expression of deep emotion, listen quietly, without interrupting the flow, and maintain eye contact and appropriate body language to show that you are interested, involved and accepting.

Inform and support the patient

Offer information at a level and pace that are acceptable and helpful to the patient. Many people offer too much too quickly, but patients can retain only so much, particularly when they are anxious or distracted by other significant issues in their life.

Support them, even if you disagree with their perceptions or values. Ultimately, it is the patient who has to adapt to change and cope with unusual demands.

Acknowledge and use your own personality

We often possess individual characteristics that can enhance interpersonal relationships. An appropriate sense of humour, specific attributes or talents, and even language codes or culturally determined behaviours can be used to promote a more genuine and warm encounter. It may take time, and some mistakes, to integrate the role and the person effectively. It is always essential to be professional, but it can help to break barriers when we demonstrate individuality and show the person beyond the uniform.

Acknowledging emotions and not personalizing the negatives

Being genuine presents its own challenges in nursing care. There are times when we feel emotionally vulnerable, confused, angry and frustrated. It can sometimes be difficult to control these powerful emotions and sometimes unavoidable. While attempting to demonstrate genuineness in care provision, we have, at the same time, to consider the consequences, primarily for the patient and secondarily for ourselves. Rogers (1961) raised the issue of 'transparency' and warns of its dangers; Mearns and Thorne (1997) use the metaphor 'lace curtains and safety screens' to acknowledge the semi-transparency that is perhaps more appropriate in helping relationships. It would be inappropriate to prescribe a specific approach in relation to such issues; the guidelines therefore should be to identify and clarify the boundaries, to clarify responsibilities towards each other and towards ourselves, and to maintain a focus on the experiencing person's (in this case, the patient's) subjectivity.

Being competent and confident, doing your best

Psychological needs are complex. There are many factors that can compromise the psychological wellbeing of patients in hospital. If these needs can be identified and addressed, the opportunities for patient empowerment, participation and the promotion of independence can be enhanced. Patients can subsequently experience a reduction in anxiety, an increase in understanding of their situation and an enhanced ability to cope with the demands placed on them.

Much of this depends on the nurse's ability to take a holistic approach, to acknowledge that psychological needs are as important as physical, social and emotional needs. This chapter has highlighted some of the needs and explored ways in which they might be addressed in order to promote holistic care. It has acknowledged the theoretical contribution, addressed a range of commonly experienced concepts and explored some scenarios.

Nursing competencies include many of the issues addressed. Nurses also have limitations and it is important to recognize that other disciplines have an equally valid contribution to make towards patient care.

Nursing is also a humanistic practice; it involves working with vulnerable people whose emotional state may be quite fragile. This practice thus demands sensitivity and a sense of genuine concern for the individual. This is where the personality can shine through and be used to help the patient to go on with life, having had a positive and fulfilling experience of the nurse–patient relationship.

Appendix: An example of how Maslow's hierarchy (1968) might be used as a framework for intervention

Safety needs (physical and psychological)

- Risk assessment may be indicated.
- Mobility assistance may be required.
- Means of maintaining nutrition may require attention.
- Information and support may be required to reduce fear and anxiety.
- Facilitate strategies that need to be identified to ensure a degree of autonomy for the patient.

Belonging needs

- Provide information and promote positive interpersonal encounters to ensure the patient feels valued as an individual.
- Maintain patient contact with significant people.
- Facilitate early return to roles, routines and lifestyle as appropriate and desirable.

Need for acceptance

- Accept and acknowledge the patient's views and feelings, even when they differ from your own.
- Accept the patient's strengths and weaknesses, potential, and means of self-expression.

Cognitive needs

- Help the patient to know and understand.
- Help the patient to make sense of information and situations
- Help the patient to work with information in a problem-solving manner.
- Help the patient to use past experience to deal with new situations.
- Help the patient to own the decisions that must be made.

Aesthetic needs

- Help the patient to hold on to the things he values in life
- Help the patient to acknowledge and appreciate the wider picture of his situation: the potential and the knowledge and experience to be derived.

Actualization needs

- Acknowledge the patient's individual potential and assist him towards goal attainment and personal fulfilment.

References and further reading

Adler A (1927) The Practice and Theory of Individual Psychology. New York: Harcourt Brace Jovanovich.

Bruner JS, Taguiri R (1954) The perception of people. Cited in Lindzey G (ed) Handbook of Social Psychology, vol 2. Reading, MA: Addison-Wesley.

Bruner JS, Oliver RR, Greenfield PM (eds) (1966) Studies in Cognitive Growth. New York: Wiley.

Egan G (1990) The Skilled Helper: a systematic approach to effective helping, 4th edn. Pacific Grove, CA: Brooks-Cole Publishing.

Freud S (1976) The Psychopathology of Everyday Life. Pelican Freud Library (5). Harmondsworth, Middlesex: Penguin.

Freud S (1984) The Ego and the Id. Pelican Freud Library (11). Harmondsworth, Middlesex: Penguin.

Gibson JJ (1950) The Perception of the Visual World. Boston, MA: Houghton Mifflin.

Goffman E (1968) Asylums – essays on the social situation of mental patients and other inmates. Harmondsworth, Middlesex: Penguin.

Gross R (1996) Psychology, the Science of Mind and Behaviour, 3rd edn. London: Hodder and Stoughton.

Jung CG (1964) Man and His Symbols. London: Aldus-Jupiter Books.

Kelly GA (1955) A Theory of Personality – the psychology of personal constructs. New York: Norton

Kubler-Ross E (1970) On Death and Dying. London: Tavistock.

Maslow A (1968) Toward a Psychology of Being, 2nd edn. New York: Van Nostrand-Reinhold.

Mearns D, Thorne B (1997) Person Centred Counselling in Action. London: Sage.

Pavlov IP (1927) Conditioned Reflexes. London: Oxford University Press.

Price B (1990) A model for body image care. Journal of Advanced Nursing 15(5): 585–593.

Ramsey R, DeGroot W (1977) A further look at bereavement. Paper presented at EATI conference, Uppsala. Cited in Hodgkinson PE (1980) Treating abnormal grief in the bereaved. Nursing Times 17: 126–128.

Rogers CR (1951) Client-centred Therapy: its current practice, implications and theory. London: Constable

Rogers CR (1961) On Becoming a Person. Boston, MA: Houghton Mifflin.

Selye H (1956) The Stress of Life. New York: McGraw-Hill.

Skinner BF (1971) Beyond Freedom and Dignity. New York: Knopf.

UKCC (1992) Code of Professional Conduct. London: UKCC.

Watson JB (1924) Behaviourism. New York: Lippincott.

Worden W (1991) Grief Counselling and Grief Therapy. London: Tavistock.

Index

Page numbers in **bold** indicate a reference to a table

309

mouth care 143, 213
multiple sclerosis 166–172
musculoskeletal system, effect of
  protein–energy malnutrition **100**
mycardium 3
myocardial infarction (MI)
  complications 23–25
  diagnosis 18–19
  health education 23
  medical management 19–20
  nursing care 22–23
  pathology 17
  signs and symptoms 18
myocardial ischaemia 20
myxoedema 224
myxoedematous coma 225

nausea and vomiting
  in MI 18
  in pancreatitis 240
need for acceptance 307
negative pressures 292
nephrons 198–199, 214
nervous system
  anatomy and physiology 146–150
  assessment 151–152
  common disorders 165–193
  diagnostic procedures 160
neurological system *see* nervous system
nitric oxide 256
nociceptors 271
non-steroidal anti-inflammatory drugs
  118, 283
nurse
  accountability 266, 269–270
  caring skills 304–306
  drug administration 280
  emotions 298, 305
  and pain control 266, 279
  personality 304–305
  self-appraisal 303
nurse–patient relationship 266, 269–270
  in holistic assessment 302–303
  patient's experience 300, 306
  in respiratory care 78, 92
  role theory 301–302
nutrition 89, 93–94
  see also malnutrition
nutritional assessment 101–104
nutritional support 104–108, 112, 124,
  212

nutritional supplements 105, 210
occipital lobes 148, 178
oesophageal disorders 110–116
oesophagoscopy 111
oliguria/anuria 206–207, 209–210
opiate analgesics 281–283
oxygen
  binding to haemoglobin 62–64
  carriage in the circulation 62–63
  delivery devices 86–87
  demand, and breathlessness 76
  exchange 57
  in metabolic processes 47–49
  requirements and saturation 85
  therapy 85–87, 90

pain
  acute 268, 276
  anatomy and physiology 270–273
  assessment 274–278
  biophysical explanation 270
  chronic 268, 276
  and culture 273–274
  factors affecting 276
  function 266, 268
  gate theory 270, 272
  historical aspects 267
  location 275
  and mental illness 277
  observing signs 266
  onset 275
  in pancreatitis 240
  in patients with learning disability
    276–277
  reaction to 157
  transmission 272
  treatment 278–289
  types 268–270
  verbal description 275
  what it is 267–268
pain control
  in brain tumours 192
  complementary methods 286–288
  in myocardial infarction (MI) 17
  nurse involvement 266, 279
  psychological approaches 289
  in respiratory disease 89
pain fibres 271
pain receptors *see* nociceptors
pain-relieving drugs *see* analgesics
palliative treatment